DELLA MEDICINA

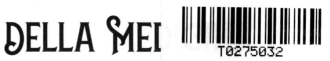

T0275032

"My immense enthusiasm for the release of Lisa Fazio's *Della Medicina* is twofold. It is the perfect choice as a required text for my university course on Italian folk medicine and magic as it will simultaneously educate and enchant my students. Secondly, as the great-granddaughter of an Italian healer, I have long lived with many of the traditions Fazio explores. Lisa Fazio's expertise as an herbalist and her meticulous research have greatly expanded my own understanding of the remedies passed down through the generations in my family. This book is a must-read for Italian Americans as well as readers from any cultural diaspora seeking to deepen their knowledge of folk healing practices."

GINA M. MIELE, PH.D., PROFESSOR SPECIALIZING IN
ITALIAN FOLKTALES, FOLKLORE, AND TRADITIONS
AT MONTCLAIR STATE UNIVERSITY

"I have been longing for this magical book my whole life. Lisa Fazio is one of our generation's greatest teachers of Southern Italian folk medicine. *Della Medicina* is for everyone drawn to plants and their healing powers and anyone in search of ancestral connection. For those of us from Italy's many diasporas, this is a pathway home, an invitation to remember."

JENNIFER GUGLIELMO, AUTHOR OF
*LIVING THE REVOLUTION: ITALIAN WOMEN'S RESISTANCE
AND RADICALISM IN NEW YORK CITY, 1880–1945*

"This book warms my Southern Italian soul! I love it! What a fascinating apothecary of history, mystical folk knowledge, tools, and inspiration for anyone wanting to draw on one of the most amazing herbalism traditions on the planet to nourish their lives and heal our world. Brava, Lisa Fazio, for honoring the ancestors in a way that shows the universality of their expansive wisdom."

MARGUERITE MARY RIGOGLIOSO, PH.D., AUTHOR OF
THE SECRET LIFE OF MOTHER MARY AND
THE MYSTERY TRADITION OF MIRACULOUS CONCEPTION

"This book dives deeply into how we of the Italian diaspora can reclaim our roots and restore our connection to the earth, which is our true nature. Lisa Fazio weaves the daily with the divine by offering rituals, ceremonies, and healing practices with reverence and wisdom."

"*Della Medicina* takes us into the deep ancestral energy of magical medicines that have long pervaded the Mediterranean regions, where folk medicine, divination, holy wells, sacred sites, and ancient rituals combined with potent healing plants to bring sweet relief and healing to the peoples of that region. These teachings are also connected to the early burgeoning practices of modern medicine and how our connection to the energetics of plants can still be used to bring about true health and healing."

"Lisa Fazio's *Della Medicina* is a deep exploration of ancestral wisdom through the lens of Italian folk medicine. Drawing from her rich heritage and herbal knowledge, she beautifully illustrates how plants can serve as sacred portals to our ancestral roots. Her holistic approach reminds us that folk medicine is for everyone, transcending cultural, political, and economic boundaries while fostering deep connections with both human and nonhuman communities. This book is a treasure for anyone who loves plants and seeks harmony with the world around them. Lisa's insights and the accessible plants featured make this a practical and profound guide to inner healing through traditional plant medicine."

"Lisa Fazio's book represents the best kind of ancestor work—connection with our beloved ancient kin, the plants; connection through cultural frameworks that are instructions from the lands of our ancestors; and connection that does not try to simplify what is deeply complex."

DELLA MEDICINA

THE TRADITION OF ITALIAN-AMERICAN FOLK HEALING

LISA FAZIO

Healing Arts Press
Rochester, Vermont

Healing Arts Press
One Park Street
Rochester, Vermont 05767
www.HealingArtsPress.com

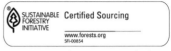

Text stock is SFI certified

Healing Arts Press is a division of Inner Traditions International

*Note to the reader: This book is intended to be an informational guide. The remedies,
approaches, and techniques described herein are meant to supplement, and not to be a
substitute for, professional medical care or treatment. They should not be used to treat a
serious ailment without prior consultation with a qualified health care professional.*

Cataloging-in-Publication Data for this title is available from the Library of Congress

ISBN 978-1-64411-753-8 (print)
ISBN 978-1-64411-754-5 (ebook)

Printed and bound in the United States by Lake Book Manufacturing, LLC
The text stock is SFI certified. The Sustainable Forestry Initiative® program
promotes sustainable forest management.

10 9 8 7 6 5 4 3 2 1

Text design and layout by Priscilla Harris Baker
This book was typeset in Garamond with Gill Sans, Gotham, Italian Oldstyle, and
Lansdowne used as display typefaces
Materia Medica artwork by Monica Basile (also used as decoration throughout
the text)

To send correspondence to the author of this book, mail a first-class letter to the
author c/o Inner Traditions • Bear & Company, One Park Street, Rochester, VT
05767, and we will forward the communication, or contact the author directly at
therootcircle.com.

Scan the QR code and save 25% at InnerTraditions.com.
Browse over 2,000 titles on spirituality, the occult, ancient
mysteries, new science, holistic health, and natural medicine.

In memory of Kelly (Colette) Louis. This dream is yours too;
I write for both of us.

Thank you to my nonno, Nicola Fazio, who never stopped me
from going off the path and up the side of the mountain and was
always willing to try my herbal concoctions. And to my nonna,
Elena Minicozzi, who always said yes when I wanted her to teach
me how to cook or knit something and for talking to me like I
was a real person and not a little kid; like I was her friend.

Thank you to my brother, Nicholas Fazio, whose explorations
and courage brought our family and me back to Calabria.

To the city of Utica, New York, which holds us now and has held
us for four generations.

To La Madonna, the Blessed Mother, who is my constant beacon
and who, no matter where I am, always leads me to her grotto.

To America: we have come as one; you call us "Italians."
To the Risorgimento: we are and always have been many.

È vietato calpestare i sogni.

It is forbidden to trample on the dreams.

A SPRAY-PAINTED SIGN IN FRONT OF THE
RUINS OF THE ABBAZIA DI SANTA MARIA
DI CORAZZO, CARLOPOLI, CATANZARO,
CALABRIA, ITALY

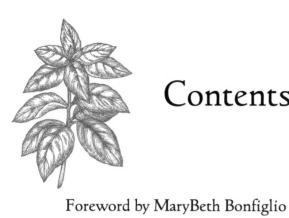

Contents

PART I

ORIGINS OF SOUTHERN ITALIAN FOLK MEDICINE

PART II

MODERN ADAPTATIONS OF FOLK WISDOM

PART III

PRACTICAL SKILLS AND TECHNIQUES

PART IV

Materia Medica

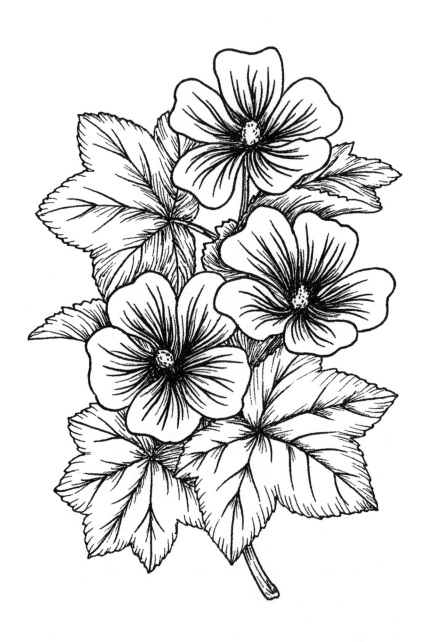

Foreword

By MaryBeth Bonfiglio

THE FIRST THING I want to say to you is this: you are about to read a book that is the only one of its kind. There is no other book like *Della Medicina*; no other written resource or reference book full of this particular wisdom in the English language. For this fact alone, you are blessed, or as we say in Italiano, *fortunato*, or my favorite in the Sicilian language, *culoso* (yes, that's derived from the word culo, which means "ass"). We are all lucky and blessed to have *Della Medicina* written, bound, and published.

There are many, *many* people out there waiting for this book—for the information and resources and stories that have been, until now, only known to us through oral tradition. We have leaned on fragmented storytelling or studies written in other languages or outside of our culture via anthropological papers, meaning written by outsiders for academic purposes.

For reasons on which we can only speculate (illiteracy, secrecy, or straight-up tradition), our people passed all information and wisdom down via word of mouth. So until now we've been left with frayed edges and bits and pieces that we have been trying to mend back together. There are very few recorded understandings of who our people were and how they practiced healing each other. That said, we also know that all of it lives within our bodies, and this is the very reason we have been longing for this book. We needed a map, a remembering. This is why we are so blessed to finally have something so many of us have spent countless hours looking for, praying for. Something to awaken us to our own medicine and keep us from total cultural amnesia.

There comes a time when someone has to step up and in, to compile everything that is out there, to sit for years with the information available, and to make the bits and pieces whole again—whether they are from personal experience, direct spiritual transmission, or extensive research and study—someone out there needed take on the task. Without a person or a community of people willing to do this, we risk a collective forgetting. We risk the loss of our oral-tradition lineage. We probably needed this book a decade ago, but we know and can be extremely grateful that it's coming out at the exactly right moment, in divine timing.

There is no better or more knowledgeable or trusted person than Lisa Fazio for birthing this book and offering it as a gift to us. The amount of love, time, organization, and devotion she has poured into it is outstanding. I am so grateful she is the one who stepped in and began compiling and writing the medicine and folk magic history of our people, so it will not be lost, and our oral traditions can still be passed on.

You are holding in your hands a huge piece of our history, our present, and our future. You are holding a spell that will keep alive a way of being—a way of being with plants and a way of being with medicine and magic that is universal and also incredibly unique to the Italian diaspora.

I met Lisa many years ago in the same way many of us—as writers and artists and as members of our diasporic community—have connected: through the wild terrain of the internet, following threads and sharing our hearts and minds out there in the ether.

I was writing extensively about being a second generation Italian and Sicilian living in the United States in North America, or Turtle Island as it is called by some Indigenous peoples. My body of work includes exploring the layers of what it means to belong to a liminal culture, to be "in between" cultures, to find the connections and poetically map how to weave our bodies back into being in relationship with what our grandparents left behind, including the land, but also to claim and to carry what they indeed brought with them as immigrants: the stories and folk magic they held close to their hearts and between their Hail Marys and their mysterious ingredients and infusions stuffed in a tied-up piece of cloth hidden in the pockets of their housecoats.

I didn't really know anybody else out there exploring Italian Americanness in this way, and I was lonely. I kept hoping that my vulnerability and longing and grief about culture loss and sharing ways of how I was "re-membering" would land with someone out there in the interworlds and that someone reading my words might feel what I was feeling, too; that somehow who and what I was seeking was also seeking me.

I had long connected with other folks around ancestral reclamation and healing, but none in the Italian-American diaspora. And though so much of this work is collective, there was an ache in me to connect with those who may have lived a unique cultural experience similar to mine. Where were my people?

In no time at all, Lisa and I met. I am sure the ancestors pushed us together. I don't remember how or when exactly, but I do know that when we met, I felt like she was a gift in my life.

Lisa and I shared similar questions and passions and life experiences. She was also a grandchild of the diaspora that had settled in an enclave in upstate New York (she in Utica and me in Jamestown). There is a simple and yet profound connection between Italians from upstate New York—if you know, you know. For one, there is that accent, that twang, that is inimitable, and when you find another who has it, there is just a connection that cannot be put into words. I was floored when I found her. Finally, a beautiful and talented human, writer, plant lover, herbalist, mother, and witch with the same cultural marrow as my own.

Lisa quickly became someone I would call a friend, or in the Sicilian language, a *cummari*, which is a word used to describe a female friendship that is more like family. Lisa felt like family, became family. The rhizomes of both the internet and the old country were moving us toward each other, bringing us nourishment through community.

Recently Lisa told me that when she first found me on instagram she thought, *Well here is a woman openly being Italian American and talking about these things and using her Italian last name, too,* and it inspired her to use her Italian surname professionally. This might sound odd if you are not Italian American, and you may ask yourself, *Why would some-one not want to use their own name?* The fact that that question is being asked is exactly why Lisa's book is of great importance and why the ongoing conversation about Italian Americanness, especially within our folk traditions, is deeply needed. To unearth the spectral and potent being-ness of who we are is imperative.

For too many years we have hidden ourselves as southern Italian Americans in plain sight. Our food has been celebrated, our mafia movies have been beloved box-office hits, and caricatures of us abound. But what about our magic? Our truest way of being who we really are deep in our bones?

How many know that we come from long lines of people who have been in deep and reciprocal relationship with the land, the plants, the spirits? How many people of the diaspora know that perhaps much of their spiritual and physical discomfort comes from not knowing the medicine of their people? And how much of their spiritual understand-ing and own personal magic and potency and intuitive wisdom come from the deep medicinal ways of their ancestors? How many have no idea what their great-great-grandparents used to regulate their nervous system or to invoke dream-space healing, or which saints were connected to which plants and which sacred and powerful words could be used to heal an ailment? How many of us don't know but somewhere inside *feel* this vibration of longing?

For so long, it was all hidden. Assimilation and the fear of being seen are real. The hiding of who we are and who we have always been has created a "culture of forgetting"—not just who we are but also how to be in good and right relationship as humans, how to show up as the medicine for others. Our ancestors were healers, witches, drummers, and herbalists—those living on the "outside." They were spectral, liminal, and neurodiverse people whose healing modalities were drawn from the unseen and whose knowledge of plants and what grows was just a part of their existence. It was not a special skill; it was the normal everyday way of being and living. We are the descendants of dreamers and protectors and essence makers. We are the granddaughters of those who knew that praying was not "just praying."

This "hiding" that we have done was most likely an epigenetic survival tactic carried on by our grandparents to aid in assimilation and to be accepted into the "Great American Experiment." Regardless of the why, there is something of importance here to remember: *our medicine needs to be seen and held and passed on.* There is dis-ease and trauma in our diaspora because it has not been seen. This book is literally a moment in time in which we all now have access to a resource we can dive into to learn about the plants and ways of being that can mend and thread our healing back together.

A book that compiles our *medicina* is one of the most beautiful gifts. It is a pathway forward for our collective healing and aliveness.

Although this is a book primarily based on plant medicines, Lisa goes beyond them to connect all aspects of folk medicine and healing together. *Della Medicina* is a connection to all aspects of life. Lisa understands that nothing is separate from anything else, and her writing brings everything back into wholeness. The plants are interconnected and in relationships with all of our other ways of being: prayer, ritual, deity worship, protection, and healing. Everything is linked, and Lisa does an impeccable job of sharing this wisdom.

Lisa also doesn't bypass the complexities of our culture and our roles as assimilated people on stolen land. And trust me, there are a lot of complexities. I have had extensive conversations with Lisa, and her thought process is brilliant and thorough, and she is always ready to dive deeper, explore more, and question even herself. We've spent many hours sharing the "fun stuff"—how we were raised, the different kinds of foods we ate on holidays, and our experiences as kids with elders and rituals—and we compared our folk ways of being that were passed on to us by our community elders. But we also have gone down many deep portals of the hard stuff. For instance, one of the biggest topics we would always circle back to is how very differently we were raised compared to other communities or populations of people—especially ones you might identify as white or more aptly, white Anglo-Saxon Protestants, or WASPs. Lisa doesn't shy away from the hard conversations. Our willingness and desire to confront our whiteness was at the forefront of many of our conversations. But our *unwillingness* to let go of our culture, our lived experiences, and the unique and magical medicine ways of Southern Italy, or Sud Italia, has been strong. And to have to dance between being white and being southern Italian in enclaves, masking for the rest of the world and having to hide, is never something Lisa tries to avoid.

Lisa understands the many layers and nuances of our historical and lived experiences, and she moves between these layers throughout *Della Medicina*. How do we live in a liminal way? In a culture between cultures? How can we be in relationships with the plants with context and symbiosis and be both true to our ancestors and also adaptive to the world we now live in?

As she was writing this book, I watched Lisa twist and turn with the complexity of being Italian American. Of being white and also being, geographically and culturally, of the Mediterranean. Together we have grappled, weaving both the ancient and recent past and the present and trying to anchor into what of the future was meeting us. Lisa, through working with the spirits of the plants and sharing them as a portal into other folk medicine, has a unique and profound way of honoring where we are now and where we have been. I know this book is a spell for those who have left us with the power of this medicine and a spell and prayer for those to come who will carry it on.

In this book, Lisa generously shares her extensive wisdom of southern Italian plant medicines and ways of being as no Italian American has done before. There is a reason why: it's not an easy task. This kind of work entails massive amounts of patience, not to mention endless hours of work translating books and documents and papers from Italian to English. It requires eye-bleeding kinds of research. It requires a lot of intensive diving within one's own epigenetic experiences and memories. It requires trust and resilience. And it requires a devotion to a role her ancestors have given her.

She has shown up.

Della Medicina is now a part of our lineage—a crucial part—and it will be something we keep on our shelves and give to our children, our grandchildren, and our communities. I think this book will change the way we remember ourselves, the way our people will be in relationship to plants, and how that relationship weaves into everything else: our health, our magic, our rituals, and our prayers.

This book will become something for us and our descendants to lean into. Because of this book, we will know the plants, the myths, the way we are, and the way we have always been.

Bless this book. And bless you as you read it.

Sá benedica,

MaryBeth Bonfiglio

Gardiner, New York | Sicilia, Italy

MaryBeth Bonfiglio is a second-generation Italian/Sicilian American writer, facilitator, and cultural community curator. She teaches online and in-person workshops in creative writing, tarot, and folk magic. She organizes and facilitates pilgrimages to Sicily to connect people with local teachers and healers and to learn about folk herbalism, music, drumming, mythology, cooking, and ritual. She received her MFA from Antioch University in creative nonfiction. She lives in the mid-Hudson River Valley with her family and spends three months a year teaching, learning, and writing in Italy and Sicily.

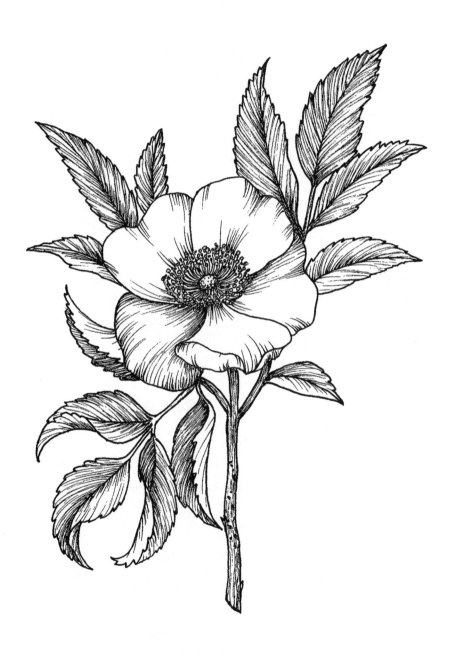

Finding Myself in Plants

THIS BOOK CAME INTO BEING as part of the process of my own ancestral reconnection and veneration. It is really a prayer and a homage to my ancestors that began with my relationship with my Italian immigrant grandparents, family, and community and became further rooted and embodied when I began my studies as an herbalist.

Difficult socioeconomic and political conditions in Southern Italy in the early twentieth century led to the families of my *nonne* (grandparents) emigrating to this country. My *nonno* (grandfather) remembered how his belly hurt from hunger when he was a boy. He related how his *nonna* (grandmother) would make bread once a week and by the end of the week it was hard, but that was all there was to eat. The villagers where he lived would wait for someone to come through selling goat's milk, and my grandfather told me, "If you had a coin you could get a cup." Many of the immigrants who left Europe during that time period came to America out of necessity to earn money for their families back in Italy and in hopes of a better life.

My nonne, along with other extended family members, were a prominent influence in my childhood, as a major aspect of Italian culture holds family and family life as the foundational center of community. The first Italian immigrants brought their cultural traditions with them when they settled in areas and neighborhoods with other Southern Italians (as did most of the other ethnic groups at that time). These Italian enclaves were also locations of cultural exchange as the immigrants came from provinces all over Southern Italy where the traditions were highly specific and unique from region to region, although they might have looked the same to an outsider.

Southern Italian folk medicine is not an organized system; it is a localized vernacular tradition with practices that are largely parochial. Evidently everyone believed that their way was the right way. For instance, my nonna was born in the city of Benevento in Campania, quite a distance from my nonno's little village in Calabria, and her family traditions, Italian dialect, recipes, ritual prayers, and crochet patterns were notably different from his. They are but one example of how families from different regions ended up blending and converging their cultural traditions. A great deal of adaptation emerged. It was a matter of survival in the New World.

As a second-generation immigrant living in an Italian-American community, the traditions and practices of my Italian family were not even thought of as "traditions" or even thought of at all; they were just a part of daily life. There was no name for what we practiced, or if there was one, no one ever used it. In later life, I heard it called Benedicaria, which literally means "Blessing Way" but is often translated simply as "the things we do." In the region of Campania where my nonna was from they sometimes refer to it as Fa Lu Santuccio, or "do a little holy thing." And this is what our practices really were; just the things my family did.

Unfortunately, as a child I did not value or appreciate any of this. In fact, I pushed back and resisted my heritage. Italian Americans were heavily discriminated against in the not-so-distant past, and "the things we did" in relation to the dominant culture seemed silly and superstitious as well as a source of ridicule and alienation. I understand now that this is a common theme among diasporic peoples. It leads to a deep ancestral disconnect and a loss of historical orientation.

I should disclose that my intentional ancestral work began with a longing to connect with my Irish lineage. My mother is of Irish descent and this heritage, being generationally further back than my Italian heritage, was far more mysterious and enticing to me. I had a greater sense of loss around these ancestors, as they had immigrated four to five generations back and experienced a longer period of assimilation. My Italian heritage, in contrast, was a living presence in my life, so it didn't seem like an "ancestry" in the same way. And yet by seeking my Irish ancestors, I came to realize the value and support I have been blessed to receive from the relative *intactness* of my Italian-American culture. It has offered me the tools, groundedness, and sense of foundational well-being that I needed to face the much more challenging work of connecting with my Irish ancestry.

Part of my work on my Italian heritage has involved extended visits to Southern Italy to spend time with other plant folks, village healers, the land, and my relatives there. Back here, I sought out and increasingly appreciated many local Italian-American friends and elders that continue to practice the old ways. I was also able to return to Ireland for a blessed pilgrimage to the land and ancestors there. Of course, I'm not the only modern-day American with a mixed heritage. It may complicate one's journey to parse the different threads, but the process of choosing one line of ancestry to connect with often leads us toward other ancestors from different lines.

All of this occurred within the guiding forces of the plants and plant ancestors that began with my first herbal studies three decades ago. Initially my interest in plants—just learning to spend time sitting with them, observing them, and noticing the way they expressed themselves—seemed unrelated to my cultural-heritage journey. But of course, it was not. In fact, it was key.

Plants have a language, they have dialects, and they had much to tell me. I would often sit with plants whose names I didn't know so I could learn about them without any preconceived ideas or expectations around their character. As I tuned in to all potential sensory information such as smell, taste, touch, and any somatic signals that occurred in my body, I was treading in the footsteps of my human ancestors—I just didn't quite realize that yet.

It wasn't too long after beginning this practice, however, that I started to notice that although I might have no idea what a plant's name or use was, the sensory information I was receiving gave me some type of uncanny familiarity with them. It was like there were just some plants that I knew, like recognizing old friends, and I couldn't explain why. At some point in my training I asked my teacher at the time, Pam Montgomery, why I was having memories of plants I had never met before. She explained that they were waking up my epigenetic/ancestral links to plants used by my ancestors. Since then I've learned that our ancestral plants are not the only ones that can share ancestral knowledge and memories, but they seem to be the ones that afford us the most direct and potent contact with ancestral information, thus making them one of the most accessible means of ancestral reclamation available.

Human relations with plants involving not only their food and medicinal uses but also their significance as living beings of patterned and transactive presence has always been a component of human community. Human and other animal life could not exist on our planet without plants and the network of other life forms with which they interact and share generative convergence of life-sustaining biological fundamentals.

This is now my understanding and my message: Herbal medicine and plants are tools for ancestral reclamation and healing, accessible to anyone. This book is for anyone who is interested in connecting with their ancestral healing practices—no matter where on Earth your ancestors originated from.

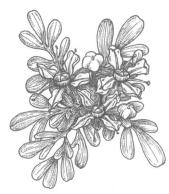

Wild-Foraged and Garden-Grown Remembrances

We can re-tell but not repeat, each storyteller must make the tradition come to life.

PETER GREY, *APOCALYPTIC WITCHCRAFT*

THIS BOOK IS NOT ABOUT going back in time to some ideal past or recreating the exact traditions of our ancestors. Instead this book is a basket, a woven bag of wild-foraged and garden-grown remembrances, as well as a collection of my own personal experience and noticing of how those traditions evolved through time, the way they are being practiced now, and their significance and potential for the current and future generations. It is also an ongoing adventure, a mythic tale from my own lived experience being born a second-generation Italian immigrant on Turtle Island. In my life I have been driven by longing and curiosity to collect whatever intact remnants of my people were given to me and others who are also doing this practice, without extracting these remnants from the entanglements of our times, weaving them instead into something embodied and real enough to perhaps lead others to their own adventures and discoveries.

In the words of Martin Prechtel,

We can no longer have our "old" origins back because we have lost that string long ago. What we can do is to begin a new string altogether which, by the blessing of the inevitability of time, will become a legitimate old origins for our descendants, and if we do it right, the one we lost as well will appear like a long-lost sprout by its own volition.

What this means in my own practice is that ancestral revival or reclamation is about deepening into the presence of now, not going back. It is also about the future and the collective visions we have for how cultural life will evolve for our descendants. My hope is that this book is both an anchor in time and a contact zone where multiple symbolic threads can come together and come alive in a new way.

Immigration in our capitalist industrial society often alienates us from our origins as the pressures of assimilation for survival demand that we shed our ethnic diversity, which results in our disconnect from collective social contracts and supports. Alienation replaces old systems of survival and adaptation with the dominant narrative, which in this case is individualistic and founded on the cultural traditions of the white Anglo-Saxon Protestant founders of the United States. Sometimes this is called assimilation, and it comes at a high price that ultimately erases and replaces our past in which our ancestors lived for thousands of years with a short history of maybe a hundred years or so.

When we reconnect to our ancestral memories and cultures, however, we begin to know ourselves as part of a living tradition beyond our political and racialized identities. This in turn grounds and centers us in our bodies, where we also begin to understand our ancestral griefs and traumas as well as to orient ourselves on the paths of our ancestors who led us to where we are now. Ultimately, our ancestor reclamation and connection can enable us to build a secure relationship or create an anchor in time with who and where we are in a way that frees us to live the creative present and leads the way for future generations.

Although this book is focused on Italian-American folk medicine and traditions, the basic methods that I describe can be applied to the reclamation of any traditional culture. That said, this is not a standardized system. Rather, it is an assemblage of my own personal exploration and discoveries along the path of ancestral reclamation.

Folk or vernacular medicine originated in small villages, and its methods were shared by oral tradition spoken in dialects by people who had lived in the same place for generation upon generation. These methods were inextricably linked to the unique and regional rituals of the people who performed them as a means of acknowledging and cultivating their sacred alignment with the mysteries of nature. This medicine belongs to the peasants who made a life from community-based self-sufficiency through practices of engagement with creation as an ongoing emergent process. Therefore, the medicine is not standardized or predictable, nor can it be reduced to repeatable proof or statistically significant evidence.

Folk medicine and traditions emerged in context with the landscape and the other-than-human world of beings, including deities, ghosts, mycelial fungi, shared history, and myths. This is part of the work of current generations seeking to reconnect to ancestral wisdom and embody it. We must ground our ancestral traditions in context and situate them in the time and space where we are now.

This presents challenges as most of us don't have teachers or elders to guide and support us. We are oftentimes starting with just a few hints of where we might have come from or none at all. This book will not replace the once-oral transmission of healing wisdom from elder to younger and shouldn't be mistaken for that.

Yet, we have to work with what we have even if all we have are remnants. Why? Because those remnants carry the holographic shreds of wisdom that, when noticed and followed, will lead us into our own origins and context starting right where we are at this moment. Our remnants call us beyond time and space into the same natural human longing that called our ancestors to devise and uphold these traditions through time. Remember, our ancestors had their own remnants that were woven into real context and cultures by necessity and longing much like we are doing now.

In this sense, this book starts in this moment, as the moveable center from where we can tap into the matrix of nonlinear time by stepping into the place where we are. From there it tracks back through some of the foundational history of Southern Italy and the Italian-American diaspora and then moves forward again into the dynamic present . . . to hopefully be continued in new and diverse ways through time. Thus, this book is not an ending or a beginning; it's a cross-section from the wild, spiral vortex of time.

This book is also not based on "expertise" in either Italian or Italian-American culture. And, in fact, I'd argue that any idea of "expertise" is antithetical to "folk" or vernacular traditions, as they are nonessentialist. This means that they are in constant creation and synergy with relational experience. Although knowledge can be transmitted via books and teachings, wisdom is something that happens through embodied experience and that cannot be taught; it must be lived. The Italian-American experience is vast and diverse, and this book is only based on my own experience. It is not intended to usurp or replace anyone else's. What I have written here is based on my lens, my personal life experience, as well as the research and teachings I've sought throughout my life. Tradition, culture, and healing are arts, not moralistic dogma. As Maggie Nelson says in her book *On Freedom*,

> The trickiness has to do with art's status as a third thing between people whose meaning, as Jacques Rancière has it, "is owned by no one, but which subsists between [artist and spectator], exluding any uniform transmission, any identity of cause and effect. . . ." Art is characterized by the indeterminancy and plurality of the encounters it generates, be they between a work and its maker, a work and its variegated audience, or a work of art and time. Its capacity to mean differently to different viewers—some of whom have not yet been born, or who died long ago—will always complicate any judgment that pretends certainty about any given work's meaning, or that purports that meaning to be self-evident or fixed.

Our vernacular healing traditions originated in place. These traditions were created by the people who were born in a particular spot on Earth that fed them from its seeds, waters, and winds for so long that the cellular blood, skin, and beating hearts of the people were made with the same elements as the trees, plants, and other animals living in the same place. Yet they are not static or immoveable. The word *place* comes from the Proto-Indo-European word *plat*, meaning "to spread," which is active. When something is "taking place," it means that something is "happening." Folk healing traditions are happening. They are "becoming with" place and the people that belong to a place and as such are a force of creation, part of the evolution of human community, and are in an ongoing process of emergence.

This process involves continuous and symbiotic regeneration of the raw, universal, and energetic forces of nature as it is happening with the current conditions of the living. Our traditions are the framework or vessel for these sacred activities of life; they are frameworks for our historical sovereignty that is not chained to the past or entranced by it but carries it as a lineage into the fold of recreation.

My access point to ancestral connection was founded in my work with plants, which are the primary focus of this book. All of us originally come from plant-based cultures, and plants and plant medicines have been in symbiotic relationship with the human community since the beginning of time. We have coevolved, and in my practice with my ancestors I have found plants to be strong mediums and allies that both awaken and hold space for our contact and remembrance of who we are and where we come from. Plants are the gathering basket, the net bag, where we connect to and collect our inherited losses, curses, blessings, and wounds.

I learned about the advantage of having such a container from Ursula Le Guin's model of the "carrier bag." In her essay "The Carrier Bag Theory of Fiction," she explains the cultural and practical necessity of having a container, or carrier bag, to hold our gatherings whether they be nuts and berries or stories, traditions, and words:

> I would go so far as to say that the natural, proper, fitting shape of the novel might be that of a sack, a bag. A book holds words. Words hold things. They bear meanings. A novel is a medicine bundle, holding things in a particular, powerful relation to one another and to us.[1]

A carrier bag or bundle or any other such container is also a receiver. It is capable of receiving and holding something to be carried somewhere, shared, or stored for later. As Le Guin puts it, this container can be "a leaf a gourd a shell a net a bag a sling a sack a bottle a pot a box a container. A holder. A recipient."[2] Even a container such as a cocoon, a cave, a meditation hut, or a compost bin can be a holder for change and transformation. Or, like the pericardium that wraps, holds, and bundles our hearts, a cloak or protector.

Plants and plant medicines are also examples of such containers, and as plant people we, too, become containers, holders, carriers, and recipients. As such, we are approaching an apex of sorts where we face the next turn of our trade as it lives within an inherited healing paradigm that has arrived at the crossroads of the current globalized industrial complex.

My expectation for this book is for each person who reads it to have a different experience and perspective with which to integrate the information. I honestly hesitate to write down and print living traditions because I don't believe they are meant to be fixed or literalized. I am also coming from a position of situated knowledge from which it is impossible to encompass the whole of *what Italian folk medicine is* for everyone either in the Italian diaspora or Southern Italy.

Each member of the Italian diaspora lived and is living their traditions in specific personal, generational, and geopolitical contexts. I say this carefully because there are certainly strong traditional components that must be fed by commitment and respect of principle amid any backdrop. This is part of why those of us doing the work of ancestral reclamation are doing it: to ground and orient us in a way that basically situates old beliefs and practices from knowledge gained through lifetimes of ancestors and makes them analogous and consistent with each person's life.

You do not need to be an herbalist to use this book. I've written it for the layperson as well as for the practiced plant folks. Our relationship with plants is constantly emerging and revealing new insights and ways of connecting. Plant relationships are no different than human relationships in that we are continuously learning about each other and growing and changing together.

You also don't need to know anything about your ancestry to use this book. One of the questions around ancestral connection that always comes up is, "What if I'm adopted or don't know anything about my lineage?" While that certainly adds a level of complexity, it's important to know that everyone has ancestors, and *they know you even if you don't know them.* The practical methods of addressing questions of unknown lineage are, of course, doing ancestral research and possibly getting DNA tested. This is controversial and not for everyone, but it can be enlightening for some.

This book is not a "how-to" book, although there are some recipes and ritual descriptions. There are enough other books and social media sites out there on how to do various practices. Italian folk medicine and magic have become so popular that basic techniques can be easily googled. Instead, this is more about what's beneath or within those practices and the trajectory they have taken through Western culture, herbal medicine, and the lateral, rhizomatic turns and twists that have shaped the way we express these traditions now from my view. As mythologist Michael Meade says, "The lost home we are seeking in ourselves; it is the story we carry within our soul."[3] My hope is that this book may help you find your own story that has been carried from human to human since the beginning of time but has now emerged in you in a unique way. This book is not meant to replace your story or experience with mine.

Another reason why I do not share many exact how-to formulas is because the ones that were given to me were given by oral transmission and, although I understand the importance of written and even videoed or recorded transmission, I believe that for now my familial practices are not ready to be shared in that way. As you will read about in chapter 8, the importance of keeping certain rituals *la segretezza*, or secret, is of utmost importance because it creates a container for the healing power. It is not to gatekeep the knowledge; it is to transmit it without leaking or losing its energetic and mythic meaning. Also, with the sharing of knowledge comes the responsibility for it and because traditional knowledge was cultivated and curated slowly through lifetimes, I believe we must be intentional and conscientious about how we choose to share it. I do not

believe that this makes the knowledge any less accessible as we are working with the same basic energies our ancestors were, and we are always
in a new place of beginning. Our ancestral traditions did not arrive on
the doorstep completely intact; they were grown from the soils and fed
by the rains and winds that our ancestors lived in. And we can do the
same as they did with what we have now. We can follow the same calls
and longings as our ancestors as those are the entry points to the eternal
where all magic emerges.

The inspiration for this book was not only a response to my work
with plants but also my work with my community as an activist and orga-
nizer. I have been involved with antiracist and other social justice movements since I was a child as my parents were both politically active, and
I was included in their organizing projects, going door to door, attending
meetings, making T-shirts for fundraisers, and so on. I grew up in a poor,
multicultural working-class immigrant neighborhood. My generation,
Generation X, was the first post-civil rights generation that experienced
integrated schools. I attended an integrated, public city school where
racial and ethnic tensions were part of everyday life. Yet, our history class
mainly provided the history of the United States and its founders, who
were not the ancestors of most of the student body. Knowing our ancestral history is a cornerstone to self-knowledge. This does not deny the
history of the places we live in now but enriches both it and us.

Along my own inner desire to learn my ancestral history, I was asked
in my direct and personal interactions with other ethnic and racial
groups, and in particular friends and teachers from the Haudenosaunee
(Iroquois) Confederacy, specifically the Kanien'kehá:ka (Mohawk)
nation, to understand myself and my people better so that we could come
to the council of all beings more self-oriented. The disconnected and lost
histories of those of European descent have resulted in continued harm
toward others as we have forgotten where we came from and how we got
here along with what the consequences of that colonialism have been and
continue to be for others. It is in our fullness, including the harms we've
caused, and not in the denial of it that we can truly meet the challenges
of the world today.

When reading this book, you may want to skip around to different chapters and sections rather than read straight through from the beginning. This is fine, but I do suggest at least reading chapter 1 first because that is where you will find the history, and as I mentioned above, our history is one of the fundamental keys to our deeper understanding.

The first section of this book starts with the origins of Southern Italian folk medicine. In chapter 1 I travel back to the ancient Mediterranean world, where the first healers divined the words of the gods at the sacred temples, and the Sibyls and oracles channeled prophecies. There are chapters on the Asclepiadic dream temples, the ancient Mediterranean physicians, and the first systems of plant medicine that have become part of modern herbal medicine practice, such as the four humors and the four elements. These foundational origins are where what we now know of as Italian folk medicine emerged and are still active principles in use by folk healers today in Southern Italy and in the Italian diaspora. This section also covers some other ancient practices such as astrology and tarot as well as Southern Italian animism.

Part 2 focuses on more recent manifestations of Italian folk medicine such as Italian witchcraft and Benedicaria. Benedicaria is is the Italian folk medicine that syncretized witchcraft animism with Catholic folk magic. It is still practiced in Southern Italy today.

Part 3 focuses more on practical skills and techniques. It includes methods of plant preparation, rituals, and recipes, tools and techniques for protecting, setting boundaries, and warding off the *malocchio* (evil eye), and material on kitchen medicine and magic.

Part 4 is a materia medica featuring plants that are native to the Mediterranean and primary remedies in Italian folk medicine. Each plant monograph provides the full multidimensional scope of plant uses from scientific constituents, folklore, and current uses in herbal medicine to magical applications.

It is my sincere hope that you will find something here that reminds you of your own center, your own lineage, or maybe even awakens an ancestral memory for you or somehow guides you toward your own direct realization. I don't believe a book is ever really complete because if we're engaged with the work on a dynamic level something new is always coming to light. I don't know everything about this topic, nor do I want to, as that would be exhausting. There may be things here that don't resonate with you, so feel free to exclude them. One of the main points I repeat to my students is that they always have the power of the word *no* in any interaction with plants or other magical practices. This includes saying no to me or my ideas. You don't have to like a plant just because I do.

As Peter Kingsley has said, "Real teachers leave no traces. They're like the wind at night rushing through you and totally changing you but leaving everything unchanged, even your greatest weaknesses; blowing away every idea of what you were and leaving you as you always have been since the beginning."[4] These words provide guidance for me and those I've taught and are something I aspire to. You already have everything, your ancestors are living in you and you in them, and there is nothing that anyone can teach you that you don't already know. All a book, a teacher, or an experience can do is light it up for you so you know it's there. Then the work is yours.

As I mentioned, this book is not just for those of Italian descent; it is for anyone who is reaching for their ancestral context and connection. Many of the cultural traditions of Southern Italy are similar to other traditions in the Mediterranean and all of Europe as well as other cultures worldwide. We all have ancestors even if we don't know who they are. And we all have ancestral plants with whom our DNA has coevolved and with whom we share ancestral and epigenetic memories. Plants are our ancestors that are still alive!

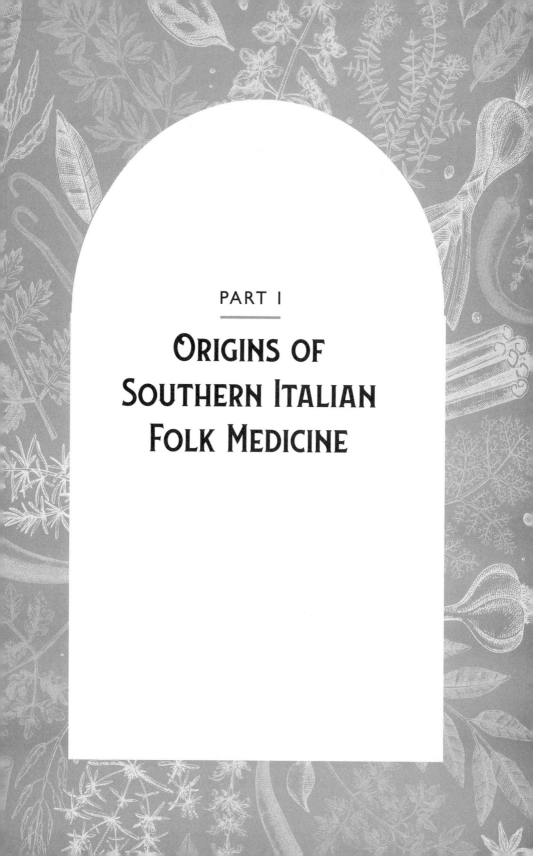

PART I

Origins of Southern Italian Folk Medicine

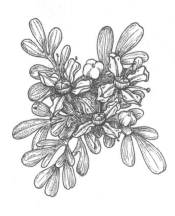

1

La Medicina Contadina

From Ancient Mediterraneans to Italian Americans

La medicina contadina che somministrava in dialetto le cure di un sapere dimenticato. La lingua delle guaritrici.

The peasant medicine that, administered in dialect, are the cures of a forgotten knowledge. The language of the healers.

CRISTIAN BONOMI, *Io Prima Di Me*

LA MEDICINA CONTADINA is an Italian phrase that means "folk or peasant medicine" with *medicina* translating as "medicine" and *contadina* meaning "peasant" or "farmer" in the feminine (note the a at the end). There are other words and phrases that describe this tradition such as *medicina popolare*, but I prefer *contadina*, or *contadini* (plural), because it brings in the peasant and farming origins of the practices. La medicina contadina, or peasant medicine, is the medicine that emerges from the heart of the common people and their continuous participation in the cycles of life and death, especially their struggle with oppressive, hierarchical systems of power.

Our folk traditions have been passed down through generations from cultures that can be traced back to before nation-states and global politics. When we practice ancestor remembrance we inevitably follow our lineage paths back through our ethnic, political, and cultural identities. While these identities make up only part of our relationship with our ancestors, they are important, as these are places and ways in which our ancestors—and we ourselves currently—interface with the world as it was and is, as well as how the world interfaces with us. Our ethnic identity points to where we emerged and from where we are continuously becoming. Political borders, nationality, and nationalism are real forces that are alive and impact how we experience all aspects of life. Yet, these are only points of reference along a timeline that goes back well before any idea of "identity."

The natural medicine that emerged from human hunter-gatherer interaction and attunement with the land did not end with farming and agriculture but was integrated with it. This is not a unique condition to Sud Italia (Southern Italy) and, in fact, it is the natural and ordinary way of being for most, if not all, indigenous peoples around the world.

Peasants or farmers, the contadini, were an integral part of society in Sud Italia and pretty much every other place on Earth. Our dominant narrative about farmers and peasants disparages them as the lower echelon of society who are uneducated, dirty, and powerless. Yet these are the people who, throughout history, have remained in the closest attunement with the undomesticated, still-wild forces of creation. As humanity shifted further and further toward domestication, the peasants and lower classes remained the most connected to survival: the need to predict the weather, the need to know where wild herds are grazing, the ways in which the wind is blowing, and therefore the ways in which the cycles were changing. They were at the contact point between the tamed and the untamed. As the imperative to transition from hunter-gatherer to farmer developed, so did a new relationship between humans and plants that required a different type of reverence and communion with natural forces.

The intentional raising of plants and animals is thought to have begun during the Neolithic era about ten to twelve thousand years ago in the fertile crescent.[1] The beginning of farming is also thought to have been the beginning of the end for humanity's unblemished, wild, utopian link to nature. No one knows exactly how or why farming began, but it's thought that it started as a way to increase food production so it could be stored and accumulated. This ultimately led to resource hoarding as a means of control and manipulation as well as an impetus for war. The adopting of agriculture practices by our ancestors has often been considered the intial catalyst of humanity's current systems of oppression and many of our dominant binary narratives about "good" and "evil." But historians and anthropologists debate how clear-cut this shift was, and our folkloric myths and cosmologies don't fit nicely into what is essentially an academic framework. Nobody actually knows exactly what our ancient ancestors' motivations were or exactly how humanity's transition to agriculture unfolded or why.

Ancestral and traditional medicine is not based in absolutes but instead is "situated," relational knowledge that, when intact, is transmitted from one generation to the next. When not intact, as is most often the case in our current times, it is forgotten, leaving us no anchors or points of reference for how what "is" relates to what "was." Reconstruction requires a great deal of theorizing and filling in the blanks, usually by employing what we currently know to be "normal" as our point of reference.

Situated knowledge, a term coined by social science scholar Donna Haraway, is knowledge gained, shared, and produced from multiple perspectives that are situated in relationship to many variables. These are always entangled with external powers and forces that include geography, ecology, the elements, and the essential conditions of "place" as well as multispecies interactions and our human networks of family and community. In other words, situated knowledge means that knowledge is based in place and time, as well as in a history that is both personal and collective and that the meaning of things changes through time and from place to place. Our traditional knowledge emerges from specific contexts. The traditions that we have now in the current times were formed based on information passed down through the generations and adapted to our lives now. This means that traditional knowledge can never be entirely objective. It's not standardized. As professor of critical psychology Wendy Holloway explains,

Whenever knowledge is thought, produced and disseminated, it's always because it is situated. It's situated in a certain time; it's situated historically; it's situated in certain places and it varies from place to place. It changes with social change. Knowledges change, social psychology has changed and continues to change in many ways. And it's also situated in terms of values, belief systems and cultural differences.[2]

Part of ancestral remembrance is to do our best to learn the way that our histories of lineage spiraled through time and place. It is often tempting to romanticize or bypass the people and events that are uncomfortable or difficult to integrate, but if we are to understand ourselves in our wholeness we have to acknowledge the shadows as well as the light of our lineages.

Italian folk medicine does not derive from one place or people but from a dynamic assemblage of cultural adaptations influenced by the entirety of the Mediterranean region. The ancient peoples of this area fall within the current borders of many nation-states that include Southern Europe and SWANA (Southwest Asia and North Africa), and all made major contributions to what is known as the Western world, particularly those nations of the Mediterranean that fall within the borders of Europe and that rose to prominence as a result of imperialism and colonization. The fullness of the history often erases the contributions and influence of the nations outside of Europe, and this is one area that is crucial for us to begin to remember. We also need to remember that our ancient peoples lived before patriarchy and capitalism and that their traditions were sacred and not secular and were not originally used to oppress others.

According to author and scholar of Western spiritual philosophy Peter Kingsley, we have been in a collective sleep in the West where we have forgotten who we are and where our sacred origins began. He says that we need to recover this knowledge in order to relate to others in a way that is nonappropriative and that can cultivate authentic connection and real oneness among peoples. This will offer us the opportunity for new and diverse traditions to evolve in a way that is creative and vital for our times.

Once we have a firm grounding in our own sacred traditions, then we can relate to other sacred traditions. And that's what

practitioners of other sacred traditions, whether it's indigenous shamans or elders or Tibetan Buddhists, that's what they want from us.
It's fine for them to discuss their sacred traditions with us but that's
not really a connection or really oneness. It's talking about oneness.
To me the real oneness comes when the different traditions come
together experientially.[3]

The Ancient Mediterranean

One day when I was standing looking out over the Tyrrhenian Sea on the
west coast of Southern Italy, I watched the waves splash up along the edges
of the hot, arid landscape and wondered how many of my own ancestors
might have stood looking in this exact same place. My eyes now looking at
the same place theirs once looked, my feet touching the same sands theirs
might have, my body a vessel of DNA that evolved beneath the same Sun,
my breath becoming one with the same air, and the gods of place whisper-
ing in my ear as they did to my ancient people. Although I have always
lived in diaspora and grew in another place, my body remembers times far
beyond my own life in all directions, especially when I'm in Italy.

Southern Italy is a land of volcanoes and hot, dry summers, yet there is
something fresh and vibrant all around in the forests grown on volcanic ash
and the fields fed by underground aqueducts and mountain washes. Before
I had ever traveled to Italy, I asked my nonno how so many delicious foods
grew in such a dry place, and he said, "Oh, everything grew!" And it was
true; the figs, lemons, olive trees, and all the home gardens were all so lush.

There are three active volcanoes in Southern Italy: Mount Vesuvius
(Naples), Mount Etna (Sicily), and Mount Stromboli (off the coast of
Calabria). Both Vesuvius and Etna are so active that they are under con-
stant surveillance by the International Association of Volcanology and
Chemistry of the Earth's Interior, or IAVCEI, a project of the United
Nations that conducts research and promotes public awareness about the
current status and hazards of the world's volcanoes. There are multiple
other dormant and extinct volcanoes formed where the Eurasian and
African tectonic plates once collided thirty million years ago. The Italian

peninsula is literally made from this collision and exists along the boundary of the two plates.

The soils of Southern Italy have been fed for millennia by volcanic ash, making the land rich in minerals, layered with magma, and fed by underground springs that rise from deep caverns beneath the surface. Italy's water comes from both these springs and rainfall, although in current times Italy is facing water shortages, like most of the world, as climate change and failing water systems impact availability.

Southern Italy is itself an element of the greater landscape and ecology that is part of the entire Mediterranean basin. When we are exploring our folk traditions, it's important to remember that the ecosystem, which includes the entire living field of interacting forces and beings, is an integral part of their formation and dynamism. All cultural systems are defined by seasonal cycles, weather patterns, geological formations, natural disasters, and, according to our ancestors, all interspecies inhabitants including mythological/spiritual gods and otherworldly spirits. Human participation in nature includes our capacity to sensorially alchemize ecological information into dreams, myths, art, and ritual that are the raw materials of cultural traditions. And, in fact, human culture emerges directly from the landscape and geography and, at the same time, becomes part of the ecology.

The area of the world that we now call Italy has only been considered a nation-state since 1861. When we look at the ancient history of the region we see that it is geographically and culturally part of the much wider region of the Mediterranean basin and beyond. One of the dominant but unproven narratives about the Paleolithic and Neolithic peoples of the Earth is that they lived in separate, isolated bands. Yet based on ethnographic evidence we also know that cross-regional cultural traditions are astoundingly similar. Our ideas about social organization now do not necessarily correspond backward in time. Our ideas around political boundaries do not have supporting evidence from prehistory, nor do our ideas about the way "primitive" people were able to trade and exchange goods and information.

In the book *The Dawn of Everything*, authors David Graeber and David Wengrow contend that in earlier centuries, forms of regional organization might extend thousands of miles. Aboriginal Australians, for instance, could travel halfway across the continent, moving among people who spoke entirely different languages. . . . "Society," insofar as we can comprehend it at that time, spanned continents.

In fact, the evidence suggests that the people of the Upper Paleolithic were quite cosmopolitan [as] "from the Swiss Alps to Outer Mongolia, they were often using remarkably similar tools, playing remarkably similar musical instruments, carving similar female figurines, wearing similar ornaments and conducting similar funeral rites."[4]

Our general concept of society becoming global and more homogenous is true in a sense, yet our borders and boundaries have become more rigid with passports, checkpoints, and immigration bans.

If we survey what happens over time, the scale on which social relations operate doesn't get bigger and bigger; it actually gets smaller and smaller. . . . Overall, though, what we observe is not so much the world as a whole getting smaller, but most peoples' social worlds growing more parochial, their lives and passions more likely to be circumscribed by boundaries of culture, class, and language.[5]

The archaeological evidence for this is solid. Artifacts of "primitive trade" have shown us that various types of "currency" such as stones, gems, and other valuable objects traveled great distances: "3000 years ago Baltic amber found its way to the Mediterranean, or shells from the Gulf of Mexico were transported to Ohio."[6]

Diversity Hot Spot

The Mediterranean Basin includes portions of Europe, Africa, and Asia. It begins in the west with Cabo Verde and spreads to the east as far as Jordan and Turkey. It includes Lebanon, Syria, Palestine, and the Balkan states as well as the entire coast of North Africa and Southern Europe as far north as the Azores.

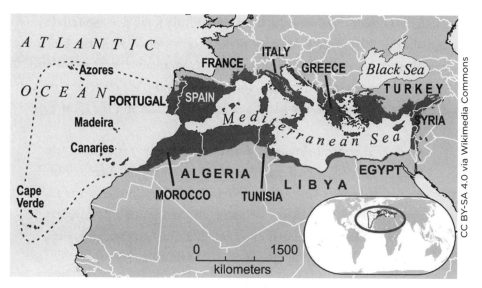

Map of the Mediterranean Basin
Conservation International

The Mediterranean Basin is characterized by hot, dry summers but bountiful winter rains. During the Last Glacial Maximum, or LGM, when the glacier was at its greatest extent, Italy was beneath the alpine ice cap, which disconnected it from the rest of Europe and protected it and the entire Mediterranean from the negative impacts of the last Ice Age, allowing the region's abundant diversity to continue to flourish. It is the second largest hotspot for biodiversity in the world and the third largest hotspot for plant diversity. There are an estimated twenty-five thousand plant species in the Mediterranean, many of which are endemic, meaning they do not exist anywhere else on Earth. The Mediterranean Sea is rich with marine creatures, including three hundred mammal species, and the forests host more diverse tree species than any other forests in Europe.[7]

The Ancient Peoples

The oldest human remains found in Italy date back one million years and were the ancestors of modern humans. The ancient hominins of Italy include *Homo erectus*, *Homo heidelbergensis* (Ceprano), and *Homo neanderthalensis* (Neanderthal). According to archaeological evidence, modern humans inhabited the Italian peninsula forty-five thousand years ago, during the Upper Paleolithic period.[8] Italy's position in the center of the Mediterranean basin made it accessible from many directions for trade, cultural exchange, and migration. Immigration and trade routes intersected Italy from the Balkans, the Black Sea regions, Africa, and the Near East.

> During the Neolithic and for thousands of years later, the Mediterranean Sea itself contributed to shortening the distances and making Italy one of the gateways to the European continent: first acting for millennia as a barrier separating the African and the European continents, and then turned into a bridge as the first Bronze Age seafarers started to travel in open water (Broodbank 2006).[9]

Many groups and civilizations are known to have inhabited the Italic Peninsula, which has a diverse genetic and cultural history. Countless people have either migrated to or colonized Italy since the Neolithic period including Near Eastern farmers and Italic tribes descended from the Indo-Europeans, Ligurians, Etruscans, Phoenicians, Greeks, Celts, Goths, Lombards, Byzantines, Franks, Normans, Swabians, Arabs, Berbers, Albanians, Austrians, and more. In fact, the Phoenicians colonized Southern Italy and Greece somewhere between the twelfth and eighth centuries BCE,[10] before either region became prominent empires, and they have been referred to as the "first rulers of the Mediterranean."[11]

There is also much evidence of prehistoric humans in Italy. The infamous goddess figurine known as the Venus of Willendorf is a thirty-thousand-year-old artifact whose origin has been traced to Italy, indicating that ancient peoples had lived there.[12] Remains and evidence of the Uluzzian culture, including human bones, shell beads, and natural mineral pigments, were discovered in the Grotta del Cavallo (Cave of the Horse) around the region of what is now Apulia. This group of cave dwellers inhabited the area during the transition from the Middle to Upper Paleolithic periods.[13] Uluzzian caves have also been identified in other areas of Italy, including Campania, Basilicata, and Calabria as well as in Greece.[14]

The Villbruna hunters and gatherers left evidence of their existence fourteen thousand years ago in the Veneto region. Burial objects such as painted stones, a chunk of ochre, propolis, and a flint knife were discovered. The grave was marked with burial drawings made with ochre.[15]

Early farmers were thought to have migrated to Italy from the Near East in about 8000 BCE, replacing or displacing the hunter-gatherers. The archaeological evidence uncovered from this early agricultural period was the foundation of the work of archaeologist Marija Gimbutas. Southern Italy was part of the region that Gimbutas designated Old Europe. According to Gimbutas, Old Europe existed during the late Neolithic period (7000–3500 BCE) and included the Adriatic, Aegean, Central Baltic, Middle Danube Basin, East Balkan, and Moldavian-West Ukrainian areas.

What we now know as Southern Italy was a part of the Adriatic region of Old Europe. These were pre-Indo-European indigenous civilizations that had a complex social organization, artistic and healing traditions, and an intricate economic system based on food production. The people of these times had written language that was primarily expressed in symbolic script and many other technologies and tools, including metallurgy and the domestication of plants and animals. It is most important to note here that, according to Gimbutas's findings, these societies were peaceful and matricentric, and no cultural expressions of war or warlike symbolism have been found in any of the archaeological artifacts.

These societies also held prolific cosmological beliefs that were intertwined with the art, ritual, and social expressions of daily and seasonal existence. Plants were a central focus of life as both food and medicine. Archaeological symbols have been discovered that reference the vegetal life cycle, the seasonal cycles, and the cycle of life, death, and regeneration. Indigenous cultures have always been plant based, which means that plants were not only valued as a food source and means of survival but that they were also an integral component of the social ecology or the social field.

People had emotional and spiritual relationships with plants that involved more than just a physical-needs exchange. Plants were often deified with the personas of gods and goddesses as well as animistic nature spirits and allies. Plant medicines were not only used to treat acute illnesses but were also invoked in ritual preparations such as smoke and used in performative art, as objects of divination, and as entheogenic substances to induce prophetic and healing trances. Healing and the use of plants in healing in the ancient Mediterranean was intricately woven into the human relationship with divine energies, as the sacred and the profane were in a constant dance within the earthly lives of the people.

Around 3200 BCE the Indo-Europeans arrived from the Caucasus Mountains and Pontic Steppe. The archaeological evidence from this invasion shows a regional transition from a peaceable matricentric culture to a more warrior-like patriarchal culture from which the tribal groups of the Bronze Age and forward emerged.

The Italic Tribes

The Italic tribes were ethnolinguistic groups that spoke Indo-European derived languages. It is likely that they merged with the microregional people that were already in Italy so, though there is great cultural diversity among groups, the Italic tribes and their modern descendants spoke from the same linguistic root.

We see that starting around 1100–600 BCE, Italy hosted large tribal groups such as the Oenotrians whose name means "people from the land of the vines" or "people led by Oenotrus." The territory of this group stretched through Southern Italy from Paestum (Salerno) to southern Calabria. These were the people who were in Southern Italy when the Greeks first colonized it. It is thought that the Oenotrians migrated from the north, pushing previous groups such as the Elymi, Itali, and Siculi into Sicily.[16]

The Etruscans and Latins

Existing around the same time as the Oenotrians, the Etruscans, a mysterious people, were prominent in the areas of the Po Valley, Tuscany, western Campania, Umbria, Emilia-Romagna, Lazio, southeastern Lombardy, and southern Veneto. Part of the mystery is that the Etruscans did not speak an Indo-European-derived language; nor did their language have any known parent languages.[17] The origin of the Etruscans is highly debated. One idea is that they were early Greek settlers, but another suggests that they were an ancient indigenous group, and recent DNA analysis supports this view.[18] It is the Etruscans who are sometimes believed to have founded Rome. A competing and more likely theory is that Rome was founded by the Latins (another Indo-European descended group), or that it was a collaborative between the two groups.

Other Major Tribes

The ethnic and cultural groups of people who have inhabited the Italic peninsula have been ever mixing, mingling, and recombining due to the constant flux of political and social conditions. Even during the height of the Roman Empire, there were diverse tribal societies that inhabited what eventually became the regional provinces of modern Italy.

Some of the most prominent tribes include the Samnites, who inhabited the southern Apennine Mountains around the area now known as Campania and Naples, the Lucani who were generally located around the areas of Apulia and Basilicata, the Brutii who occupied what is now Calabria, and the Sicani, who lived on the island of Sicily.

The Italian Diaspora

From these ancient roots what we now know as the nation-state of Italy was eventually formed. In fact, the formation of this republic occurred quite recently, as mentioned in the beginning of this chapter, and has been called the Risorgimento, or the unification of Italy. This event combined the south and north of Italy. Before this, Southern Italy and Sicily were known as the Kingdom of the Two Sicilies and were under Bourbon rule.

The unification of Italy has been considered by many, particularly Southern Italians, to have been an all-out conquest, an invasion from the north that ousted the prosperous functioning monarchies of the Kingdoms of the Two Sicilies. Southern Italy is also known as *mezzogiorno*, which means "midday" and refers to how hot the Sun gets there. The Kingdom the Two Sicilies was a sovereign state that included all of mezzogiorno, the island of Sicily, and the island of Sardinia. It was formed from the merger of two previous kingdoms, the Kingdom of Naples and the Kingdom of Sicily and was one of the last remaining feudal societies in the world. Land was owned by nobles and the church or was communal. The peasants didn't own land and primarily lived in towns and villages and farmed the common land outside of the villages.

The Risorgimento did not ultimately bode well for the south as the invading expedition led by Giuseppe Maria Garibaldi, an Italian general, moved thousands of troops into mezzogiorno, overthrowing the capital cities and absconding with the wealth held there. This included the possession of the southern banks that sent the vast fortune of the overthrown Bourbon monarchy to support northern agendas. The north sent its system disparities to the south by implementing and enforcing northern laws and economic policies that were not applicable to the agricultural- and communal-based methods and conditions that drove the southern prosperity and cultural cohesion. The feudal land system of the south was dismantled, with the north confiscating and dividing monastic lands, breaking up communal farms, and transferring land ownership to the elite members of the northern regime. This left southern farmers to sharecrop for northern landlords amidst increasing taxes and little-to-no profit margin. Overall, the unification of Italy was a disaster for the south and resulted in the severe oppression of its peasant people, ultimately leading to mass emigration.

The unification of Italy did not unify the people of the south; it destroyed their villages and communities, as individuals and often entire families fled abject poverty and political violence to become refugees in the United States and other places worldwide while most of the industrialization and its resulting wealth remained in the north. The unification and the subsequent economic disparities it created is what directly led to the mass emigration from Southern Italy. The small-scale agriculture, subsistence farming, and traditional shepherding practices of the south led them to an economic disadvantage that still exists there today.

Southern Italy is distinct from Northern Italy, and there has been an ongoing divide between the two regions for eons. Although there is no physical divide, it is quite obvious economically and politically. The south is statistically much poorer than the north. For instance, in 2018 the unemployment rate in the province of Calabria (the toe of the boot in Southern Italy) was 21.6 percent as opposed to the northern province of Tuscany at 7.3 percent. The distribution of wealth is most noticeable along the north/south divide, with the majority of Italy's wealth being generated in the north and only 22.5 percent of the nation's entire GDP for 2017 coming from the south. Northern Italy is far more industrialized than Southern, and this adds to the divide as Southern Italy remains an agrarian culture. There are several other distinctions between the two that are often cited, including differences in food styles, lifestyle, music, and many other aspects of culture.[19]

Immigration

The Italian immigrants left Southern Italy to find work in many places, including Australia, Canada, and, of course, the United States where they were welcomed as part of the American call for mass labor during the late 1800s and early 1900s. An important but largely unacknowledged aspect of Italian immigration is that the primary motivation of most of the immigrants was to find jobs and send money back to their families. Many Italians went back and forth several times, living in both places. It was not necessarily because they wanted to leave their homelands for a better life or "streets paved with gold," but that they were doing what they had to in order to help their families survive.

The Italian diaspora in the United States today is its fifth largest ethnic group,[20] as many did ultimately remain in America. Still the Italian immigrants tried their best to maintain their strong sense of family and cultural traditions by living in the communal ways they were accustomed to in their homeland, while also trying to adapt and survive in a new country. They faced widespread discrimination and oppressive violence including the lynching of eleven Sicilians, which was one of the largest mass lynchings in US history.

The pressure to assimilate and acculturate was powerful. Most Italian homes insisted upon their children speaking only English and acting and dressing according to American ways at least outside the home. The desire to blend in and belong was a means of survival where access to resources and economic stability depended upon the standards of white, Anglo social systems.

The Italian immigrants lived in enclaves, or segregated sections of the towns and cities where they settled. This supported the continuation and transmission of their cultural traditions to the following generations. Some of the most prominent facets of Southern Italian culture have been carried on in the Italian-American diaspora down to second- and even third-generation Italian Americans. There was strong pressure for Italian immigrant children to marry other Italians, so often the first generation born in America had both parents of Italian descent. Although the pervading tendency was to speak English, many older immigrants never learned it or spoke with accents, and their children and grandchildren grew up hearing "broken English" laced with common words of dialect from their local regions.

The traditions that the Italian immigrants brought with them included their regional dialects, foods, cultural customs, and folk healing methods. A major aspect of Southern Italian culture, as with all indigenous cultures, was plant based with the use of specific native plants in the preparation of foods and herbal remedies as well as in facets of worship, ritual, and deeply embedded folk Catholicism.

Ultimately, the food, folk Catholicism, and "superstitions" of the Italian immigrants were integrated into what became a distinct Italian-American culture. These very customs that made them different in a new country were also a means of orienting and adapting. This means that Southern Italian culture and folk medicine have been successively preserved as well as adapted in a unique way outside of the country of Italy.

What Is a Tradition?

Knowing something's origins does not determine what happens next.

DONNA HARAWAY, *FOR THE WILD (PODCAST)*

Although this is not a treatise on immigration and culture loss, it is an act of cultural recovery and adaptation as well as what I believe is an important practice for facing the current crises of our times. It is necessary here to consider the meaning and our understanding of the nature of what we call traditions. The word *tradition* literally means "transmitted thing." The basic definition of *tradition* is "the transmission of a custom or belief from one generation to the next," and a tradition can be created between as little as two generations. *Traditional* is defined by ethnobotanists as "something that has been an integrated part of a culture for more than one generation."[21]

Another important aspect of traditions is that they are not fixed or static. Traditions are fluid, flexible, and mobile. Traditions travel and are an inextricable part of both personal and collective human evolution. They emerge from practices and methods of survival that have evidently worked for previous generations in relation to the conditions they engaged with during their lifetimes and what they learned as a result.

In this sense, traditions are not arbitrary but innovative and intentionally formulated to ensure the transmission of information between people of the present and the future. In a sense, traditions are a language of communication through time. They are historical records that form a continuous thread around the Earth from the vast reaches between diverse cultures and peoples where exchange and convergence has occurred to the familial and individual shared experiences of each of us.

This movement is being reflected internationally in response to the effects on local and regional culture due to large-scale globalization and mass-media culture. In 2003, the United Nations Educational, Scientific, and Cultural Organization, or UNESCO, held the Convention for the Safeguarding of Intangible Cultural Heritage, which began the process of recognizing and protecting what they have called "intangible cultural heritage." This is defined as

> the practices, representations, expressions, knowledge, skills—as well as the instruments, objects, artefacts, and cultural spaces associated therewith—that communities, groups and, in some cases, individuals recognize as part of their cultural heritage. This intangible cultural heritage, transmitted from generation to generation, is constantly rec-reated by communities and groups in response to their environment, their interaction with nature and their history, and provides them with a sense of identity and continuity, thus promoting respect for cultural diversity and human creativity. For the purposes of this Convention, consideration will be given solely to such intangible cultural heritage as is compatible with existing international human rights instruments, as well as with the requirements of mutual respect among communities, groups and individuals, and of sustainable development.[22]

This program has designed five main domains that list the specific areas of culture that are included. Plants have been recognized here under the domain of "Knowledge and Practices Concerning Nature and the Universe" as "knowledge about local flora and fauna" and "traditional healing systems."

According to sociologist Edward Shills in his book *Tradition,*

> a tradition includes: material objects, beliefs about all sorts of things, images of persons and events, practices and institutions. It includes buildings, monuments, landscapes, sculptures, paintings, books, tools, machines. It includes all that a society of a given time possesses and which already existed when its present possessors came upon it and which is not solely the product of physical processes in the external world or exclusively the result of ecological and physiological necessity.[23]

Not only is tradition a "transmitted thing," it is also a thing in the process of being transmitted. It is a living, dynamic, and emergent expression of how a people form and organize relationships with each other and the more-than-human world as well as their understanding of their position and influence in it.

Traditions are meant to create stability and webs of connection through time and space that ground each generation in the present while enabling them to have access to the full database of ancestral knowledge, from where their current situation evolved. This enables them to orient, center, and create the dynamic equilibrium necessary for generative and holy engagement with life as well as to carry and shape these wisdoms with the information gained by their experience until they can be passed forward to the next generations.

Although traditions generally emerge within the collective, the unique expression of the individual is where the meaning of each tradition is expressed, and each person and generation will interpret and modify them as necessary. This means that although they are built on past representations, new versions of old ways emerge in every person and every generation. Therefore, traditions are adaptable and subject to change.

We see this clearly in the Italian-American diaspora where individuals, often separately from ancestral villages and family, carried their community knowledge with them and used it to creatively develop new versions and expressions of this knowledge, combined with that of the other Italian immigrants in the new world. This often meant imaginatively using ingredients that they weren't used to, intuitively adapting old formulas and remedies, making new prayers that could address the concerns of living in a foreign land, and creating new ways of expressing traditional knowledge that could be shared locally and produce similar webs of connection to the way they once lived but in a new place.

As Donna Haraway has said, our cultural traditions are practices of knowing and living now that include their historical and ancestral connection as a combination of events that are not separate from their "complex historical embeddedness of the things known and the knowers." Our traditions are "strong truths and a profound relationality in historical conjuncture . . . a profound relationality."[24] And according to Per

Binde in his *Bodies of Vital Matter,* "a tradition of knowledge is handed down from the past to the present, from one generation to the next, but it is also subject to constant modification."[25]

The way that traditions are expressed from one generation to the next is not necessarily predictable, and there are always aspects that will cease to be transmitted for various reasons, including cultural assimilation and oppression and the need for reformed knowledge. This can look like cultural and tradition loss, but it is more accurate to say that traditions are modified from two basic perspectives: the micro-perspective, which involves the way that the imaginal and intellectual processes of the individual give meaning to applied cultural symbols and collective knowledge, and the macroperspective that includes social change over time.

This means that our traditions from the past, even many generations back, are entwined with the new traditions we all participate in here and now, although they may be changed beyond recognition. Even so, if we look deeply at ourselves and our personal history, we can often find traces of where our own worldview and cultural perspectives originated. This is not in an effort to go back to an idealized time and place where we were all part of intact indigenous communities and everything was wonderful. That is not even possible and there is, in fact, no conclusive way to know exactly how our ancestors lived, thought, prayed, or connected with healing and the sacred although there is often good reason to mourn these great losses, especially now as our world becomes more and more globalized and standardized. And in fact, we need to mourn and use that feeling of grief and loss to guide us toward our remembering of who we are and where we came from.

> *My teacher always said that, if there is to be any hope whatsoever of living well on this earth, we have to take the ancient root and put new sap in it. That doesn't mean we need to do something new, but to do something old in a new way, which takes great courage.*
>
> MARTIN PRECHTEL, "SAVING THE INDIGENOUS SOUL"

Ethics of Transmission:
Ancestral Reclamation

As I have progressed along my personal path with my ancestral work I have been in a continuous state of self-examination and questioning as well as in continuous conversations with others about the ethical concerns of ancestral reclamation from the position of the Italian diaspora. While I don't have exact answers, and I certainly don't have answers for everyone, I have occasionally found solid ground to move forward from, which ultimately leads to more questions.

There have been many inspiring people along the way, but one person in particular I'd like to mention here is Alexis Pauline Gumbs. While listening to a podcast interview between Alexis and Prentiss Hemphill, I found a beacon of truth in Alexis's words. She described her work with her ancestors as a way for her to become a "compass of ancestral light" and a "knowing where we are." The question is less about knowing *who* we are and more about knowing *where* we are. This work creates an expanded view of ourselves beyond our individual or separate identities that puts us in contact with a greater matrix of being with others. "I'm not an individual, I'm a multitude," Alexis says.

Because of the recent increase in popularity of ethnic folk healing traditions, one of the issues that continuously comes up in my own work with ancestral revival/reclamation is how to receive, transmit, share, collaborate, and steward our ancestral traditions. When there has been such profound culture loss it is imperative that cultural transmission is made accessible collectively without so-called gatekeeping. *Gatekeeping* by definition is "the activity of controlling, and usually limiting, general access to something."

Yet these very traditions were originally embedded in place and in communities as well as families where they were facilitated via long-standing social contracts. At this time, particularly in diaspora, those social contracts no longer exist for many of the younger generations. There are no intentional rites of passage or initiations being guided by responsible elders.

It is becoming more and more common to find the techniques and methods of Italian folk medicine shared widely on social media and otherwise, yet they were not originally intended for mass consumption. These traditions were transmitted orally and in real life between specific people. Not everyone in the community would be transmitted the knowledge of every healing technique or formula. This knowledge was considered potent and powerful; therefore it was passed on carefully, sometimes after years of training and relationship building between an elder and a younger.

Sometimes healing methods were considered "secret" and never shared outside of the sacred relationships between those who were specifically chosen to receive the knowledge. This is because knowledge is powerful and not everyone has the psychosocial-neurological capacity to be in contact with it. The elders were responsible for determining when a person was ready to receive *il potere* (the power). It is also thought in some regions of Italy that the elder loses their power when they pass it on, so they would not do so until they were about to die. In other cases, the younger person receiving the healing methods and formulas were held to secrecy because if their elder was still alive and practicing, they could lose their power if it was shared.

At the same time, it is true that the transmission of knowledge in Italian folk medicine followed specific frameworks. It is also true that most of those past means of sharing no longer are in effect. This is partly what led to our culture loss. It's a bit of a double bind and begs the following question: How do we continue to remember and regenerate our ancestral traditions in a way that is sincere and genuine while also keeping intact the power and fullness of the potential energy of our healing methods without bypassing important initiatory steps and trainings that make a sacred and cohesive container?

Gatekeeping can be interpreted in multiple ways but it generally has a negative connotation in that it suggests that only certain people are holding the knowledge and wisdom and are doling it out as they see fit based on their own ego desires and agenda, as well as for monetary benefit. Basically, it's a colonial, capitalistic expression of greed and scarcity. So we don't need gatekeeping, but we do need stewardship. Even our fragments of cultural knowledge must be held in reverence and combined with close communication with our ancestors. Along the way of ancestral remembrance, we have to continually ask ourselves if our work is in alignment with our heart and with what our ancestors are asking of us, as well as what we hope to pass down to the future generations.

Our cultural traditions and transmissions are sacred and bound to context and place in many ways that makes it unethical to just pour them out all over the place or make them into a marketing strategy. One thing about traditional cultures—Italian or otherwise—is that there is a process that one would go through to become a mature, proficient, and respected member of the community. It included specific stages as well as initiations, some formal and public, others informal and carried out in the daily moments of family and community life. Skilled proficiency in healing or cultural magics had to be practiced and demonstrated before others, whether that be zie (aunts) and nonne or the neighbors and parish.

For instance, in Italian culture the Catholic sacraments would mark the phases of spiritual development, and one had to meet the requirements of each sacrament to proceed to the next. Much of this was abandoned by subsequent generations as assimilation to secular life took hold, and the Catholic church became a source of much abuse, scandal, and powermongering.

Another aspect of traditional culture is that it was largely self-regulating. Italian villages, and to some degree Italian-American enclaves, were insular and self-sufficient. Cultural transmission was passed on within the community in the following five basic ways:

1. Knowledge was familial and shared between generations based on the discretion of the elders in the family. Family life was extended and nonnuclear, and personal identity was centered on the family not the individual. There was a great deal of yielding to the collective that meant the individual's wants or desires might not be met.

For me this was one of the most challenging aspects of growing up Italian as interdependent family or communal life was in direct opposition to the Western cultural paradigm I was living in, which held the individual and their independence at the center of social and economic life. Access to resources came from the ability to compete in the market as an individual not from the ability to cooperate interdependently with others in a family or community group. Access from resources didn't come from our ability to form consensual and reciprocal relationships where we were held accountable for how we interacted with power dynamics.

2. Knowledge was shared among village or neighborhood members and again often at the discretion of elders. Certain types of knowledge could only be shared among family members while others could be exchanged between families. Often this happened as a result of friendship or marriage relationships.

3. Elders were trusted based on lifelong transparency and reputation. Trust was earned over a lifetime. Transparency was at the heart of this type of trust. In traditional cultures people talked among themselves. They talked to each other. They lived in close proximity and met outside of the family regularly. If someone was lying or hiding something it didn't take long for everyone to know. Word got around. Now we call this gossip, and it's used a weapon to outcompete, cancel, or otherwise disparage others, often and especially in social media spaces, when we really don't have any in-person knowledge of each other and where there are not adequate containers for conversation with one another.

4. Younger folks were sometimes told that they did not have the skill or mastery to be given certain types of information. There was no entitlement to knowledge, especially spiritual, healing, or sacred knowledge. You had to demonstrate that you had the capacity for it. This was not the same as getting a license or certificate. Credibility came from the expression and practice of the individual as well as how they were observed handling their own energy and their relations with others.

5. Everyone was held accountable by both the family and community. If you did something that did not align with the shared values and social mores of the village or neighborhood there were consequences usually doled out by parents or other adults. These consequences could exclude you from certain aspects of cultural life, usually temporarily but sometimes not. It could include exile.

An example from my own life is that my great-grandfather left my great-grandmother and had another family. When he wanted to bring his new wife and children to his village in Italy to meet his family, he was told that he could not come. He had broken a communal agreement as well as a spiritual/Catholic one.

Please don't mistake these points to mean that I think we should go back to this style of knowledge transmission. I honestly don't know what the best way forward is, but I do know that we need to steward our traditions somehow and that in a society of hyperindividualism it is a great challenge to determine how to share and facilitate knowledge ethically and sustainably. I hope this becomes a greater conversation as we all move forward toward a better world.

Overall, I believe that we need to be able to hold a paradox in order to regenerate a culture that can carry diverse traditions respectfully and ethically. The paradox being that we live in the climate of capitalism, white supremacy, and so on while attempting to revive ways of being that are intentionally and strategically destroyed by such. Going forward amid all of these considerations is an uncharted path where we are bound to make mistakes, but we must try to do our best by taking it slow, asking for help, and being in community with others who hold similar values as much as we can.

I don't think there is one answer, and every situation is highly nuanced and complex. Reading the book *Sand Talk* by Tyson Yunkaporta, I found that I really resonate with how he explains the necessity of respect for our own cultures as well as others. He says,

> Respectful observation and interaction within the system, with the parts and connections between them, is the only way to see the pattern. You cannot know any part, let alone the whole, without respect. Each part, each person, is dignified as an embodiment of the knowledge. Respect must be facilitated by custodians, but there is no outsider-imposed authority, no "boss," no "dominion over."[26]

In this sense each of us is a custodian or facilitator of our traditions, which requires that in our ancestral work we form ethical relationships within our traditions, with our ancestors, and with others within the culture and with those from other cultures that we are in the field of experience, or the ecosystem, with.

Yunkaporta says this requires cultural humility as a "useful exercise in understanding your role as an agent of sustainability in a complex system." When we use this framework for discerning the differences between cultural appropriation and cultural exchange, gatekeeping and respectful facilitation, what to withhold and what to share, it's quite clarifying.

Asking ourselves how we can become the ethical stewards, as opposed to owners of, our present culture and our ancestral cultures as they are emerging in the present is a moveable and adaptive inquiry that can aid our attunement with changing conditions, if we can hold both respect and ethics while maintaining an open system that allows the flow of adaptable knowledge to the benefit of the past, present, and future.

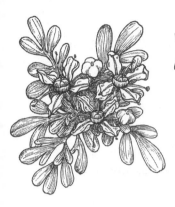

2

A Fusion of Knowledge

Western Herbalism and Italian Folk Medicine

When you know the fourfoil in all its seasons root and leaf and flower, by sight and scent and seed, then you may learn its true name, knowing its being: which is more than its use.

OGION IN URSULA K. LE GUIN'S
THE WIZARD OF EARTHSEA

OUR CONCEPTION OF HERBALISM in the dominant culture is derived from the world's major traditional healing systems such as Traditional Western Herbalism, Ayurveda, and Traditional Chinese Medicine. Each of these include vast bodies of knowledge about healing that evolved as a result of thousands of years of cultural, social, and ecological shifts and transformation. Medicinal healing technologies are an intrinsic component of human culture and, before the rise of modern science and allopathic medicine, were remedies based in whole plants, natural magic, and shamanic arts. All cultures, large or small, now and throughout history, embodied their own unique healing customs created to meet the distinct needs of the local people.

Traditional Western Herbalism, as one of the prominent herbal medicine systems, includes a variety of methods that originate in many cultures including those from the Mediterranean, North America, and Northern Europe.[1] Also, of significant influence to Western Herbalism has been North American Black Herbalism—a synergy of African, Indigenous, and European folk traditions, with an added element of folk Catholicism.[2] All peoples around the world lived in plant-based cultures at one time, and much of the world continues to do so. According to the World Health Organization (WHO), traditional medicine, including herbalism, is the primary source of health care for many developing countries, and it is estimated that plant-based medicine serves up to 80 percent of the population worldwide.

Traditional medicine is defined by the WHO as

> the sum total of the knowledge, skill, and practices based on the theories, beliefs, and experiences indigenous to different cultures, whether explicable or not, used in the maintenance of health as well as in the prevention, diagnosis, improvement or treatment of physical and mental illness.[3]

The ancient physicians, philosophers, and village healers of the Mediterranean made a major contribution to both Traditional Western Herbalism and Western medicine, which we will discuss in depth in this chapter. The full scope of mainstream herbal medicine today cannot be defined by one standardized set of criteria or qualifications and there is, as of yet, no centralized regulatory organization that determines what is or isn't the practice of herbalism. In this way, herbalism remains a relatively dynamic, self-organized traditional healing modality that functions autonomously within the field of "alternative medicine."

Italian folk medicine as a tradition is a fusion of knowledge spread by the ancient herbalists and doctors in the Mediterranean. In turn, the ancient herbalists and doctors, who had significant prominence and access to resources, were informed by the local village healers who lived in their regions. Although the entirety of Italian folk medicine involves many elements, plants are a central component. Plants have always been at the locus of human community as a source of medicine, food, and tools for ceremonial and spiritual magic and ritual.

What Is Folk Medicine?

Italian folk medicine is called *medicina popolare*, which translates to "medicine" and "people" making it the "medicine of the people," or simply "folk medicine." It's not institutionalized in any way and is accessible to everyone, distributed from village to village or neighborhood to neighborhood by practitioners who live there. It's either free, paid by trade, or very low cost. It's subcorporate health care. In other words, folk medicine can be described in much the same way Ani Defranco describes folk music: "It's an attitude, it's an awareness of one's heritage, and it's a community. It's subcorporate music that gives voice to different communities and their struggle against authority."

Any of the larger systems of traditional medicine that we speak of today emerged from these types of decentralized, bioregional healing practices that were aspects of collective survival, sustainability, and resilience. According to herbalist Phyllis Light, "Folk medicine is defined as a system of medicinal beliefs, knowledge, and practices associated with a particular culture or ethnic group."[4] This alludes to the fact that traditional medicine is also an aspect of culture, one of the ways that the natural qualities of the community are expressed and shared.

Folk medicine is relational knowledge as opposed to individual knowledge. As artist and writer Rachael Rice says, "the smallest unit of community is not the individual but it's the relationship." This does not mean that members of a community don't have individual agency; instead it means that the individual receives knowledge from being in relationship with others, human and other than human.

In this way, we learn about the nature of something and how to attune to it and ourselves by means of direct realization. Direct realization requires no intermediary; it occurs through being in communication and interaction with a variety of forces, including other humans, plants, trees, rivers, and so on. A teacher, "guru," or priest can't give the knowledge to someone without that person having been in practice with it. The knowledge comes from within them as a result of their practice. The teacher can only share techniques to help cultivate the receptivity needed for that person to step into the webs of associations where they can have the direct experience of knowledge. This may sound complicated but it's actually quite simple and an innate human propensity. We are a communal species.

In regard to plant medicine, this is a relationship between plants and people and all of the associations that they are linked to. It's much more than just knowing the uses of a plant; it's knowing the plant itself and forming a long-term, often multigenerational, relationship with that plant as an entity or being. This is ultimately an aspect of the process of coevolution whereby people and plants are changing in response to their relationship to each other as well as to all of the other ecological and more-than-human beings that they are interdependent with.

> *Every carbon atom in our bodies has at one time passed through the chloroplast membrane of a plant.*
> DALE PENDELL, *PHARMAKO GNOSIS*

Folk healers and folk healing methods always arise within a regional ecosystem as an expression of the unique character of a specific group of people, their physical, social, and spiritual needs, and how these needs are affected and transformed by the facilitation of local corporeal, energetic, and elemental forces. This means that folk medicine is emergent and thus is impossible to standardize in its essence. It cannot be replicated on a mass scale with effective, predictable results, nor is it intended to be. If the relationship between the practitioner and the practice is not present, the medicine will lose its meaning and potency.

Emergence is defined as "a process of evolution that creates new properties," and it is the result of synergy, or *sympoiesis*. Sympoiesis occurs when two autonomous agents, beings, or forces combine, cooperate, and converge in mutual interchange, and the consequence is an emergent or new property. This new property does not belong to either component separately. It is also generative and more complex, meaning that it does not expend or drain the energy of the separate components but instead increases it. It makes more for all involved, and it is self-organized, self-regulated, evolutionary, and creative.

In her book *Emergent Strategy*, Adrienne Maree Brown quotes the following definition of emergence by Nick Obolensky: "Emergence is the way complex systems and patterns arise out of a multiplicity of relatively simple interactions."[5]

Emergence occurs as a process of simple interactions, which is why it does not require complicated skills, tools, or knowledge. An example of a simple interaction that results in emergence is when two people share an exchange of ideas and, in the information gained from what the other has shared, a new idea becomes known. This is what might be called an insight.

Folk medicine as an aspect of culture emerges in communal containers. In Southern Italy during traditional times, villages were quite insular and life was centered in them. People didn't travel, and when they did it was on foot so they didn't go far. Adherence to local customs was valued and expected, and every region of Italy had its own unique dialect. This meant that there were strong bonds and cohesion among the locals, making the village a vessel of traditions, yet these traditions were flexible.

Folk healing techniques were transmitted informally and orally, as most people were not literate. So although these traditions were facilitated within a communal container, they were open to adaptation based on any change in circumstances, and according to Per Binde, "new beliefs and practices [could] easily emerge as a bricolage of elements already employed."[6] And the knowledge gathered in this type of system is cumulative from generations past, so an individual can have access to vast experiences from many lifetimes.

Folk healing, developed in communities of those that would once have been considered peasants or ordinary and common people, is also known as "demotic medicine." Demotic medicine, or *demoiatria* stems from the Greek word *demos*, which means "the people" and "of or belonging to people," which was Latinized from the Greek word *dēmotikos*, which means "of or for the common people" and "in common use." Therefore, demotic medicine is the medicine of the commons.

The commons as a structure of society has long been lost to privatization and centralization, yet it still exists within our folk traditions and, in some respect, is an important aspect of survival for groups that have been excluded or displaced, as well as oftentimes harmed, by hierarchical power structures, oppression, and colonization. We can also think about this as the difference between "hegemonic" culture and "subaltern" culture. The word *subaltern* was coined by Italian philosopher Antonio Gramsci to define the common people living in disparate systems of power and wealth.

One of the major discussions around herbal medicine right now is about licensure and legitimacy for herbalists. Perhaps this seems like the natural trajectory given the way our health care system operates, and in the paradigm of the medical industrial complex it is. But if our intention is to allow herbal medicine to be accessible to common people and preserve the ancestral traditions of folk herbalists, it has to remain demoaitric or it will not function as folk herbalism.

La medicina contadina, or peasant medicine, is the medicine that emerges from the heart of the people and their continuous participation in the cycles of life and death, especially their struggle with oppressive systems of power that often impact them negatively. This is not the same as health care in the way that we think about it today, although it is certainly a form of it. The difference is that it is decentralized and not distributed from a state institution or governmental agency. It's not given to people; it comes from the people. This makes these practices adaptable, improvisational, and subject to modification based on changes in the environment or any aspect of the social field.

Peasant medicine occurs worldwide cross-culturally and appears in many ways, but the function stays the same: to provide healing and care for the community. This function does not include profit; it operates in a different paradigm. Peasant medicine includes the forces of magic whether they be ultimately sourced in biological reality or in the mythological narratives of the *popolani* (common people) who have to adapt and survive in a subaltern culture. According to Francesco Scaroina, emeritus head of internal medicine at Ospedale S. Giovani Boscomedical,

> to approach the knowledge of folk medicine, we have to consider the possibility of a coexistence between rational and irrational elements,

thus creating a modus operandi which is not always attributable to superstitions, but which results from millennia of experiences, traditions and beliefs. The origin lies in a time when magic, religion and science were so close that they seemed to be a single reality.

Today we define folk (or demoiatrica) medicine as a tradition capable of recomposing, symbolically, and then practically, the balance between human-nature in compliance with the rules of a mythical-biology that was made part of the collective cultural heritage for centuries. It includes beliefs and practices on individual ailments, resulting in experience and benefits even for the whole family and community.[7]

Ancient Greek and Roman Physicians

Folk medicine as a traditional practice is being continually influenced and modified by the surrounding culture. As mentioned above, it is the accumulation of ancestral wisdom that has been shaped by time and circumstances. For the medicina contadina of Southern Italy, this includes knowledge from the ancient Greco-Roman philosophers and physicians along with the pagan spirituality of both cultures.

Healing and medicine were originally divinatory arts that, in ancient times, didn't mean predicting the future but instead meant connecting the corporeal world with the divine world. This has also been called both magic and "sapiential medicine," whereby ritual and prayer were used to invoke miraculous and spontaneous healing. Prophecy or prediction could also be used but always in collaboration with the divine.[8]

The very first ancient physicians of the Greco-Romans were known as iatromanteis. An iatromantis was a specific type of healer that used trance, incantations, and channeling during the dream/sleep state, a practice otherwise known as dream incubation, to bring about healing. *Iatro* means "doctor" and *mantis* means "magic, divination, oracle"; these were physician-magicians, or physician-seers.

One of Greek history's most famous physicians was Hippocrates, whose oath, known as the Hippocratic oath, is still recited by modern-day physicians and is considered to be the central moral code of professional biomedicine. It does, in fact, invoke the gods and goddesses in the first sentence although it has been revised many times since it was first written:

ὄμνυμι Ἀπόλλωνα ἰητρὸν καὶ Ἀσκληπιὸν καὶ Ὑγείαν καὶ Πανάκειαν καὶ θεοὺς πάντας τε καὶ πάσας, ἵστορας ποιεύμενος, ἐπιτελέα ποιήσειν κατὰ δύναμιν καὶ κρίσιν ἐμὴν ὅρκον τόνδε καὶ συγγραφὴν τήνδε.⁹

I swear by Apollo Physician, by Asclepius, by Hygeia, by Panacea, and by all the gods and goddesses, making them my witnesses, that I will carry out, according to my ability and judgment, this oath and this indenture.

Plato even gave Hippocrates the title of Asclepiad in his writings, alluding to the divine link between the doctor and the gods. The Asclepiads were a guild of healers thought to be directly descended from the God Asclepius, who we will discuss further in the last chapter.

Hippocrates founded the Hippocratic School of Medicine at Kos, the Greek island where he was born. This school was a healing sanctuary where both medicine and worship were practiced and from where the *Hippocratic Corpus* was written. This is a collection of treatises on medicine from which the vast majority of our modern herbalism as well as biomedicine evolved.

Sanctuaries such as the one at Kos included temples built to honor the gods and goddesses and became centers for healing, ritual, and celebrations of worship in the Greek and Roman world. Some of these temples housed the sibyls and Pythia, the ancient oracles, and others were dream temples or incubation centers of healing. Both of these will be discussed in upcoming chapters.

Most of what has been documented in writing about ancient Greece and Rome, however, does not give credit to the folk practices of the common people. This is quite typical within our dominant paradigm whereby those with access to resources, such as scribes or the printing press, were the ones who were able to transmit their version of history and receive acclaim for it. The written information we have from the ancients emerged from patriarchal societies. Therefore, the voices that were heard were only those that had obtained some manner of social and economic status, which was primarily only afforded to elite men. Access to paper and printing tools and technologies was rare and there was, and still is, always competition to gain success and acknowledgment for one's achievements. This means that politics were always involved and were directed by those in power, and that led to the implementation of unscrupulous and corrupt means of acquiring information that could be deemed compelling and useful in the written doctrines of the time.

This, of course, doesn't mean that these texts and the associated folklore aren't valuable, for they are full of clues and some real truths about life during those times as well as traditional healing methods. It's also true that our famous treatises on medicine and society from ancient Greece and Rome contain the indigenous knowledge of the common people, as the elites often gleaned the knowledge they claimed from them. They can also be considered ancestral archives. Many of the early European physicians gathered their knowledge from village herbalists, who were often women who could not read or write. These women are rarely even mentioned in the published literature of medical history.

An example can be found in the book written by Dr. William Withering (1741–1799), the man who is said to have "discovered" the medicinal use of foxglove. The very first page of his book makes a short mention of a village wisewoman who used it in a formula for dropsy: "I was told that it had been a long-kept secret by an old woman in Shropshire, who had sometimes made cures after the more regular practitioners had failed."[10]

The village healers were not elite or favored by the ruling classes and, in fact, were historically perceived as a threat as we all know from the tragedy of the Inquisition, during which the local herbalists and folk practitioners were killed for their skill in encouraging the reliance and self-sufficiency of their people.

Over time, a divide developed between elite practitioners and the village healers, but the divide was not clear-cut, and its spectrum and knowledge continued to move between the two poles. The early philosophers were often common people themselves who gained status as masters of alchemy and magic. They were magicians and mystics and were called *physikos*, a word from which our modern term *physician* is derived, though our modern idea of physician includes a much narrower scope of practice. The early physikos were concerned with all realms of existence, not merely the physical.

In his book titled *In The Dark Places of Wisdom*, Peter Kingsley says,

> For a long while now the beginnings of western philosophy have been presented as purely a matter of intellectual speculation, of abstract ideas. But that's only a myth. Especially in Italy and Sicily the reality was very different. Their philosophy had developed as something all-embracing, intensely practical. And this included the whole area of healing, except that healing then wasn't the same as it's now understood.
>
> In fact, you wouldn't be wrong if you were to say that the western rational medicine we're so familiar with came into being as a direct reaction against the earliest of those philosophers. . . . Our modern image of doctors and healing was first shaped by Hippocrates; and the famous school he founded soon felt the need to define its aims by excluding from medicine anything that didn't specifically have to do with medicine. So it lashed out at those philosophers, attacking them because of the way they insisted that before you can really heal anyone you first have to know what men and women are in their deepest nature—what human beings are from the beginning, not just how they react to this or that condition.[11]

Southern Italy and Sicily became centers for philosophical medicine as well as the location of many Greek and Roman healing sanctuaries. Two of the most well-known philosophers of ancient history lived there: Pythagoras (570–490 BCE), who lived in what is now Calabria in the city of Crotone, and Parmenides (c. 515–450 BCE), who lived in the Greek colony of Velia in what is now the province of Salerno, Italy. From Pythagoras we of course have named the Pythagorean theorem. As for Parmenides, it is believed that he founded the dream temple there as well as the Eleatic school of philosophy. Parmenides is also the author of an epic poem in which he describes a journey he took to the underworld, guided by the "daughters of the Sun," or kourai, where he encounters a goddess he does not name. Parmenides was taught by this goddess about the practice of logic from which he developed his own teachings on logic and metaphysics.

While the Hippocratic physicians were writing medical tomes and building teaching schools and healing centers, the folk healers, from which many of the physicians' practices evolved, were continuing to practice within the same cultural framework as the physicians. Although the folk methods were passed on by oral tradition, many of their techniques were recorded in various medical texts by the physicians as well.

The folk tradition at the time was pluralistic, meaning that many practitioners worked within one system, using various skills and specialities. There was a great deal of crossover between groups as the idea of a "specialist" was not the same as our reductionist idea of what a specialist is today. These practitioners were often part of various healing cults that moved within the cultural landscape of the time, syncretizing medicinal folk methods with the scientific and biological. One prominent group were the *rhizotomi/rhizotomoi/rhizotomoki* or "root gatherers," who were essentially the herbalists of the time. In his book *The Herbal Lore of Wise Women and Wortcunners*, Wolf-Dieter Storl states, "Rhizotomi, root gatherers, roamed the field and forest for simples. The deities of the netherworlds were propitiated with magic and sacrifices, and herbs were thought of as the 'blood' of chthonian animals."[12]

The rhizotomoki were rhizomatic practitioners of underground and lateral energy patterns as found in the plant kingdom. According to Christian Rätsch, "the rhizotomoki still spoke with the plant spirits." He adds, "These root-gatherers observed the gods sacred to the respective plant. They made use of the Moon's energy and knew the particular oath formulas for each plant. Witchcraft medicine belongs to the spiritual and cultural legacy of the rhizotomoki."[13]

The rhizomati were carriers of traditional healing knowledge and have emerged at various points in time just as a rhizome would—going underground for a time and sprouting their legacy up to the surface in another place or time. Renowned modern-day herbalist David Hoffmann has compared herbalists of our time to the Greek rhizotomoi who held a very special place in the hierarchy of health care practitioners during ancient times. He asserts that, now as then, herbal healers "breach so many realms."[14]

Other groups of folk practitioners included the pharmakopolai, or "drug sellers," the maiai, or "midwives," and the goai, or "sorcerers," who were wordsmiths and used both written and verbal incantations to heal.[15] There were also the pharmakos, who were shapeshifters and wizards such as the herbalist and witch known as Mestra who could turn into a variety of animals.[16]

In addition to being influenced by folk-healer wisdom, Hippocratic physicians also derived their knowledge from the Greek and Demotic magical papyri, a collection of Greek, Roman, and Egyptian texts of healing wisdom that included rituals, spells, prayers, recipes, and healing formulas. According to Leanne McNamara, they were

> written by magico-religious practitioners themselves, hence these texts provide a unique insight into the beliefs and clinical practices of folk healers. However, it must be noted that although the magical papyri contain many parallels with earlier Greek magico-religious literature, they originate from Graeco-Roman Egypt, and also contain Babylonian, Jewish and even Christian features.[17]

The rhizomati were members of a sacred healing tradition that included the use of magic and connection with the divine as well as providers of medicine to local and lower-class citizens. We can see here how the ideas of healing and medicine were beginning to divide between the spirit and the body. The idea that this is a divide is not quite accurate, however, as the healing methods of this world remained interlaced, coming in and out of contact, merging here and there through the generations. The magico-religious nature of medicine formed and reformed throughout history, merging the folk and academic knowledge from ancients that created the recent folk traditions of Southern Italy and took root in modern folk herbalism all over the Western world.

Moving forward in history we can find that many of our most famous Western doctors and herbalists were healers from the Mediterranean region including Pliny the Elder, Pedanius Dioscorides, and Galen of Pergamon.

Pliny the Elder (23/24–79 CE)

Gaius Plinius Secundus, also known as Pliny the Elder, was a Roman lawyer and army commander who died on a ship in the Bay of Naples when Mount Vesuvius erupted. He also had a passion for the natural world, which drove him to write the multivolume work *Naturalis historia*, or *Natural History*. The thirty-seven volumes of ancient knowledge range in topic from math to astronomy, physiology, mineralogy, and magic, with volumes twelve through twenty-seven being about botany and healing herbs. In the books he gives the ingredients and doses of numerous remedies to treat a wide range of ailments. Pliny's contribution to the recorded history of herbal medicine has been immeasurable, and his book is still referenced by modern herbalists.

Pedanius Dioscorides (40–90 CE)

Pedanius Dioscorides was a Greek physician who was employed by the Roman army and wrote a five-volume botanical materia medica titled *De materia medica*. This work includes the uses of about six hundred plants and how to prepare them. It is still consulted by herbalists today and considered one of the most reliable sources of traditional remedies available.

Galen of Pergamon (129–c. 200/216 CE)

Claudius Galen, born in present-day Bergama, Turkey (then known as Pergamon), was the official doctor of Emperor Commodus and was on the frontline of the plague that hit Rome in 166 CE, which became known as the Plague of Galen and is believed to have most likely been smallpox. Galen of Pergamon's work dominated medical theory in the Christian West and the Muslim East.[18] Most notably, he gave us the theory of the four humors, which is the primary foundational theory of elemental energetics from which all traditional Western herbal systems have evolved. We will go into this theory in depth in chapter 6.

Ancestor Knowledge

Overall, the influences I've shared here about the origins of Italian folk medicine are well documented, but there are far more cultural intersections that were not codified or otherwise integrated into the dominant paradigm. What we now know of as Southern Italy was part of the greater Mediterranean world that was a major point of intersection between the West and the East as well as Egypt and Africa. Because folk medicine and magic were transmitted orally by the majority of the populace, we can only begin to fathom what we don't know. It is here that the practices of ancestor reverence and plant spirit medicine (working directly with the spirit of the plants) are our greatest sources of knowledge as we carry the genetic memories of our ancestors in our DNA, and so do the plants.

Erased History

Southern Italy has been profoundly shaped by both Arab and African—in particular Egyptian—healing, spiritual, and cultural traditions. In fact, Italy was the home of two Arab emirates—one in Palermo and one in Bari. A great deal of this history has been erased because the Greek and Roman empires and later the British and American empires took preeminence over the political and economic resources of both Italy and Greece, essentially erasing the SWANA contributions to the intellectual and spiritual elements from which both countries emerged.

Greek scholars and philosophers drew a great deal of their literature, science, and healing practices from Persian and North African influence. According to Alice Sparkly Kat in her book *Postcolonial Astrology*,

> The first Greek astrologers had a strange relationship with the older cultures that surrounded the new nation-state. Before Alexander the Great, Greeks felt culturally inferior in comparison to the richness of the Persian traditions that surrounded them. They compensated by mimicking the Persians in their religion, cosmology, and arts. It is customary for Greek philosophers to credit their theories to an ancient Persian source.[19]

For instance, the tradition of Hermetic astrology, which arose during the Hellenistic age, is essentially the progeny of Babylonian astrology. Both mathematical astronomy and genethlialogical astrology (natal chart casting) migrated westward from Babylon to Greece probably sometime during the last three centuries BCE. During this period, in 334 BCE, the old Persian empire was conquered by Alexander the Great and the entire Near East became accessible to Greek culture.

Another prominent Greek state during the same time period was Hellenistic Egypt, which was one of the most prominent cultural centers in the history of astrology and was considered to be the "badge of legitimacy and authority" for astrological studies:

> The Greeks were aware that compared with the cultures of the ancient Near East theirs was a young culture much indebted to "alien wisdom." To be sure, they were quite capable of cultural chauvinism—less so of out-and-out racism, since being "Greek" was not so much a matter of ethnicity as of speaking the language and assimilating oneself to the culture. Nevertheless, respect for other cultures and their legendary sages ran deep in the Greek philosophical tradition. If there was a perverse side to this respect, it was the readiness of admiring Greeks to pass off their own works as that of the alien sages, not so much with the intent to deceive as to place themselves within an admired tradition.[20]

We can trace many of the roots of astrology, medicine, or any other of the ancient healing and philosophical arts back to SWANA origins. One of the world's most brilliant and revolutionary doctors was Muslim philosopher and physician Ibn Sina, born 980 CE in Afshana, Bukhārā (Uzbekistan). His name was Latinized as Avicenna, and he was responsible for writing 450 works on medicine, philosophy, and metaphysics, drawing from Persian, Greco-Roman, and Indian texts that he studied extensively. Ibn Sina's theories and practices have influenced world medicine, as he defined Unani Tibb medicine. Unani Tibb is an integration of traditional practices from the Mediterranean and the Near East. According to Ibn Sina, Unani Tibb is "the science of which we learn the various states of body, in health, and when not in health, and the means by which health is likely to be lost, and when lost, is likely to be restored."[21] Unani Tibb expounded on humoral theory and the four elements to more succinctly identify the ways in which these energies interface with the human body and how it relates to its ecology. According to Dimitri Gutas on the Stanford Encyclopedia of Philosophy website, Ibn Sina

> combined the disparate strands of philosophical/scientific thinking in Greek late antiquity and early Islam into a rationally rigorous and self-consistent scientific system that encompassed and explained all reality, including the tenets of revealed religion and its theological and mystical elaborations. In its integral and comprehensive articulation of science and philosophy, it represents the culmination of the Hellenic tradition, defunct in Greek after the sixth century, reborn in Arabic in the 9th.[22]

All of these early contributions fed into the emerging prominence of Western medicine that became more and more defined in Italy during the early medieval period through to the Renaissance. Around the tenth century CE, the Scuola Medica Salernitana (Salerno Medical School), located in Salerno in Southern Italy in the region of Campania, became the foremost medical school in Europe.

The school, originally a monastery, rose to prestige along with the expansion of Greco-Roman thought and philosophy all over Europe. It was here that many Greek and Arabic texts were translated into Latin making the doctors trained at Salerno some of the most accomplished in Europe. One of the most famous doctors of Salerno was Constantine the African, an Islamic practitioner who is accredited with having translated many Arabic medical books into the Latin. The "Schola Salerni" was a center for healing the sick as well as educating the physicians and people who traveled there from all directions.[23] The school offered not only medical teaching but also courses on religion, politics, law, and philosophy. Generally, the students were men due to the patriarchal structure of the times, but there was one woman, known as the Trota of Salerno (sometimes called "The Trotula") who became a leading physician and is thought to have written "The Trotula," a compendium of women's medicine:

> Trotula of Salerno (also known as Trotula of Ruggerio) was an eleventh-century Italian doctor, who is frequently regarded as the world's first gynecologist. Her many achievements in the male-dominated specialty of gynecology both educated her contemporaries and advanced progressive ideas about women's health care.[24]

Other Notable Female Italian Healers

Matteuccia da Todi or Matteuccia de Francesco, a highly skilled herbalist and village healer, was born in Ripabianca and was the first woman in Europe to be tried for witchcraft and burned at the stake. She was tried before the Tribunale dei Malefici on charges pressed against her by Bernardino da Siena who accused her of flying on a goat to the walnut tree of Benevento to cavort with the streghe (witches) there. Her execution was carried out on March 20, 1428. She was forty years old at the time.[25]

Giulia Tofana, born in Sicily (possibly Palermo), was an expert at poisoning people, a skill that has fallen out of practice in our modern age.

She is most well-known for providing poisons to women who wanted to kill their husbands and forming a network of poisoners that stretched from Rome to Naples and down to Sicily between 1630 and 1655. It is thought that she was a lineage poisoner who learned her trade from her mother.

Poisoning is not always a sinister or violent practice and, in fact, using low-dose poisons is a potent healing modality even in modern medicine; for example, chemotherapy. And although Tofana is generally considered to have been a criminal, her clientele were primarily lower-class abused women in much need of help. She was also an all-around cunning woman who sold remedies for a myriad of ailments, managed a full apothecary, and became a major contributor to what is known as the medieval "magical underworld" of those who provided medicinal alternatives to their communities during a time when medicine was being co-opted by elite doctors and clergy. Tofana's network likely employed hundreds of people, and according to historian Mike Dash, it included

> wise women, astrologers, alchemists, confidence men, witches, shady apothecaries, and back-street abortionists who between them told fortunes and cast horoscopes, sold love potions and lucky charms, cured toothache, and offered to dispose of unwanted babies and unwanted husbands.[26]

Tofana's signature poison elixir was known as Aqua Tofana, and it is believed to have been based in arsenic and to have included other poisons such as belladonna[27] and toadflax, though the name Aqua Tofana became known at the time to refer to any poison elixir at all.[28]

It's important to note here that the two sources about the life and work of Giulia Tofana considered to be most reliable were written by men: the book *I misteri dell'acqua tofana* was written by Alessandro Ademollo (1826–1891), and the article "L'acqua tofana" was written by Salvatore Salomone-Marino (1847–1916) and published in the book *Nuove effemeridi Siciliane*. Because men were the target of Tofana's poison elixirs, we have to imagine that these accounts might be biased.[29]

Overall the tradition of folk medicine in Italy and the Italian diaspora has ancient roots in the political, environmental, and cultural history of both the Italic peninsula and the greater Mediterranean. Those roots have grown and sprouted throughout the Western world influencing the way we now understand both modern medicine and Western herbalism as well as witchcraft.

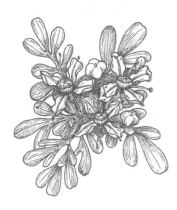

3

Animism, Totemism, Oracles, and Chthonic Gods

Healing as a Divinatory and Spiritual Art

IN THIS CHAPTER we will trace the roots of healing as both a divinatory and spiritual art, as well as a way of being. As briefly discussed in chapter 2, even before our human ideas of a God of religion, our ancestors were aware of the existence of forces beyond the physical or beyond what could be understood and communicated using ordinary perception. These forces are often called "divine."

According to Nicola Luigi Bragazzi, et al., "Divination, in fact, was the most genuine form of knowledge, a sort of half-closed door or bridge that connected the human world with the divine one."[1] And to the ancients—and to many of us today—divination was a healing tradition that aligned humans, both individually and collectively, with the words and will of the sacred forces that intersect our physical realm. The word *sacred* refers to that which is "made holy by association with the divine."[2]

Divination identifies the sacred so that we can become aware of its presence and communicate and interact with it. In ancient Greece and Rome, divination was often a means of contact with the gods and goddesses or other animate forces in what is sometimes called the "otherworld." Divination helps us understand how that world exists in coherence and dynamic exchange with matter.

The methods of divination have changed over time, and they continue to change. At one time, the distance between spirit and matter was nonexistent. But through time humans became more "civilized" and human-centered, or secular. This increased the abyss between spirit and matter, making our ritual and divinatory needs more complex and, perhaps, ultimately leading to the need to symbolize what would have at one time been integrated forces into shapes and forms that began with nature spirits becoming gods and goddesses and, ultimately, led to organized religious systems.

Before formalized religions, paganism, Christianity, and even what might be considered spirituality, the people of Southern Italy were animistic, as were all indigenous cultures at one time. Human healing, divination, and our links with the more-than-human world, including the divine, were likely much less segregated when the world of humans was consciously integrated into the network or web of animated forces on Earth. The landscape of healing was part of the social field. Herbal or plant medicine was an extension and expression of this landscape as plants were considered beings with agency as opposed to taxonomical objects that contained chemical constituents and biologically active compounds. Plants were/are alive in the same way that humans are, and we can interact with them socially and spiritually and as allies in healing.

The Social Field

The idea of the social field is an important element of Italian folk medicine because it is where it emerged from and continues to emerge from. The *social field* is a term currently applied in the field of sociology and is based on the work of French sociologist Pierre Bourdieu. In sociological terms, social field theory examines the position of the individual within their social environment and how their actions affect the field as well as how the actions of others affect them. However, the term has been expanded to include the entire gestalt of ecological forces including human and more than human. As dancer and choreographer Alkistis Dimech has described in her essay "Dynamics of the Occulted Body," the social field is where the animate body has the capacity for sensory receptivity and expression in every cell. The body is a channel for ecological energies, including unseen or divine, and is capable of kinetic resonance that is the

> evolution of an expansive, rich and fluid lingua franca composed of sound, sign, signal and gesture—elaborated in song, dance, play and ritual—enabled communication with peers, with neighbours and strangers, and with an entire ecology of spirits, ancestors, flora and fauna sharing a common habitat, "a single social field" which is vibrantly animist in character.[3]

Divination is our "lingua franca," or common language, that can enable our communication and collective growth across the entire field of experience. The social field, as I'm applying it here, is the field within which humans not only inhabit a shared life place with plants and the fundamentally healing evolutionary propensity of nature but are also all part of the essential architecture and expression of it. The relationship between plants and human communities, as well as the folk healing practices that use them, are implicit functions of Earth's relational field and, therefore, no human community or ecosystem will ever exist without them. In this way, Italian folk medicine, whether pagan, Christian, or otherwise, is a continuous thread that has adapted, changed, and shapeshifted, an entity of its own through time.

Animism

The kernel of the old Roman religion and the greater part of its belief and practice, before its extension, which was also its contamination, owing to foreign influences, belongs to the phase or stage to which modern anthropology has given the name of "animism."

CYRIL BAILEY, *PHASES IN THE RELIGION OF ANCIENT ROME*

Animism is an academic term that came out of Western anthropology and was originally coined by the writings of Sir Edward Burnett Tylor in the nineteenth century. It is a term that represents and describes a pre-religious pattern of human behavior. The term does not predate religion, but the behavior does. Anthropologists gave it this label or container and in that there is an intrinsic academic bias that we need to be aware of.

Animism is not a religion or even a spiritual belief; nor is it a culture. It is a method for identifying certain patterns in the way humans relate to the more-than-human world around us. Animism is defined as

> both a concept and a way of relating to the world. The person or social group with an "animistic" sensibility attributes sentience—or the quality of being "animated"—to a wide range of beings in the world, such as the environment, other persons, animals, plants, spirits, and forces of nature like the ocean, winds, sun, or moon. Some animistic persons or social groups furthermore attribute sentience to things like stones, metals, and minerals or items of technology, such as cars, robots, or computers. Principles of animation and questions of being are thus key to animism.[4]

Animism has been associated with the concept of the "vital force" in Traditional Western Herbalism. This is the vital or immanent principle that is inherent in all living things, although the word and its categorizations have been recently constructed. It is important not to confuse it as a system or practice; instead, it is an element of relating that can be found in what are called "primitive" cultures around the world. More simply it is a way of being that is held and facilitated by culture so that humans may socially and spiritually interact with the world as a living organism expressed in sentient and diverse forms including ourselves.

Animism is not hierarchical in the conventional sense; it is far too improvisational and creative for religious hierarchies. Instead, as Morten Pedersen attests, it typically occurs "where societal relations as a whole are horizontal in character."[5] And in some shamanistic systems, Troy Linebaugh says, where any being has the potential to mediate between the spiritual and material realms, animist sociality between persons occurs in an egalitarian fashion. Humans communicate with the spirits of ancestors, plants, and animals and vice versa in a "boundless whole" of society, according to Pedersen's Swiss-Cheese-Universe Theory. . . . In such a universe, the "whole" of the universe is all of the same unified substance, the "cheese," and the "holes" in the "cheese" are different social positions to be occupied by animate beings ranging from geographic features and weather phenomena to plants, animals, and humans. Moreover, the socialization or shifting between the existing categories is horizontal, meaning it is egalitarian and perhaps anarchic.[6]

During the initial phase of animism, in ancient Rome and the Italic peninsula, the universe was believed to be infused with *numina*, a type of spiritual force that could dwell in objects and vessels such as rocks. This particular spiritual worldview has been often called the Religion of Numa, where the unseen force that influences human and earthly life was called by the "numen."[7]

Numina, in the original sense, was a manifestation of power and energy and was not in the form of a god/goddess and was certainly not gendered. From here we see the development of diverse and more specific beings, or what we might now call mimetic entities, that inhabit particular places, objects, and ideas, and it was even believed that words contained numina/spirit: "This force is not an independent power; it is thought of as residing either in natural objects themselves or in the actions and words of man, which are supposed to control events."[8]

δαιμόνιος ὁ τόπος
The place has a daimon in it.
HERBERT JENNINGS ROSE, "NVMEN INEST"

A daimon, δαιμόνιος in ancient Greek, is another word used for a spirit or being, or an entity that is not human and may not even fall under the category of "alive." It's important to note here that the ancient idea of being alive was probably much different from ours and that even spirits were considered as having a "body" of some type; in other words, spirits had density but less than humans have. Sometimes daimons are perceived as ghosts, gods, and other noncorporeal beings that have subtle agency and power in the corporeal realms. A daimon can also be considered the force of an individual or family's good or bad luck as well as their "genius," or their inherent unique intelligence and blessings.

Herbert Jennings Rose says that in discussing the question "bodiless existence,"

> it is well to begin by ridding our-selves of certain irrelevancies. It is not to the point to insist that, so far as our material goes, the ear-lier generations of Greeks, at all events, and presumably the earlier Italians like-wise, were incapable of conceiving bodiless existence. The Homeric ghosts, for example, lack solidity (φρένες οὐκ ἔνι πάμπαν, they have no "insides"); but they are not altogether without body, having apparently a sort of misty structure and being capable of absorbing literal and material blood, which a wholly spiritual creature could not do. Ghosts which are animate corpses appear now and then in Greek tradition, and even such an apparent abstraction as Death is so solid that, in the legend of Alkestis, Herakles overcomes him in a literal wrestling-match. The Homeric gods are so far from being disembodied that they are not really invisible; only there is a mist over men's eyes which prevents the divine figures being seen and known unless they choose to reveal themselves.[9]

The pregnant vegetation goddess, who we will discuss more about in chapter 4, is one of the earliest manifestations of the idea of spirit imagined into human form. She has also been worshipped in the shape of various animals such as deer, bear, bird, and snake. The Earth-based relationship between humans and the divine was anchored in humans' solidarity with all beings, including the elements and other species. The purpose of animistic ritual was to generate and regenerate mutualistic connections that would enable the continued sustainability of natural cycles on which humans' very existence depended. This all points to not only animism but also totemism as being a central cosmology in the origins of Italian folk medicine.

Another Western academic who popularized the term *animism* was John McLennan, a nineteenth-century Scottish anthropologist who was studying the totemic practices of both North American and Australian indigenous peoples. It is important to note animism as a concept that came out of elite academia as a way to categorize the cultural elements of the original peoples who were colonized by the very people doing the categorizing, the same people who failed to see, or were unconscious of, the animism (and totemism, which we explore below) that their own culture emerged from. Any deeper exploration of animistic principles and cultures should include this awareness.

Totemism

We find totemism in many instances of Italian spiritual, religious, and folk practices. Sometimes totemism is considered a category of animism and sometimes it's a separate framework that not only considers the natural world to be animate but also that humans are in relationship or entangled with the spirit, soul, and diverse beings that we share the ecospiritual landscape with. Both animism and totemism orient humans to the social field, but totemism defines affinity groups or categorizes different species and spirits as opposed to "self" within the field of animistic energies. This orientation is relationally adaptive for survival because it determines categories and boundaries as well as contact zones, where mutual and cooperative behaviors become symbiotic tools for accessing natural resources. Totemism in this sense creates a multispecies culture and "clan-based ecology" from which human communities generate mythologies that can be transmitted from one generation to the next, thereby communicating essential information for survival as well as social life within the place-based social field.

When communal human groups or clans identify with specific totemic animal species they are able to tap into long-held multispecies alliances that link them to historic relational agreements between humans and other species as well as agreements between nonhuman groups, such as the wolf and the crow:

> In the severe fight for survival within nature, the wolf and the crow are two inseparable "comrades" who skillfully cooperate with consideration for one another. The crow always crows "caw, caw, caw" when it flies, thus providing the wolf, who runs on the ground, with the information necessary for knowing the whereabouts of potential prey. In return, the wolf, after having eaten its fill, leaves the rest to the crow.[10]

Totemism is defined as the social-spiritual relationship between humans and other species, usually plant or animal spirits. Totemism is a set of relational practices that can only be truly understood and embodied by being in those relationships. Studying them from the perspective of an observer will not produce the same effect as does being in present, lived engagement with the natural world. And as with any academic or outsider study of indigenous people past or present it will include the intrinsic biases of the researcher.

Italian folk medicine and all of our folk or *demoiatric* practices, including folk Catholicism, still contain practices and beliefs that can be identified as both animism and totemism. Many Catholic prayer, ritual, and ceremonial practices are focused on relationships with the spiritual essence of many objects and beings such as the cross, holy water, candles, saints who have power over certain aspects of life, and so on. One place we see this association through time from ancient to the present is around protection magic where certain items are considered to be one form of a specific elemental force:

> A number of naturally occurring stones and found objects were thought to have apotropaic qualities, and were carried in the pocket as protection or incorporated into other amulets. For example, arrow

or spear points from Paleolithic sites, known as *pietre della saetta*, were believed to be the physical manifestations of lightning, and to be both the cause of and a form of protection against strokes. In some areas of southern Italy, women would find round or kidney-shaped stones of iron-rich clay that rattled from the loose minerals trapped inside. Through sympathetic magic, these became known as *pietre della gravidanza*, or pregnancy stones, and were believed to protect pregnant women and allow them to carry to term successfully.[11]

Many of our Catholic saints and sanctuaries have what could be considered animal totems. One of the places we see this quite clearly is at the Santuario di Montevergine, or Sanctuary of Montevergine, in Avellino, Southern Italy, which is the region of the Hirpini (Wolf) Samnite tribe who were a branch of the Sabellian peoples that lived in the Apennine Mountains. The Latin *lupu* or *lupus* also means "wolf" and the well-known festival of Lupercalia that began in pre-Roman times with the Sabine people who were another one of the Sabellian groups.

The festival celebrates the "lupercal cave" where the mythological beginnings of Rome occurred. It is in this cave that Remus and Romulus were abandoned by their mother, Rhea Silvia, and survived because a wolf mother suckled them. After the twins were born they were exiled by King Amulius of the ancient Latin city Alba Longa who saw them as a threat to his reign. The king had them left on the banks of the Tiber River in a basket. The river carried them away until they were caught by a wild fig tree where they were soon found by a she-wolf who took them to the cave on Palatine Hill (now one of the seven hills of Rome) and fed them her own milk.

The festival began as a method of penance to absolve Remus and Romulus of the violence they caused each other in the founding of the city of Rome. They had had a dispute about which hill to build the city on that led to Remus being killed by Romulus. The original ritual involved the sacrifice of goats and a dog. The ritual knives were then purified with goat's milk, representing the milk of the she-wolf, and placed on the heads of two members of the Sodales Luperci (wolf cult) representing

Remus and Romulus. This is an act of atonement as well as accountability. Although the original Remus and Romulus cannot be there to make amends, their descendants can take on that responsibility ritually.

Mario Alinei, in his article "Evidence for Totemism in European Dialects," points out many other such totemic relationships:

That Italics were conscious of their "totemic" relationship with some animals is, in certain cases, beyond doubt: ethnonyms such as Hirpini from hirpus (Samnite name for "wolf"), or Picentes from picus "magpie," are usually presented as "totemic" in essence by most historians and linguists. In fact, as late as the eighth century, Paulus Diaconus, in his epitome of Festus, could still say: "Irpini appellati nomine lupi. . . . eum enim ducem secuti agros occupavere" (where the totemic function of the wolf, ducem "leader," is still explicit). The she-wolf, milking Romulus and Remus; the luperci, priests disguised as lupi "wolves," and their lupercalia festival; the geese who "saved" Rome; the snakes protecting the lares as genii familiares; and the sacred role played by innumerable animals, in Latin as well as in Greek ancient mythology and culture, are less often presented as developments from totemism, but the burden of the proof should fall on those who try to deny the evidence.[12]

We see instances of totemism all across Italy even to this day. In the region of Abruzzi the remnants of a snake cult continue to exist with the yearly festa di San Domenico, or the "serpari" festival, when a statue of the saint is carried through the town covered in snakes. This festival goes back to the ancient worship of the Roman snake goddess Angitia.

Another prime example is the Cinghiale (wild boar) of Benevento, the symbol of the city that is engraved on the outside of the main cathedral. We also see the connection between certain gods and goddesses as well as kings and other prominent figures with specific animal totems. For instance, La Casa Dei Leoni (the house of the lions) at the temple of Aphrodite in Locri, Calabria, is a hall of worship believed to have been dedicated to Adonis, the first king of Cyprus.

Chthonic Deities and the Oracles

Along with the sacred relationship between humans and other animals was the relationship between humans and the other forces of nature, such as daimons and the numina as mentioned above, but also with the chthonic (pronounced "thon-ic") deities. *Chthonic* refers to that which dwells or inhabits the underworld or that which lives within the soil of the Earth and comes from the Greek word *khthon*, meaning "earth" or "soil." It translates more directly from χθόνιος, which means "in, under, or beneath the earth," and can be differentiated from Γῆ, or "ge," which speaks to the living surface of land on the earth. Here we can think of the original creator of the world from Greek mythology, the goddess Ge—Earth itself.

The importance of the understanding of the gods/goddesses as dwelling and inhabiting the Earth is that it offers a perspective shift from our pagan and Abrahamic gods who live in "heaven" somewhere in the sky. When our deities live with and among us, we have a different type of relationship with them as well as with the afterlife. When we die and expect to go into the ground of Earth, to the underworld, or to remain on Earth in an altered form or dimension, we are not leaving to go somewhere better or more holy. When our gods live with us we do not have to die to be with them. We are always in contact with them and can access them directly. Often this access was made by visiting openings in the earth: caves, wells, volcanic cones and volcanic fissures, tree trunks, or any place where the earth is turned over such as places where crops were planted.

Temples were often built around sacred places where it was believed that a deity resided so that people could enter and be in communion with them. Although patriarchy shifted the focus of spiritual contact off of the Earth, we still continue to find examples of chthonic worship to this day such as all the holy wells devoted to the Virgin Mary and holy wells, chapels, and monuments devoted to other saints.

The way that we relate to the divine shifts when we are in its presence as opposed to it being a reward that we get after we have behaved a certain way. Chthonic worship or devotion is something that is a presence in daily life as a part of the ecological landscape, and the oracles of the ancient world were thought to be those that had an innate propensity to bring awareness to the holy that permeates the living world and become containers/channels for humans to be in conversation with that holiness.

The Pythia and the Sibyls of the Mediterranean are thought to have been either fully human or part human/part god, or both. They are often recorded to have been female, but it's likely that they were many gendered people with a feminine propensity to be receptive and deeply connected to the cycles of the Earth. These oracles that once spoke amidst the Greco-Roman landscape have roots in the mythos of Old Europe and the pre-pagan "mother" worship where Earth and the entire cosmos were born from the womb of the goddess. The modern region of Italy still runs rich and deep with sacred serpentine rivers, blessed mountain sanctuaries of worship, ruins of dream temples, and caves that reverberate with the ancient prophetic language of the oracles. Although the power and agency of feminine forces on Earth and in the otherworlds was usurped by first pagan and then Christian-based patriarchal rule that leveled itself upon the dark, volcanic soils of the Mediterranean world, the ritual arts and healing practices of the goddess culture continue to entwine with the changing culture.

The oracles inhabited caves and sanctuaries built in places where the chthonic gods abided. Although there is no way to know when and where the first oracles began to channel and speak for the divine, it is likely that the practice first originated in Africa or possibly Mesopotamia. There are multiple origin stories.

Oracles in North Africa

There is much evidence that the oracular tradition was brought to ancient Greece and Rome from Africa:

> There is a rock rising up above the ground. On it, say the Delphians, there stood and chanted the oracles a woman, by name Herophile and surnamed Sibyl. The former Sibyl I find was as ancient as any; the

Greeks say that she was a daughter of Zeus by Lamia, daughter of Poseidon, that she was the first woman to chant oracles, and that the name Sibyl was given her by the Libyans.[13]

There is also a theory that the first oracles established in the Greco-Roman world and the greater Mediterranean were brought there by early Ethiopians. The Ethiopian dynasty was vast and as documented by Egyptologist E. A. Wallis Budge as well as Diodorus of Sicily (circa 80–20 BC), there is a direct link between them and the founding of the oracle at Delphi: "The early Ethiopians—whom Homer describes in his Iliad as being cherished by Zeus above all others—sailed down the Nile to colonize Egypt and continued to establish colonies in Crete, in Greece and elsewhere."[14]

Although this part of Mediterranean history has been erased and usurped by empires as well as white supremacy, if we want to understand the history in its full complexity and richness it's important to learn about the complete history. There are few resources easily available, but there is a comprehensive book about the African origin of the oracles by Mama Zogbe titled *The Sibyls: The First Prophetess' of Mami (Wata)*. Mama Zogbe says, "For 6,000 years, Africa was ruled by a powerful order of Sibyl matriarchs. They produced the world's first oracles, prophetess and prophets, known as "Pythoness," they worked the oracles in the Black Egyptian colonies in ancient Greece, Rome, Turkey, Israel, Syria and Babylon."[15]

Another origin story begins with the first mother of the world mentioned earlier as Ge (pronounced "y-eh aa") or Gaia (the Romans' Terra Mater, or Mother Earth) or who is sometimes equated with Eurynome whose temple was located at Delphi where it is believed that the first oracle channeled her words and was seated. The Greeks regarded Delphi as the spiritual center of the world and, in fact, *delphus* means womb.

Ge was born out of the primordial chaos and was the great mother of all creation. She was a parthenogenetic being. *Parthenogenesis* means "reproduction without sexual intercourse" or "virgin creation." Scientifically it's a phenomenon that induces meiosis, or the splitting of a cell that then fuses with another split cell, basically fertilizing itself. Ge, in this sense, was a multigendered entity who contained both masculine and feminine, was beyond duality, and gave birth to everything: the stars, the heavens, the soil and rocks, and the cosmos within, without, and everywhere. Ge even gave birth to the sky gods and her husband Ouranos, or Uranus.

Her lineage includes the birth of a family of giant gods and goddesses known as the Titans that included six male Titans (Oceanus, Coeus, Crius, Hyperion, Iapetus, and Cronus) and six female Titanides (Theia, Rhea, Themis, Mnemosyne, Phoebe, and Tethys). Her grandchildren were the first generation of Olympians: Zeus, Hades, Poseidon, Hestia, Demeter, and Hera.

The Pythia

At Delphi, Ge had a python that guarded her temple and oracle, which was called the Pythia, a name that is derived from Pytho and refers to the mythical serpent thought to be either the daughter of Ge or her water serpent/ *drakaina* (she-dragon), whose name was Pytho. The python inhabited the temple at Delphi where Ge's priestesses lived and served the goddess and Pytho. That is until the temple was taken over by Apollo who slayed the serpent and took control of the Pythia to be the channel for his voice.

The hostile takeover of an Earth mother goddess by a male sky god is the mythic symbol of the shift from feminine source and consciousness to masculine. The goddess Ge, as represented by her snake, was earth-bound, underground, and chthonic. This story elucidates a major shift for humanity. The takeover of the temple at Delphi is thought to have occurred some time during the eleventh to ninth century BCE and at the latest the eighth century BCE until 393 CE when the last response/ prophecy was recorded. It was then that the emperor Theodosius I ordered pagan temples to cease operation. The last words of the oracle are thought to have been "all has ended."[16]

Many and different are the stories told about Delphoi, and even more so about the oracle of Apollon. For they say that in

earliest times the oracular seat belonged to Ge (Earth), who
appointed as prophetess at it Daphnis, one of the Nymphai
(Nymphs) of the mountains.

PAUSANIAS, *DESCRIPTION OF GREECE*

Many believe that these original oracles emerged from the same
archetype as Jesus Christ and were able to perform healing miracles long
before he did. Or, looking at it from another perspective, Jesus was the
oracle of the god Yahweh. Jesus was the "voice of god" and was in a long
lineage of divine oracles and healers. When we consider Jesus as an oracle, it provides us with access to the continuum of how medicine and
healing shifted from pagan into Christianity.

The Sibyls

Long before the Savior was born of the Virgin, and up to
around the time of His first Advent, there are said to have
lived wise women who inhabited shrines, temples, and
caves, and who, being blessed "by the gods" with the gift
of prophecy, read the signs of nature in order to foretell the
future. We call these seers "Sibyls," after the Greek word for
prophetess ("sibulla").

TRACY TUCCIARONE, FISHEATERS WEBSITE

Another name for oracular seers of the ancient Greco-Roman world is
Sibyl. Although it's not really a name; it's a title and one of the titles given
to ancient prophets who divined the will of the gods by entering some type
of trance state. The word *Sibyl* comes from the Greek word *Sibylla* meaning "prophetess" or, according to the ancient Greek historian Diodorus of
Sicily, "to be inspired in one's tongue." It's not clear exactly where the first
Sibyls began their prophetic practice but, according to the Sibylline Oracles,
a series of twelve to fourteen books that contain a collection of prophecies
from the Sibyls, there were a total of ten Sibyls. There were many people in
a lineage of seers that fulfilled each of those ten roles.

The Ten Sibyls

1. Chaldean or Persian (of the line of Noah)
2. Libyan
3. Delphian
4. Italian
5. Erythraean
6. Samian
7. Cumaean
8. Hellespontine
9. Phrygian
10. Tiburtine

The Sibylline Oracles are not believed to have been written by the Sibyls and are considered to be pseudepigraphical, or written under false names, and/or are falsely attributed to them. They were written from a Judeo-Christian* perspective in around 150 BCE–180 CE. These books have been historically attributed to the Sibyls and said to be their direct prophecies, but historians contend that they likely are not. More probably they originated from Hellenistic communities as an iteration of the much older Sibylline Books.†

The books describe a historic account of the creation of humanity and the first five generations of people on Earth, including the story of Noah and the great flood. The account of the sixth generation is told in the present tense and chronicles the prophecies of the Sibyl that were told during that time, including the birth of Christ. Based on this, historians have

---

*It has come to my attention, from folks in the Jewish community, that the use of the term Judeo-Christian draws an erroneous connection between the two religions that is inaccurate and that reading texts translated into Greek have an intrinsic Christian bias that is anti-Semitic. The source that I've noted here does say in the text that "the book is primarily rooted in the Jewish-influenced tradition, but Christian-influenced people appropriated the oracle for themselves in a few places."

†The Sibylline Oracles are often confused with the Sibylline Books that are believed to have been directly written by the Sibyl. This was a collection of nine books written by one or more of the world's Sibyls, eventually ending up with the Sibyl of Cumae, who brought them to Roman King Tarquinius who reigned between 535 BCE and 509 BCE.

surmised that the author, the Sibyl, lived during the generation immediately following the flood.[17]

The Sibyl of Cumae

Arrived at Cumae, when you view the flood
Of black Avernus, and the sounding wood,
The mad prophetic Sibyl you shall find,
Dark in a cave, and on a rock reclined.
She sings the fates, and, in her frantic fits,
The notes and names, inscrib'd, to leaf commits.

VIRGIL, *THE AENEID*, BOOK 6

Cumae, Cuma in Italian, was an ancient Greek colony whose ruins lie several miles west of modern-day Naples. It is not far from the ancient Phlegraean Fields (or "burning" fields), the caldera of a volcano that is mostly under the Gulf of Pozzuoli. One of the craters is filled by the infamous Lake Avernus. The area also includes many hot springs and fumaroles where volcanic steam rises up from under the surface.

The Cumaean Sibyl has been written about in many famous works including Ovid's *Metamorphoses* and Virgil's epic poem *The Aeneid*. It is said that she lived until she was a thousand years old and then turned into dust. According to Ovid, she lived this long because she lost a deal with Apollo. He was in love with her and wanted to marry her, and she agreed but picked up a handful of sand and told him that, in return, she wanted to live as many years as there were grains of sand in her hand. Apollo agreed and granted her wish, but the Sibyl then refused to marry him. Apollo was so angry that he told her she would live as many years as there were grains of sand in her hand but not with eternal youth. Consequently, she lived and lived getting older and older, drying up and withering until she became so small she lived in a jar.

'Maiden of Cumae choose
whatever you may wish, and you shall gain
all that you wish.' I pointed to a heap

of dust collected there, and foolishly
replied, 'As many birthdays must be given
to me as there are particles of sand.'
For I forgot to wish them days of changeless youth.
He gave long life and offered youth besides,
if I would grant his wish. This I refused,
I live unwedded still.

METAMORPHOSES, BOOK 14

The infamous Sibylline Books were brought to the Roman king, Tarquinius, by the Sibyl of Cumae, though they are thought to have been a compilation of writings by several Sibyls and were presumed to be their direct prophecy in regard to the future of Rome and the rest of civilization. The books were written over time, probably starting around 630 BCE. This circumstance has become one of the most legendary tales of Roman history. It begins with the Sibyl of Cumae trekking to Rome with all nine books and bringing them before the king to sell for the price of nine bags of gold. The nine books foretold the future of Rome, which would have been of great benefit to him as it would have allowed him to plan defensive, political, and battle strategies. But he refused to pay the high price.

Upon his refusal, the Sibyl burned three of the books in front of him and left with the other six. She returned the next day and offered him the remaining six for the same price: nine bags of gold. He again refused, and she burned three more of the books and left. The king then went to consult his augurs (those who prophesied by divining the patterns of the birds) who told him that the books were authentic and that he must pay whatever price the Sibyl asked for the remaining books.

The next day when the Sibyl returned, the king bought the remaining three books for the price of nine bags of gold. These books were kept at the Temple of Jupiter and consulted for major state decisions until they all perished when the temple burned down in 83 BCE.

Tarquinius, wondering at the woman's purpose, sent for the
augurs and acquainting them with the matter, asked them

what he should do. These, knowing by certain signs that
he had rejected a god-sent blessing, and declaring it to be
a great misfortune that he had not purchased all the books,
directed him to pay the woman all the money she asked and
to get the oracles that were left.

DIONYSIUS OF HALICARNASSUS,
ROMAN ANTIQUITIES, BOOK 4

The Oracular Trance

There are several theories about how the oracles were able to commune, channel, and prophesize the words of the divine. Some sources contend that they were simply gifted mediums or psychics. It has also been surmised that they used mind-altering or hallucinogenic plants such as oleander or bay laurel.[18] These were most likely burned and inhaled as smoke. Another possibility is that the oracles inhaled the smoke from *Cannabis sativa*.[19] There are some suggestions that they may have taken a type of hallucinogenic preparation made with honey and possibly bee venom. Of course, there is a long history in European shamanism, witchcraft, and prophecy that involves the use of ointments and salves as modes of delivery for hallucinogenic substances.

It's also possible that trance-inducing substances included the volcanic vapors, or steam, that rose up from fissures between rocks. Archaeological excavation has uncovered two geological fault lines beneath the ruins of the temple at Delphi that are formed in such a way that they release petrochemical (hydrocarbon) vapors that have been identified as methane, ethane, and ethylene.[20] Ethylene, in particular, is considered a "narcotic gas" as determined by the pioneering work of anesthesiologist Isabella Herb, who found that giving a dose of 20 percent ethylene or less to patients induced altered, euphoric, and trance-like states.[21]

Other indications strongly suggest that the oracles induced a trance by using snake venom. There is solid evidence of snake worship, snake tending, and divinatory rites that involved live snakes as well as mythical serpents. Many sacred temples and centers of worship housed various species of snakes that were cared for by the priests and priestesses who operated the temples:

> Among the Romans a serpent-cult is mainly connected with the animals as embodying the genius, and snakes were kept in large numbers in temples and houses. The Greek cult of the serpent Asklepios probably influenced the Romans. . . . A more native aspect of the cult is seen in serpent cave Lanuvium, whither virgins were taken yearly to prove their chastity.[22]

The evidence for the snake venom theory is primarily in the form of snake imagery found on artifacts from this time period in and around sacred temples. The few written sources that exist point toward the use of cobra or krait snake venom, both of which can produce hallucinations. Also, it is speculated that the ancients knew how to inoculate themselves from the deadly effects of a snake bite by exposing themselves to small amounts of snake venom. This would allow them to be bitten and survive but still receive the hallucinogenic effects of the venom.

The practice and art of divination and prophecy in the ancient world happened in every culture on Earth and was a primary aspect of social and spiritual life. The oracles of the Mediterranean were one of many ways that humans sought to communicate with powers beyond their own and to further understand themselves. As the inscription outside of the temple at Delphi says:

γνῶθι σεαυτόν

Know thyself

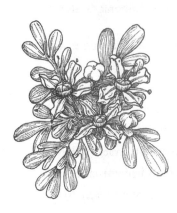

4

Mothers of Grain

The History and Cycles of Farming and Parthenogenesis

FROM THE ORIGINAL animistic relationships that humans had with the living landscape of the Mediterranean comes the emergence of place-based engagement with the spirits that our ancestors were in cyclical conservation with. These cycles were often concentric with daily ritual and routine as the center around which the larger cycles spiraled in and out. These cycles included the seasonal cycles, the family cycles of generational experience, and the human life cycle of birth and death. The Southern Italian peasants practiced attunement with these cycles in a way that allowed for change and adaptation while maintaining the ongoing ancestral conversation they were in with the land and their regional needs of survival.

The word *peasant* has a few nuanced meanings, and many of them are derogatory. An initial google search for a definition brings up a "rural person of inferior rank or condition,"[1] usually engaged in agricultural labor. But this idea of inferior rank is a capitalist overlay that has erased the sacred experience of peasanthood as well as the depth and fullness of life that was potentially experienced by people who work the land. If we look at the etymology of *peasant* we find it derives from Latin *pagus*, meaning "country or rural district," which is also the root of the word *pagan* or the Latin *pagensis*, which means "inhabitant" of a specific region or native of one's own country. From this view a peasant is one that is indigenous to a certain place. Peasants worldwide are nonelite farmers, gardeners, and community members who are intricately related to place through multiple generations.

The peasants of Southern Italy were the native people of place who were born along the continuum of lineage that coevolved with the chthonic forces of the land. If we view life as bound to the divine and to spirit, if the material world is the physical, animate expression of "god," then we humans are one of the many forms it takes. And our indigenous ancestors were the original shapes and characters who emerged from and with spirit into matter. As we discussed in previous chapters, the first humans began the unfolding process of lineage through time from which the chthonic and celestial realms interface on Earth. This process is essentially rhizomatic (we discussed the rhizomati in chapter 2), has no beginning or end, and can be entered at any point in the system. This means that even someone who was not born into a certain place or culture can join in and participate in the ongoing relationship and even influence and cocreate with it.

The farmers and agricultural peoples didn't appear out of nowhere; they were, as we are, carrying the constantly recombining genetic helix that has been passed from person to person since the beginning of time. This is a continuum that transcends the singular lifetime of an individual and ties us each to the eternal, even beyond human existence. Our DNA evolved from the first single-celled organisms on Earth and from the beginning of all creation. In this sense, each incarnation and generation is sacred as it is tied to what many call "god" or the divine, the force that drives the processes of creation. The peasants had methods and practices that allowed them to maintain the conscious awareness of the divine and the sacredness of life. The fields, the seeds, and the plants were all part of the sacred nature of life, and those who tended to them were the priests of the fields, the wisdom keepers of the spirits of place and the carriers of the skills needed to live sustainably with the land and nature as the human expression of both.

The emergence of agriculture has been sometimes interpreted as the first "fall of man" from the wild life of hunter-gatherers. But agriculture didn't take over all at once, and it didn't become severely damaging to the Earth immediately. In other words, it didn't go off like a bomb; it was a gradual process along a continuum that included the transmission of generational knowledge. The wisdom and relationships that were created by prefarming people was not simply discarded; it was modified and adapted for sure but still linked to the past. Agrarian life was originally an extension of hunter-gatherer lifeways. It was an ongoingness as well as means of responding to the demands of survival.

The peasant farmers, or contadini, of Southern Italy were, as are all peasants and other indigenous people, the holy people of the land who were in tune with the seasons and cycles of birth and death. They were adept at divining the landscape, reading the patterns of the seasons and elements, and preserving the divine mysteries of life for the community past, present, and future. Martin Prechtel elucidates the sacred path of farmers in his book *The Unlikely Peace at Cuchumaquic*, which tells about the farming rites of the Tzutujil Maya in what is now known as Guatemala:

> But no matter what they were known for, every single adult Tzutujil man and woman considered themselves to be Farmers. By definition, farming was neither a choice nor a career, but was what it meant to be human. . . . Farmers are priests; farmers must be our scholars. Farmers are ecstatic lovers of the long story of the seed.[2]

Even within an ancient-empire framework, farming was a central component of political, social, and religious life. Pliny the Elder, in book 18 of *Natural History*, describes how the Roman religion developed around farming:

> Romulus at the outset instituted the Priests of the Fields, and nominated himself as the twelfth brother among them, the others being the sons of his foster-mother Acca Larentia; it was to this priesthood that was assigned as a most sacred emblem the first crown ever worn at Rome, a wreath of ears of corn tied together with a white filet.[3]

These were the *fratres arvales* (brothers of the field), or arval brothers, a council of twelve members who were responsible for ensuring a good harvest by honoring the goddess Dea Dia, a grain mother goddess. This group also invoked and worshipped the god Mars and the Lares, who are Roman ancestral spirits of the home and place. The priests of the fields were also responsible for keeping the balance between the human realm and the plants:

> Amongst other duties of this priesthood should especially be mentioned the expiatory sacrifices in the grove. These had to be offered if any damage had been done to it through the breaking of a bough, the stroke of lightning, or other such causes; or again if any labour had been performed in it, though ever so necessary, especially if iron tools had been used.[4]

Gods and goddesses were associated with various food crops and especially with emmer wheat (*Triticum dicoccon*) and spelt, a hybrid of emmer and a wild grass (*Triticum spelta*), both grains on which the early Romans depended. As a food it was commonly made into porridge. Emmer, roasted in a ritualized manner, was made into salted cakes and offered to the spirits on holy days. The very process of roasting was given a sacred day, which was called the Feast of the Ovens.

Emmer was cultivated and harvested ritually outside the city but incorporated into all aspects of daily city life as a food and in sacrificial practices. It was even considered in the political organization of Rome. The agrarian, civil, and religious aspects of life were linked by this sacred plant and those that tended it from seed to food to spiritual offering.

> *Nothing is more prolific than wheat—Nature having given it this attribute because it used to be her principal means of nourishing man.*
> Pliny the Elder, *Natural History*, book 18

The ritualization of farming was also a death practice that mimicked the complete creation pattern of birth, death, and rebirth/regeneration. The fields and crops were viewed as an expression of the continuity and cyclical nature of the universe, and the life cycle of the seed was associated with the life cycle of humans. This birth-death-rebirth pattern was honored from the micro to the macro level, from the simple practice of planting a kernel of grain to the celebration and honoring of the mother goddess, or Earth mother, within whom the seed is germinated, and even as it is expressed in the turning of Earth within the cosmos and the entirety of creation.

> [With farming], the earth itself is made symbolically female. "Mother Earth" becomes the focus of ploughing, crop sowing, and the burial of the dead—a creature who can be made to bear fruit and receive, at the proper time, her human children back into her womb. . . . One's ancestors invested their labor in tilling the earth, and when they died they were physically incorporated back into it. . . . The earth itself was now considered as a sort of womb, with the buried body awaiting rebirth. . . . At Jericho, new faces were plastered onto skulls using the fertile foodplain mud, and cowrie shells to represent the eyes. Cowries are a near-universal "natural symbol" for female genitalia, and suggest the female power of birth required for rebirth.[5]

These cyclical patterns are nonlinear systems from which Italian folk medicine is formed. Health, healing, and overall well-being and happiness, from the view of this tradition, are the results of an ongoing participation in the balance of many living systems that go through repetitive regenerative phases. Much archaeological evidence has been found that shows us how humans in this region of the world related to cyclical and seasonal life. The evidence begins in the Upper Paleolithic era and runs up to the Neolithic. Pottery and sculptures have been recovered in Old Europe that tell us pieces of the living narrative our ancestors experienced.

Old Europe includes several Neolithic archaeological sites in Southern Italy that support the evidence of a prehistoric society that was devoted to the divine feminine as the source of all life. Many Venus figurines, such as the Venus of Willendorf we discussed in chapter 1, were found in this region and are thought to have been the personification of the many cycles, including the aspect of death and destruction. Though the goddess figurines and other artifacts that point to mother/goddess veneration have often been merely considered symbols of fertility, more evidence suggests a much broader scope of meaning than that:

The Pregnant Vegetation Goddess

According to Marija Gimbutas,

> it is inaccurate to call paleolithic and neolithic goddesses "Fertility Goddesses." Fertility is not a primary function of the prehistoric Goddess Creatrix and has nothing to do with sexuality. The goddesses that we can reconstruct were mainly life-creatresses, not venuses or beauties, and most definitely not wives of male gods. They are creations of a matristic era.[6]

I would add to this that the ancient goddesses weren't even gendered. They were pregender from where all forms and functions, including ideas about gender, emerge and regenerate. The pregnant vegetation goddess is a multidimensional force that hosts the birth-death-rebirth creation pattern. The death phase of her character is often neglected in patriarchal imaginings of her as no more than a source of sex and babies. Although fertility is a function of the goddess, as is sex, only as an element of the sacred cycle of what Gimbutas calls "eternal transformation, constant and rhythmic change between creation and destruction, between birth and death."[7]

The pregnant goddess is both chthonic and lunar. The lunar symbolism corresponds to the Moon's phases of waxing, waning, and renewal, and as we discussed in chapter 3 *chthonic refers to that which dwells or inhabits the underworld or lives within the soil.* We also talked in chapter 3 about the creation story of Ge, who birthed the world from within herself with no male counterpart. She contained everything, and this concept has been reiterated throughout time in what have been called "virgin births." Though the understanding of how the divine was perceived as chthonic living on and in the earth, it's also important to understand how the sky, the stars, and the heavens, as equally potent forces of creation, converged with the earthly powers to form new life.

One of the first things I learned from my astrology mentor many years ago was about parthenogenesis, a means of reproduction without sexual intercourse, or a "virgin creation." Scientifically it's a phenomenon that induces meiosis, or the splitting of a cell that then fuses with another split cell basically fertilizing itself. The concept of a "virgin" goddess or priestess evolved from the idea of parthenogenesis, and my teacher said, "There were always virgin births. All the gods were born that way." It blew my mind for sure having been raised to believe that the conception of Jesus was out of the ordinary. On the contrary, however, Virgin birth myths are part of many cultures including the Haudenosaunee (Iroquois) story of the Peacemaker who was born of a virgin birth. This did not diminish my reverence for the blessed grain mother at all; in fact, it deepened it.

Virgin, in this sense, does not necessarily mean "chaste" or describe someone who has never had sexual intercourse. It means that they refrained from sex in order to conceive via parthenogenesis, which is considered divine or immaculate. It's the way humans believed they could give birth to a god or divine being. Although there is no scientific evidence that this can happen in humans, there is plenty of it in nature. Bees are one species that do this as are snakes, birds, ants, and more.

There are two methods that have been considered virgin births in humans via mythology. One is the hieros gamos conception ritual whereby a human and god unite in sexual union, or "sacred marriage." If a child is conceived from this, it is considered an immaculate conception. Another form is pure parthenogenesis whereby a god, goddess, or human becomes pregnant from within through self-fertilization. This idea is linked back to many ancient Greek and Roman cults.

These cults were centered around worship held in temples that were the homes of parthenogenetic priestesses who were believed to be living in such a way as to be able to give birth to the divine on Earth. One of the most popular trends right now is to recenter our spiritual narrative from "sky" gods to the underworld, the soil, the mycelium. I see this as an important element of the universe, but it is also becoming an over-compensation for millennia of patriarchy and gods who only live above us. It's also not all about the roots, and I don't think we really want to simply switch poles, making an opposing imbalance.

According to our ancient myths, the underworld, or the chthonic realms, meet, interact with, and procreate with the full spectrum of the universe. The stars, the heavens, and the cosmos are within, without, and everywhere. Parthenogenesis was one practice that brought them together. Across Mediterranean cultures, there are multiple uncanny links to one particular complex of stars called the Pleiades, also known as the Seven Sisters and associated with the seven nymphs of Artemis.

The Pleiades were a cosmological point of focus for many cultures around the world from the Vikings to the Mayans and the Babylonians. In many of our ancient goddess temples and sanctuaries it was believed that the priestesshoods "have been seen as special women who mirac-ulously incarnated holy beings from the Pleiades." And according to Pythagoras, "Souls are assembled in the Milky Way [galaxia] which derives its name from 'milk' [gala] because they are nourished with milk when they first fall into genesis."[8]

Certain openings in the earth were considered places where the realms could meet. Caves and springs in particular are known to have been places of ritual as well as portals where both the chthonic and stel-lar energies could be channeled and merged. I understand the motivation to move from the hierarchic and solar/masculine dominant narrative, but we can't forget that there really is no such thing as up/down. A binary is only one of many tools to navigate a polar landscape. The stars, the Sun, and the "upper" worlds are also part of the synergy that generates creation. It's true we are a holy mystery of star seeds and mushrooms, soil, darkness, the Milky Way, and everything else.

The mother goddess giving birth to creation via parthenogenesis that is generated by the interaction of the demiurgic properties of the Earth and sky is the core principle of how embodied life continues to originate. Those born from this union were of every aspect of creation and all physical forms including humans, other animals, and plants. In particular for agricultural people, the raising, tending, harvesting and all activities around our relationship with plants is one of the most significant points of access to the divine in both its earthy/chthonic and cosmic forms. The pregnant vegetation goddess embodied the union of the soils, the seeds, and the rising up of the sprouts and how they related to the "above," in particular the Moon.

> The Pregnant Goddess is one of the stereotypes among the upper paleolithic divine images repeatedly produced through time. However, we do not know whether it was associated from very beginning with earth fertility (uncultivated plant life). I assume that she was then a lunar goddess, an analogy to a waxing moon, and only later, in the agricultural era, she was transformed into a chthonic deity, rising, growing and dying with plant life. Her fatness was now synonymous with the lushness of nature, with good crops, with abundance of bread. Her images of rising, growing and dying were inseparable from changing seasons, spring, summer-autumn, winter.[9]

In ancient Greece and Magna Graecia the pregnant vegetation goddess was known as Demeter, the goddess of corn and grain as well as Persephone (daughter of Demeter) and Proserpina (Persephone's Roman equivalent and daughter of Ceres) who modeled the yearly agricultural cycle. Festivals to these goddesses were held during different phases of the growing cycle such as Thesmophoria, the festival at sowing time, and Skirophoria, the festival at threshing time.

The myth of Persephone describes her apparent abduction by Hades/Pluto to the underworld where she is "god's unwilling bride." During this time her mother mourns her loss, and the crops do not grow as a consequence of her grief. People become hungry and starving, which leads Zeus, her father, to make a deal with Hades to return her. The twist comes when Persephone eats some pomegranate seeds while in the underworld, which binds her to it so that she must return for half the year.

This myth, of course, has been superimposed with patriarchal ideology that removes the potential agency of the goddess and therefore nature, subjugating both to the will of masculine forces and male gods. But if we look more deeply we see an ancient acknowledgment and expression of the cycles and transitions of life and the growing season as the goddess transitions between worlds.

As our ancestors transitioned from hunter-gatherer into an agrarian way of life the seed became a central aspect of survival, and we see the pregnant goddess symbolizing the conditions required for germination and growth as well as transformation and regeneration/replanting. The seeds are planted/implanted in the soil, beneath the earth—they must descend to the underworld. They are buried, as the human dead are, and must remain dormant, waiting, and pregnant until the time is right for them to rise. But in that rising, the seed is still rooted in the underworld as Persephone returns to her home and family, still committed to returning back to the underworld beneath the earth.

The turn of each season is portrayed here with a knowing that for life to continue, for people to eat, for the world to go on, there must be an ongoing return process, a remembering of commitments, a reactivation of the stem cells within the seed, and a willingness to descend and allow for endings and the destructive phase of the creation cycle. It's no wonder that plants and the cycle of seasons became understood as sacred and divine aspects of human life.

Plants have long been considered not only intermediaries between the human and divine realms but also as channels of the divine and even as divine beings themselves. The Earth was considered by many ancient people to be the womb of the world and the heavens and what fell to Earth from above, rain and sunlight, fertilized the seeds within. The plants become the children born of this union. When humans engage with plants whether as food, medicine, or as allies in ritual and magic, their wisdom can be accessed. As John M. Allegro describes,

this idea of the heavenly and subterranean founts of knowledge is that since plants and trees had their roots beneath the soil and derived their nourishment from the water above and beneath the earth, it was thought possible that some varieties of vegetation could give their mortal consumers access to this wisdom.[10]

The Grain Goddess/Earth Mother

Early in history, we find the triad of an Earth Mother, who becomes impregnated by a male Sky God and begets a child identified with vegetation—thus corresponding to the Christian God, the Blessed Virgin Mary and Christ. The pair of the suffering Earth Goddess and her child, the young God, who dies and resurrects in the springtime and is connected with vegetation, is a related religious constellation of ancient origin.

PER BINDE, *BODIES OF VITAL MATTER*

The grain goddess is a plurality of regional grain entities who takes on many names and forms depending on the local culture and is clearly exemplified in the Christian narrative of the Virgin Mary and Jesus. Wherever she is found she represents the germinating energy of the seed, and her son/child is the grain. His death brings life and he/they descend/fall to the underworld as the seeds are planted in order to rise again to be harvested/sacrificed in a continuous cycle.[11]

When humans participate in this creative process through cultural practices they are brought into rhythm with nature. Our rites and rituals anchor and link us to the greater or more-than-human patterns of creation in the same way that all creatures are linked. We find some form of veneration of natural cycles in most, if not all, intact traditional cultures on Earth. It is as natural for us to participate in the generative cycles of nature as it is for the butterfly or the worm, albeit we humans have our own unique qualities and gifts to add to the process.

Our sociological, spiritual, and even scientific narratives often focus on the polarity of forces such as masculine and feminine or yin and yang. Scientifically, we can think of physics with positive and negative atomic particles that magnetize the base elements of life, bringing them together or pushing them apart. The destructive and constructive phases of creation are a certain truth of nature but not the entirety of it, and our traditional cultures developed rituals and systems to acknowledge and participate in the awareness of how polar forces combine and commune to bring into existence the full spectrum of possibilities that live between them.

Sacred ritual and devotion, particularly on the local, seasonal level, can put us in tune with otherwise subliminal presences and meanings around us. Ritual embodies the awareness of the expanded meaning of why we plant, grow, tend, and harvest throughout the seasons. These rituals often include the emergence of a being, spirit, or deity that represents the form of some aspect of the seasonal cycle. Creating imagery, feasts, prayers, songs, dance, and so on as expressions of our human response to our experiences with these presences places our bodies, our minds, and our spirits in direct contact with them.

In psychological terms, this has often been perceived as anthropomorphizing or projection and to some extent it is, yet it is a natural capacity of human beings to project our inner experience outward by making symbols and images that reflect it. But it is not all anthropomorphic or projection. It is often reflexive, like a mirror that can see itself in itself or like being in communion with what's on the outside, listening and responding to the actual energetic imprint of what's going on around us. It is not just our inner experience being projected onto something outside of us; that is a monologue. Instead, it is our inner experience in communion with beings, elements, and forces outside of us—in essence, a dialogue.

The creation of shapes, forms, and beings that have human characteristics is the symbolic art and expression of an unseen exchange between seemingly polar fields of experience. In the case of gods and goddesses, it is one way of bringing together the seen and unseen, the physical and the spiritual, the material and immaterial, or this world and the otherworld, using imagery and symbolic expression to converse.

The local, land-based spirits of the agricultural communities of Italy were often associated with the sacred planting, growing, and harvesting of grain. The pregnant vegetation goddess as deities such as Persephone and Demeter were reiterated in local grain mothers or *madri del grano* (mothers of the wheat). There were many so-called Venus or goddess figurines uncovered during archaeological excavations in the area of Old Europe. They were not all pregnant; many had enlarged breasts or buttocks as opposed to an enlarged belly, again symbolizing that fertility was not her only function.

Pregnant goddess figurines show up in archaeology around 7000 BCE in Southeastern Europe. These figurines were often placed near or next to bread ovens. Prehistoric bread ovens have been found with grain goddess shrines as a symbolic form of the grain goddess herself; the oven being the womb where the grain is alchemized into bread/nourishment.[12]

Bread ovens, uncovered in the excavations at Vinca, now modern-day Serbia, were the center element of shrines built to the grain mother. At this time in history it is believed that, in the area of the world considered to be Old Europe, the human communities were largely peaceful and matriarchal. Things changed with invasions by presumably patriarchal societies from the East and Northeast, but the grain goddess remained a central figure of society in the forms of Persephone, Demeter, and others through the pagan period and up until the Christianization of Europe.

Once Christianity became dominant, these madri del grano took on the form of La Madonna/the Virgin Mary and sometimes Christian saints. This is one of many examples of the power of agential animist forces to adapt and syncretize themselves with the narratives of the over-culture even when they may contradict each other. Grain as an entity has so bonded with the animist forces of humanity that it has always managed to arise in some form throughout time. Grain and all seeds, whether fruit, vegetable, or medicinal, are the bearers of life on Earth for humans. Because our lives are dependent on them, because they give us life, it is not hard to draw a symbolic correspondence between seeds and the great mother-father god—that which gives life.

Seeds themselves, appearing inert, hold the entire cycle of creation within them and in a manner with which humans can directly partici-pate. And although we know the damage caused by not only patriarchy but the dogma and institutions of the Catholic church, we can still see the ancient core of animistic goddess/mother worship in the theology, albeit with changed names.

> *Verily, verily, I say unto you, except a corn of wheat fall into the ground and die, it abideth alone: but if it die, it bringeth forth much fruit.*
>
> JOHN 12:24–26

Grain here symbolizes the eternal, never-ending cycles of creation as seen in the sacred act of planting, the birth-death-rebirth cycle that hap-pens constantly throughout the seasons, right on the land where we live every day. As a Christian symbol it is the birth, sacrifice, and death of Christ as well as his rebirth that is clearly expressed in the unleavened bread offered as the Eucharist, the body of Christ, during holy commu-nion. And his mother, of course, becomes the grain mother.

In this context, farming becomes an act of holy ritual and farm-ers themselves—the priests of the fields, the *paesani* (peasants), the holy contadini. We can see the grain mother in this role in much of Christian iconography as well as in feast days and celebrations all over Southern Italy and other parts of the world. The sections below provide a few examples:

La Madonna of the Sheaves

This wheat mother was portrayed in a famous silver statue (now destroyed) of the Virgin Mary in a Milan cathedral where an anonymous parishioner adorned her with a cloak made from ears of wheat. She can also be found at folk festivals all over Southern Italy.

La Madonna di Polsi or Madonna della Montagna

This grain mother is found in Calabria in the Aspromonte mountains. The name Polsi comes from the Greek word *pulakos*, or "door":

Here, the ancient inhabitants of the Greek colonies came once a year to consult the oracle of Pule. "Pule" in ancient Greek means passage, someone who knocks on the door. The Pulakos is the keeper of the door. The door leads you to Olympus, to the kingdom of the gods. People arrived in Polsi not only to interrogate the oracle, but also to settle disputes between the different tribes, to divide up the territory, forge alliances, and prepare for new wars.[13]

This Madonna is a grain goddess associated with the nearby ancient Greek settlement of Locri where the ruins of the sanctuaries of both Aphrodite and Persephone can be found. La Madonna di Polsi is celebrated on September 2, though pilgrimages are made to her throughout the summer months. Her feast was originally an agricultural festival to mark and honor the harvest of grain and meats whereby wheat sheaves and flowers were showered around the statue of La Madonna and sacrifices of goats were made into meat for the feast. This location continues to be a very important pilgrimage and festival site today.[14]

La Madonna del Monte a Racalmuto

This grain mother is celebrated in Sicily, in the province of Agrigento, from the beginning of May until her feast day on the second Sunday of June. Feasting, games, music, and dance are part of her celebration, all with roots in ancient agricultural rites as described by Barbara Crescimanno:

> *si ricollega a un arcaico orizzonte di propiziazione agraria, come del resto il complesso dei riti in cui si articola la celebrazione di luglio. Questa è tuttora caratterizzata dall vivace competizione fra i giovani maschi celibi per aggiudicarsi uno stendardo (bannera), collocato in cima a una imponente struttura lignea di fattura barocca raffigurante un "cero" (ciliu), e dal viàggiu (pellegrinaggio) fino al Santuario del Monte per recare offerte votive alla Madonna.[15]*

[They are] linked to an ancient understanding of agrarian propitiation with the land, as indeed the series of rites in which the July celebration is articulated. This is still characterized by the lively competition between young unmarried men to win a banner (bannera), placed on top of an imposing wooden baroque style structure depicting an ear of wheat (cìliu), and by the viàggiu (pilgrimage) end to the Sanctuary of the Mount to bring votive offerings to the Madonna.

What she is describing here is the awareness our agrarian ancestors had of the way human activity, in this case farming, impacted the landscape and ecosystems. These rites were created as a way to bring energetic/spiritual balance.

Harvest and Fertility Madonnas

In Basilicata, during the month of August, there are many feasts and celebrations to a variety of saints and Madonnas all dedicated to the harvest of the wheat and fertility of the season.

Multilayered arrays of candles are created for the purpose of making offerings to the local saints in many parts of southern Italy. In past times, however, candles were an expensive commodity that was not within everyone's means. Peasants would instead create these arrays by tying ears of wheat together using a similar wooden frame but without the candles. Thick with ears of wheat, these offerings, often called gregne or scigli, weighed several kilos and would remain the property of the church after the festival. In some places, the name used to refer to the wheat offerings continues to be cirii, which in the local dialect means, literally, candles.[16]

Throughout Italy, August is an important agricultural month as is noted by the national holiday of Ferragosto on August 15. This is currently a worker's holiday where everyone takes time off to relax, eat, and celebrate as well as participate in community festivals such as the ones mentioned above. It was started by Emperor Augustus as a way to relieve the contadini from their work in the fields and to celebrate the successful harvesting of the wheat.

The sacred grain mother as symbolized in her animistic, mythic, and religious iterations is the weaver of human fertility, farming, and the seasonal growing of food as nourishment, and the union of the fecundity of the Earth with the divine. The divine being the mystery, the unseen, and that which is beyond our normal sensory perceptions. The sacred grain mother is the emulation of the holy in the seeds that give us life and goddess of the plants that give us medicine. Folk medicine reimbibes the daily labor and down-to-earth necessities of living a common life, of being a peasant, of being contadini within family and community with the awareness of our connection to and conversation and energetic exchange with creation.

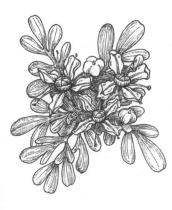

5

Birth-Life-Death

Household Representations of the Cycle of Life

FROM THE ANCIENT CYCLES our ancestors practiced in honor of the pregnant vegetation goddess to the still-happening feasts and celebrations honoring the Virgin Mary with sheaves of wheat, the cycles of life are a central component of Italian-American and Italian folk medicine to this day. The acknowledgment of the phases and patterns of creation, marking the shift from birth to death to rebirth, is often what's beneath some of our very common traditions.

One of the most obvious examples can be found right in the organization of the household. The family unit is the foundational center of life in Italian culture, and it's from the family that all other social relationships extend into the local community, the region, and only after that beyond to the dominant overculture. Family, in this sense, usually includes extended family even if they live in a different home, forming a sense of transhousehold belonging between those with a common ancestor. From the sphere of the family comes a strong sense of collectivism whereby bonds of both blood and locale, village or neighborhood life, generate a strong solidarity among members from which emerges many characteristics of what is commonly called "mutual aid." In other words, systems of equity and reciprocity are embedded in the context of daily existence.

Collectivism, in Italian culture, is notably nonindividualistic to such a degree that an individual is not only a "self" or an ego but is

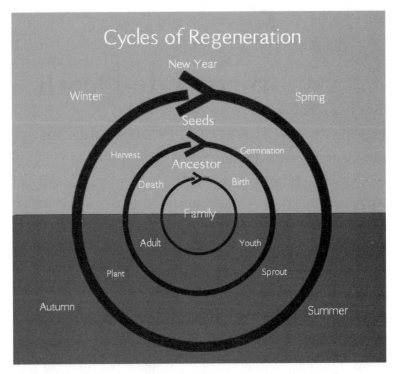

Alignment of cycles of regeneration for humans and nature

part of a larger organism: *la famiglia*, the family. Being part of a family in this way means that all decisions and actions made by one person impact all members of the group. The strength of the family in Southern Italian culture is likely due to the long-term impact of unpredictable social institutions and authorities. The peasants in this region have had to adapt to multiple invasions, constant economic oppression, war, and even many environmental disasters (often due to living on several volcanoes and fault lines).

In a society characterized by weakness of formal social organization, the sense of belonging that it inspired in the individual was unparalleled by other institutions. It has been observed that "an adult hardly may be said to have an individuality apart from the family: he exists not as 'ego' but as 'parent,'" and that "children were perceived as organic parts of la famiglia rather than as persons."[1]

The Vital Force/Vitalità

The vital force, or *vitalità*, is a term often found in Traditional Western Herbalism, and it is one of the primary sources of healing and nourishment needed to continue the circulation of cyclical creation. It is one of the "four vital faculties" that we will discuss in depth in chapter 6. In terms of the relationship between the cycles of life and Italian culture we can define the vital force as the primal, evolutionary, kinetic force that inspirits nature. The vital force is fueled by nourishment whether it comes from food, energy, or the spiritual realms. In other cultures, we might call it chi or prana.

The vital force is the movement of life that feeds and animates all life; it is the drive to grow, to heal, and to evolve. The vital force can't be stopped for long, and anything that obstructs it can cause imbalance and even lead to illness, whether that's within an individual body or a larger system such as a family or nation. Based on this idea, all healing involves the balanced facilitation of the vital force through nourishment and removing obstacles to its innate flow. When the vital force is functioning and circulating optimally, healing naturally occurs and the cycles of life continue to remain creative and regenerative. In Italian folk medicine great focus is placed on ensuring that the vital force is moving equitably and cyclically through our life system and that it's not being held up or blocked or over accumulating in some areas that will lead to a lack in others.

The Naming of Children and the Human Life Cycle

One method of continually refreshing and revitalizing health in Italian culture is through the generational naming of children. The way that children are named is a means of symbolically transferring the vital force from one generation to the next as well as a means of acknowledging the cyclical nature of the family. Any child born was named for an older relative, often the most recently deceased, although this varies from region to region. Usually the name is one that belongs to a grandparent, but it could be from any relative, living or dead, of an older generation. Another option is to name the child after a saint. The idea is that the youthful/vital energy of the deceased relative or the natural *grazia* (grace) of the saint are a means of transferring vital energy from within the birth-death-rebirth cycle to the child.

Here is an example of one way this works:

Child Born	Person the Child Is Named After
First boy	Paternal grandfather
First girl	Paternal grandmother
Second boy	Maternal grandfather
Second girl	Maternal grandmother
Third and following boys	Paternal uncles, then maternal uncles
Third and following girls	Paternal aunts, then maternal aunts[2]

Not only does the naming of a child convey vital energy to them, it also commemorates the elder or deceased relative. It places the child in the ongoing multigenerational matrix of life that stretches in both directions from ancestors to descendants. In other words, the energy goes both ways. In one area of Greece where this is practiced, "Grandparents say that namesake grandchildren 'resurrect' their names and ensure their physical continuity after death."[3]

Also, according to Caroline Oates, in her review of *Bodies of Vital Matter*,

the symbolic transfer of vital force is also identified in cyclical family-naming traditions and mortuary practices, especially mummification and double burial (disinterred bones were transferred to an ossuary). When the remains were dry and cleansed of flesh, the soul left Purgatory for the permanent hereafter, and mourning ceased. Slow decomposition, signalling excessive carnality in life or a "bad" death and a desire to return to the flesh, meant longer purgation and more grief for the bereaved. But death was also denied; the dead lived on in grandchildren named after them, in a family cycle analogous to the agricultural cycle: as beans are planted in Autumn, "die" in winter and put forth new growth in spring, the deceased rested in the earth, decomposed and were replaced by the new generation. Death was as necessary for renewal as winter was for spring, the Lenten Fast for Easter resurrection.[4]

Ancestor Worship and Practice

Ancestor veneration is another aspect of Italian folk medicine that enables us to engage with the birth-death-rebirth cycle. It's a method of communicating between worlds—the living and the dead—and it also acknowledges that birth and death are in fact part of an ongoing cycle and not beginning or end points. Birth and death are both aspects of life, and the so-called living world is actually only one possible state of being; however, it is a state that requires a particular type of vitality, or vital force, to sustain itself. The generation of the "living" state of being requires Source energy, and the practices of ancestor veneration are methods of facilitating and communing with that energy.

As we will see in the next chapter in the section about the elements, certain elements are required in greater amounts at different stages of life and death. At both conception and birth the newly incarnating soul requires large amounts of "juice," or water element, along with deep nourishment in order to grow and thrive. These essential nutrients are derived from basic elements and, energetically and spiritually, from the compost or liberated energy of those that have died, whether human or not. The death cycle of life is what provides the foundational compounds for regeneration. In order for this system to maintain dynamic equilibrium, the death phase must be attended to constantly. And it is not a one-way loop; the living and the dead are always in conversation with each other to ensure that awareness is present at all points along the spectrum.

One way to view this is that what happens on one side, happens on the other. Any action taken in the living world affects all worlds because all worlds are forms of the divine. All worlds arise from the same source and are aspects of it. When we venerate, feed, and remember our ancestors, we are ensuring that we are participating in the continuum of time that, although it seems linear to us, is multidimensional and infinite. When we lose the sense of this we lose contact with eons of wisdom and connection as well as the knowledge of ourselves as infinite beings. And the cycle needs our participation. The living have a significant role in maintaining contact between the worlds.

Italian culture has several ancestral veneration practices, many of which are linked to Catholicism and those that are much older but aligned with Catholic feasts and celebrations. One such practice is the preparation of sweet cakes to offer the witch La Befana, who arrives on the eve of the Epiphany. La Befana is an old crone spirit who represents the dead. She delivers candy and other sweets to children at night while they sleep. In exchange the children leave cakes for her. In this tradition we see how the older generations or those who have passed on feed the living with their vital energy. The sweet taste is an indication of nourishment, so sweet foods are passed on to the next generation.

La Befana not only represents the transmission of food from generation to generation but also the annual cycle and wheel of the year. La Befana rides her broom at night during the winter to bring Source essence to the living. Of course, we can see here the obvious similarity to the Santa Claus myth. Winter is the time of the year when resources are most scarce and practicing rituals of nourishment reminds us that we are part of a greater system that is in motion and will change toward a more abundant phase.

The Day of the Dead, or Il Giorno dei Morti, is another annual celebration that honors and feeds our ancestors. This is a day when the "thirst of the dead" is addressed with various practices of leaving vessels of water out. The thirst of the dead is connected to the idea that dryness is an aspect of death or illness. As mentioned, sweet and juicy is necessary for the living to thrive, and the dead must succumb to dryness. But once a year they can be watered from the living. This watering is an act of care and blessing that extends beyond our deceased relatives to all areas of life that are lacking in abundance. This often includes offering some type of alms to the poor:

Water and food were often placed on a table in the home so that the dead could refresh themselves during the night. The graves of deceased family members were visited and taken care of, and Masses were read in church for the salvation of their souls. Beggars roamed the streets and asked for alms to be offered as a suffragio (suffrage) for the dead.[5]

Suffragi are specifically offered to the dead who are thought to be trapped in purgatory. In Catholic mythology, purgatory is the place where souls who weren't bad enough to make it to hell but not good enough to be allowed into heaven are held. Generally, their release from purgatory is dependent on the living. Often those in purgatory are waiting for their deaths to be honored in some way. All Souls' Day is a day to annually attend to those who were thought to be in need of release or transition because they are stuck or trapped in one area of the cycle.

Edicola Votiva

Offering suffragi and remembrance as a means of participating in the cycle of life includes many varied traditions. One method is to simply pray for those in need. Other, more elaborate rituals are also practiced. One such tradition is that of building an *edicola*. The word *edicola* literally translates as "newsstand" in Italian, but it stems from the Latin word *aedicule*, which stems from *aedes*, meaning "small temple or chapel." An *edicola votiva*, then, sometimes referred to as an *edicola sacra* or just an edicola, is a small temple devoted to reverence. It is also a shrine to honor the dead or sometimes a saint. These shrines are usually small and contained in a corner or a small niche. In Italy you can see them near the front doors of houses. They are basically small altars specifically dedicated to the deceased or other spirits.

Foods Associated with Suffragi and the Cycles

Ceremonial consumption of whole legumes and grains, such as the traditional Calabrian dish *cuccia* as well as broad beans, chickpeas, and so on, occurred at mid-winter and autumn celebrations when these food/seeds were thought to be blessed and when the dead were nearest to the living. Food was left out for the dead so that the dead and the living were eating the same meal, creating a communion.

Beans and grains are themselves seeds, and seeds, being associated with the dead and death, are believed to hold the regenerative and life-giving potential that when eaten, revitalizes and reinvigorates the living and honors the deceased. The eating of whole grains and legumes by the living as a means of feeding the dead and feeding *on* the dead is another representation of the recyclable, regenerational nature of life. As discussed in chapter 4, this is also tied in to the reverence of the grain mother and seeds as symbols of creation. The seed cycle goes from plant to seed to plant and the human life cycle goes from birth to death to birth, or rebirth.

As Per Binde describes it, "This would then be the creation of the ideal 'good death,' in which the dead are placated by the promise of regeneration and their vital principle is recycled and received by the living—it is good for the dead to be consumed, and it is good for the living to consume them."[6]

All of this is ultimately a recycling process whereby the death phase of the cycle is quickened and vitalized in such a way as to increase fertility, again a connection to the agricultural cycle. The burial of the dead, specifically how it's done, is another important aspect of death practice and ancestor veneration. Our ancestors lived for many generations in the same place, cultivated the same fields, and buried their dead in the same place they lived. The buried dead become the protectors of the subterranean world, where our seeds are buried, and they become the essence of fertility as their decomposition enriches the soil.

🌿 Cuccìa

Cuccìa has many variations and is a traditional dish made to celebrate the feast of Santa Lucia in December. It is also commonly cooked around Christmas, for good luck on New Year's Day, and anytime during the winter for a warm bowl of deep nourishment.

The name either comes from *cuccìa*, meaning "cooked" and referring to a legend about the arrival of wheat during a famine whereby the food was cooked as quickly as possible so the hungry people didn't have to wait any longer. Instead of taking the time to make bread, the wheat was boiled into a quick porridge. As soon as it was ready the cook shouted, "Cuccìa, cuccìa!," "Cooked, cooked!" Or it may stem from the Greek *Ko (u) kkìa*, which means "wheat."[7]

There are multiple versions of cuccìa with some being sweet and some being savory. It's basically boiled wheat berries with whatever else sounds good added to it. The below recipe is more on the savory side and includes lentils because that's my favorite way to make it. In some recipes it's more of a pudding and includes ricotta.

> 1 cup of wheat berries—traditionally farro, a type of emmer, is used*
> 1 cup of cooked lentils or other legume such as chickpeas or fava beans (see instructions below)
> Olive oil
> 1–3 cloves of garlic, chopped
> ½ to 1 teaspoon of salt
> ½ teaspoon of pepper
> Spices for seasoning (e.g., fennel seed, rosemary, turmeric, cumin, nutmeg, or cinnamon)
> 3 tablespoons of tomato paste or ¼ cup of diced tomatoes
> 1 tablespoon of lemon juice
> A splash of red wine

1. Cover wheat with about 1 inch of water.
2. Bring to a boil, then turn down heat and simmer for about an hour or until the grain opens and is soft. The cooking time will depend on the variety of wheat you have and whether you soaked them overnight.
3. Cook the lentils separately by putting ½ cup of lentils and about 1 cup of water or vegetable broth in a sauce pan. (You may want

---

*While the wheat berries/farro do cook fairly quickly, it is often recommended to soak the them overnight to speed up the cooking time even more.

to add a little more water or broth depending on the consistency you want.) Bring to a boil then turn down heat and simmer until soft.

4. Meanwhile, heat olive oil in a separate medium pan, add chopped garlic, salt, pepper, and any other desired spices.

5. Add in tomato paste or diced tomatoes, lemon juice, a splash of red wine, and the lentils and warm all together.

6. Add lentil mixture to the wheat, stir together, sprinkle with parmesan cheese, and enjoy!

Optional ingredients to add: nuts, fresh pomegranate seeds, dried cranberries, raisins, chopped figs, honey to add sweetness, or greens—in my family we use escarole. I add this to the lentil combo and cook it with them and the tomato paste in the pan.

Lutto

Contributed by Kara Wood

Lutto: Bereavement, publicly grieving/mourning

The Italian-American traditions around the death of loved ones can be traced back to the "old country." The death rituals begin with food preparation, a full mass, an open casket where the body is kissed, touched, and prayed over with holy water, a funeral procession, and a burial. Public mourning by wearing black clothes or arm bands for a certain amount of time continued after the burial. All of these are extensions of ancient death rituals and rites of Mediterranean ancestors. These ceremonial acts done together in community traveled with Italian immigrants on the boats with them.

Veneration of the dead is a vital piece of tradition carried with the Italian diaspora. Practices such as visiting and decorating graves, especially on the Giorni Dei Morti (Days of the Dead) on November 1 and 2 still exist, but many of these other lutto traditions ceased in the mid-twentieth century. The word *veneration* comes from Venere, which refers to devotion to the goddess Venus.

Italian Catholicism is dominant in the diaspora (there are of course, Jewish Italians and non-Catholic Italians) and central to this cultural Catholicism is devotion to Mary. Specifically, the aspect of the sorrowful mother. Mary publicly grieves her son, his torture and murder. She mourns, and she is *still* our Mother. She shows her broken heart, lets us in, and this provides a comfort.

This is the continuation of the goddess Isis publicly grieving the death of her partner, Osiris, or the goddess Ceres grieving the loss and separation from her daughter Proserpina, or Cybele, the Magna Mater of Rome (whose temple was once where the Vatican sits now), mourning the death of her consort, Attis. This is the connection with the mother who publicly shows her sorrow, who continues to hold us *while she grieves*; it is a profound comfort.

All across the world, in many cultures, there have been public (hired) grievers. In Italy they are called *prefiche*, women who held and moved the grief energy for the community. They wailed, chanted, sang, made specific hand gestures, and waved fabric in communication with death. They released the grief so that it would not become stuck. They prayed for the dead so they may travel to the next realm safely and peacefully. They alchemized for those who were unable. It was a deeply embedded, ancient form of collective care.

Sharing and Social Reciprocity Systems

Once we understand the way that Italian folk medicine has shaped itself around the various cycles of life, how the vital force is facilitated for optimal health through the phases of the cycles, and how those cycles are connected to spirituality and animism as historical and cultural foundations, we can begin to look at how some of our practical techniques operate within them. Italian folk medicine is based on establishing harmonious relationships between natural forces that are understood as cyclical and reciprocal. The vital force, from this perspective, inhabits the collective fields of experience from the individual body to the family system, the village or community, and nature's cycles as expressed in the seasonal cycle. In terms of folk medicine, healing begins with identifying places where the vital force is blocked in some way, resulting in too much of it in one place and not enough in another. Either of these situations can lead to illness, but they can both be remedied through sharing.

Sharing is a simple word we all hopefully learn about as small children. In collectivist societies sharing is a core value, though it is often unspoken. It's an innate quality of being human that when cultivated by socialization and practice becomes autonomic. Sharing methods are ways in which the vital force is distributed from those who have more than enough to those who need it. One of the most practical examples of this is the giving of alms to the poor and making donations to charities, but sharing is about more than just economic resources; it's about energy as well.

Sharing is one of the central elements in removing the *malocchio*,* or the evil eye. The malocchio is an act of sharing whereby the receiver of the malocchio has been stolen from. When someone is given the malocchio, their vital energy has been taken, and the evil eye must be repelled or removed in order for their energy to return. This is why children, babies, and pregnant people are considered to be some of the most susceptible to the malocchio. They are full of vitality, sweetness, and life force and those that lack it will try to take it from them. Although the evil eye is thought to be cast unintentionally, the impulse to do so comes from a desire for something that one does not have.

Sharing also involves the understanding that energy moves around and that it can't be destroyed. Examples of this include the traditions around leaving bad luck at a crossroads or disposing of a curse or the malocchio somewhere that composts it. The concept of sharing involves not only the loss and recovery of vital nourishment but also the elimination of unwanted energy such as in malocchio. One common practice is to leave the materials or substances used in healing work at a crossroads or some other location whereby it can be either permanently dismantled,

---

*The grammatically correct way to spell this word is "mal'occhio," and there are many other variations depending on the dialect, but since it is so often spelled "malocchio," this is how I've rendered it throughout this book.

such as by burying, or passed on to someone else. In other words, energy cannot be created or destroyed, so it must be rendered.

> Vital force, the source of health, fecundity and prosperity, was construed (following humoral theory) as essential moisture, mainly manifest in blood, milk and semen; people's supply of vitality was limited, gradually diminished with age, and dried up in death. As dry sponges absorb fluids (a key image here), others' desires soaked up vitality, causing sickness, infertility, deficient breast milk. . . . Sharing was the best protection. Stolen vitality could be ritually retrieved from the taker, or replenished by a gift, especially from saints, whose cults are compared to evil eye traditions.[8]

When living in the Sicilian village of Milocca ethnologist Charlotte Gower Chapman wrote about how generosity was considered one of the utmost virtues one could express.[9] Sharing enables social cohesion as well as ensures the ongoing survival and thriving of the community by acknowledging the needs and dis-eases of each individual. Sharing is a social reciprocity system that understands an individual as part of a whole intertwined system and that system cannot ignore even one of its members living in scarcity because that scarcity belongs to everyone. Vitalità was circulated throughout the community and the ecological landscape as well as regenerated within it. Another source of vital energy could be bequeathed from the saints and is called grazia. This is divine grace. Grace could be petitioned through prayer and ritual to alleviate some form of illness or energetic imbalance.

All of our rituals and practices in Italian folk medicine work on some level with both divine and mundane techniques to govern and transfer the vital force where it is needed either from the mutual sharing between community members or by grazia, or the grace of the divine. Yet it's not about manipulating natural forces to our will; it's about looking at nature or the energies of the cosmos from a wisdom point of view and doing what is needed to align ourselves with that. Examples of sharing practices vary and are adaptive but include exchanging gifts, making donations, collecting food or other objects, and making petitions/prayers to saints.

Mother's milk is considered one of the most nourishing sources of vitality there is, and therefore it is often considered to be an energetic elixir and as such is also susceptible to being stolen. The loss or insufficiency of milk could be replaced by either actual food and/or a symbol of another nourishing source. There were also social customs that could prevent such losses:

> In Grottole (Basilicata), a mother with an unweaned child who visited another nursing mother was not allowed to leave the house with her child at the breast, since leaving in this way was believed to take the milk away from the woman visited. If this rule was ignored, the mother risking the loss of her milk called the visitor back, calmly and firmly saying to her:—"Please, give me back the milk that you have taken away." The visiting woman was then to enter the house, again with her own child at her breast, in this way bringing the milk back.[10]

There are abundant examples of techniques or "cures" that elucidate the way that sharing can be applied to alleviate various ailments. Most of them involve the collection of "donations" that are often merely symbolic tokens of vitality given to the person in need. The donations are gathered and often combined with a prayer or some type of petition to the divine, usually a saint, and then applied either internally or externally.

It's important to note here that sharing is not transactional; vital nourishment is given as a donation with no expectation of return. It's also important to understand that the focus here is not pathological, meaning that we're not looking for where things are wrong or sick or "not enough"; we're looking at where the nourishment or vitalità is most abundant, and we're practicing generating and regenerating that abundance in a way that is aligned with the natural healing propensity of creation:

> The mother suffering from agalactia is troubled by not having enough food for her baby, which is a state possibly caused by an insufficient

diet, and her baby suffers directly from the life-threatening lack of milk. A person who is ill needs vital force and food is a direct source of strength and vital force; hence he or she is given food. In one case, however, hog's fat was collected and smeared onto an emaciated child. Hence, the fat which the child had lost through its illness was symbolically replaced.

In many procedures involving "donations" asked for from neighbours, there is an invocation of divine grazia. The Virgin Mary and other saints were prayed to, and women named Grazia or Maria were specifically sought out as donors of food. The name Maria suggests the Blessed Virgin Mary, and the name of Grazia evokes the concept of divine grazia. The Virgin Mary was seen as a source of abundant grazia—for instance, in the Hail Mary, one of the most common of prayers, she is said to be piena di grazia (full of grace).[11]

The concept of sharing is a framework for a gift economy that supports and cultivates cooperative social behaviors. When we consider Italian folk medicine from this view, we can see how many of our healing practices make sense. Our nonni and village healers are carriers of a tradition that identifies patterns of imbalances as well as techniques for facilitating vitality that invoke the self-healing potential of the body, mind, and spirit. Our cycles of regeneration represent how the vital force circulates, as well as ebbs and flows, through all areas of life, death, and rebirth and is connected to our past, present, and future cultural experience through our ancestors.

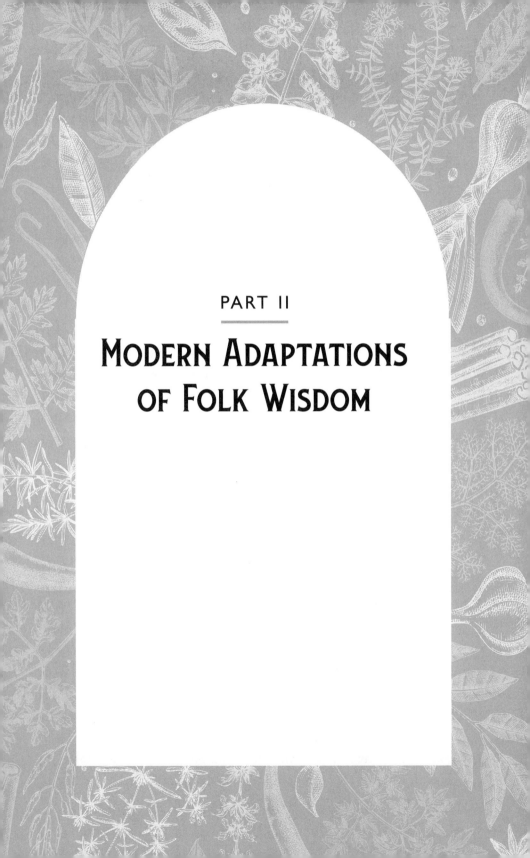

PART II

Modern Adaptations of Folk Wisdom

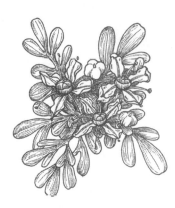

6
Renaissance Medicine

A Bridge to Modern Herbalism

AS ALREADY MENTIONED, Italian folk medicine is not a standardized system, but there are many systems that have been developed from the same foundations. Because the Mediterranean world was one of the Earth's major centers of trade and economic exchange it became a haven for philosophers and physicians, alchemists and magicians from all corners of the world. Many cosmologies and modes of thought and medicine converged in the Greco-Roman world, and these ideas and technologies became the prominent, and eventually, dominant narratives of the West.

It is imperative that we acknowledge here, as we did in the first chapter, that the ideas and practices claimed to be from Greek and Roman antiquity come from other regions of the world; specifically, North Africa and Southwest Asia. Because the Greek and then Roman empire became so preeminent, they appropriated the knowledge and codified it in their own language, leaving out that much of it originated from other cultures and other empires.[1] For instance, the Ottoman empire expanded through Greece, the Balkans, and almost to Vienna, culturally, intellectually, and spiritually influencing the entire area. And of course, both Greek and Roman expansion covered much of the Near East and Northwest Africa. It's well documented that many physicians from Greece and Rome, as well as those from all over the Eastern Mediterranean, went to study at the Alexandria school of medicine in Egypt.[2]

110

Much of the Arabic influence on Greco-Roman thought and narrative has also been ignored:

> During the 12th and 13th centuries, the European intellectual tra-
> dition experienced a dramatic surge, brought about by an influx of
> Greco-Arabic influence. Many of the ancient Mediterranean texts
> lost to medieval Europeans had in fact been preserved by the Arabic
> tradition. Beginning in 750 and lasting through the 10th century,
> Baghdad emerged as the intellectual (and political) capitol of the
> Islamic world. Under the patronage of the city's elite, numerous
> scientific and mathematical texts were translated from Greek into
> Arabic. Among these texts were the works of Aristotle, Euclid's
> Elements, and Ptolemy's Almagest. These, especially the works of
> Aristotle, had formed the core of Arabic scientific and mathematical
> thought during this time period.[3]

That is not to say that the same knowledge was not influenced and shaped by Greece and Rome; it was and significantly so, but if we are to understand this knowledge in its fullness we need to understand that it did not belong solely to them and that the historical erasure of these and other prominent contributions to any of our modern medicine practices only serves to further the reach of colonialism and empire. If we are to believe that there is wisdom in the universe, in the heavens, in the many realms of experience, and in nature, then we have to acknowledge that no one owns it and that it emerges everywhere and is accessible to everyone, albeit in different forms and iterations.

With that in mind the below are facets of what we now know of as Traditional Western Herbalism and Western medicine in general. These are based on the basic laws of nature, philosophy, math, and physics as they developed in the Mediterranean. At the foundation is also the cosmology of the people whether that be in the universal, spiritual, or religious sense. During the Renaissance period when much of this became further developed into modern systems and sciences, it was profoundly influenced by Christianity.

The Cosmos

One of the sources for learning about the cosmology of the Renaissance period is Dante Alighieri, the thirteeth-century Italian philosopher and poet born in Florence. Though he lived just before the Renaissance period, his work was one of the most important influences that informed it. In fact, the modern Italian language was partly chosen because of his influence and the writings done in his Florentine vernacular language. Dante's famous poem, *La commedia* or *The Divine Comedy*, is considered to be the foremost compendium for the worldview of the Medieval period. It has even become known as "Dante's cosmology" and led to the development of the Ptolemaic system by Claudius Ptolemy (100–170 CE), a Roman mathematician and astrologer born in Egypt.[4]

Although through time, as the scientific method evolved, we obviously learned that this cosmology was logistically wrong in many ways. Yet, it was still the basis for many branches of study including alchemy, physics, and even our modern technology. Dante's cosmology has been synthesized with a more complex understanding of the universe and nature, and it provides us with many keys to understanding the history of Western civilization. In terms of Italian folk medicine, this cosmology was iterated on every level of life, reached through hierarchies and monarchies, and transcended economic status. And, in fact, much of this information was extracted from common ways of life to be categorized and thereby specified during the Renaissance when "scholarly" and mechanistic perspectives were valued over the more "primitive" folk traditions.

As Wolf-Dieter Storl says in his book *The Herbal Lore of Wise Women and Wortcunners*,

> These carefully formulated systems of causes and effects of planetary powers, stellar influences, signatures, and so on were actually the first step toward a conception of the universe as mechanism. Fixing the living wisdom of peasants, wise women, and wandering folk into books of natural philosophy and herbalism is similar to moving tribal

weaving, shields, and artifacts into orderly museum exhibits, marking the end of free-floating, living tradition.[5]

Dante's cosmology explains with much depth and complexity the way in which the four elements—earth, air, fire, and water—operate with the "spheres," or realms of experience, to create form. Renaissance cosmology was geocentric, which means that the Earth was viewed as the center of the universe amidst multiple spheres of existence. The four elements are at play in different ratios within the universe and are all sourced from the *primum mobile*, the primary source of all life. From here the idea of the "four humors" was developed. The four humors are a manifestation of the elements in the form of hot, dry, cold, and damp:

> Like most of his contemporaries, Dante believed in the doctrine of the four elements, which Empedocles had formulated at Acragas (Agrigento) in the fifth century B.C. These elements were the result of the various dual combinations of four fundamental properties: coldness, heat, humidity, and dryness.[6]

Another concept similar to Dante's view is the holographic view of the universe as expressed in the old hermetic adage, "As above so below." This idea is based on the holographic view of life as described by physicist David Bohm that acknowledges that each form, from simple to complex, is an iteration of every other and that each small part contains all of the information and wisdom of the whole. This macrocosm is contained in the microcosm, and the microcosm is contained in the macrocosm. As Fritjof Capra says in his *Tao of Physics*,

> The universe is an interconnected whole in which no part is any more fundamental than the other, so that the properties of any one part are determined by those of all the others. In that sense, one might say that every part "contains" all the others and indeed a vision of mutual embodiment seems to be characteristic of the mystical experience of nature.[7]

From this perspective, the petals of a flower or the stem of a plant each contain all of the elemental, archetypal, or macrocosmic sources that created them. And, to dive even deeper, every cell, every molecule, and every atom, down into the quantum foam (the source, or primum mobile), is a fractal, or microcosm of the macrocosm.

The Four Elements

The four elements are the cornerstones of Italian folk medicine as well as Traditional Western Herbalism. Long before Dante's cosmology or even the ancient Greek and Roman philosophers, our animist ancestors understood the elements as part of the social field and having animistic sentience and agency. The polar opposite of this view might be considered modern science, yet our most famous physicists have been able to identify and are continuing to explore the quantum interactions of these brilliant creative forces. The human body is essentially made from earth, air, fire, and water on the molecular level, and these molecules have been combining and recombining since the universe was created. The only difference between our flesh and bones and the base elements of the universe is the complexity with which they are combined.

The four elements are the base material and energetic forms that many holistic herbal healing traditions, including Traditional Western Herbalism, developed their systems from. There are many variations of elemental theory to be found in the history of almost all healing traditions across the world. Ayurveda in India, Traditional Chinese Medicine, Greek medicine, and the European alchemical tradition are just some of the ancient methodologies that incorporate these elemental energies in various arrangements. In ancient Europe, the definition, identification, and origin of the four-element theory is attributed to Empedocles, a Greek philosopher from Sicily (circa 490–430 BCE), but there is strong evidence that it was originally the Persian prophet Zarathustra, called Zoroaster by the Greeks (600–583 BCE), who developed it.

Each of the four elements corresponds to the scientific phases of matter as follows:

Earth: Solid
Water: Liquid
Air: Gas
Fire: Radiant or plasma (The plasma/radiant/combustion phase is the most obscure and least dense of the four material forms.)

According to Empedocles, the four elements are considered to be the roots of all life and the way they either combine or separate is the way all natural processes manifest. He said,

> When a flower or an animal dies . . . the four elements separate again. We can register these changes with the naked eye. But earth and air, fire and water remain everlasting, "untouched" by all the compounds of which they are part. So it is not correct to say that "everything" changes. Basically, nothing changes. What happens is that the four elements are combined and separated—only to be combined again.[8]

There is also a fifth element, which was included by Aristotle as he expounded on the material substances. In studying the original attributes of the four elements, it seems likely that Aristotle actually separated ether out of fire as many of fire's ancient qualities resonate with what is now considered ethereal. The fifth element is known as ether (or aether) or the quintessence. This element is not, however, thought to be earthly or solid but, instead, the divine essence or, as the alchemists called it, the prima materia, or first matter, from which all forms are created and to which all forms are unified and ultimately return. The four elements exist purely and balanced in the ethers but are inextricably bound to each other when condensed into form with each not only having an effect on the other but also required to be present in some ratio in all material structures including human, animal, plant, and mineral.

Fire is thought to affect or transmute all other elements. Everything that exists on Earth is a combination of the elements, and so each being that we consider a separate entity is, in actuality, an arrangement of the same exact forces of nature that occur in a diverse range of complexities.

In scientific terms, the elements can be observed in the manner in which matter relates to space along a spectrum of mass, volume, and density. The form is assigned based on atomic and molecular proximity, which is dependent upon the laws of attraction and repulsion.

Basically, without getting into a quagmire of physics, the distance the molecules are from each other determines the state that they form. Earth is the most dense form of matter and, as mentioned above, corresponds to the solid phase of matter, while water corresponds to the liquid phase, air to the gas phase, and fire, as the least dense, to the plasma phase, although some alchemical traditions place fire before air.

Each person or living being contains all of the elements in various arrangements, but usually there is one dominant element that becomes the substance for the unique energetic architecture of every individual. Imbalance or disease occurs when there is excess or deficiency of one or more elements in relationship to their dominant architecture. Often there is both excess and deficiency, as one leads to the other. In other words, an earth element person will exhibit many earth qualities that belong to their inherent nature and are in just relation to the other elements. Each of us has a proportion of each element that is distinctive to us, and when these are in balance we are healthy, creative, and able to facilitate our own resilience. Balance does not mean equal, because one is often more present or dominant; instead it means that we are in dynamic equilibrium where the elements within us are aligned with our true nature. Disease, discomfort, or imbalance occurs when there is excess or deficiency of one or more elements in relation to our inherent nature.

The Four Qualities

The four qualities are hot, cold, damp, and dry. Aristotle described them as follows:

> Hot is that which associates things of the same kind . . . while cold
> . . . associates homogeneous and heterogeneous things alike. Fluid is
> that which, being readily adaptable in shape, is not determinable by

any limit of its own, while dry is that which is readily determinable by its own limit, but not readily adaptable in shape.[9]

The four qualities are the basic fundamental expressions, the embodiment if you will, of the four elements in nature whether we're talking about the human body, plants, or any other physical form. They are the shape as well as the action that results from their physical manifestation. The four qualities are an integral part of Traditional Western Herbalism as well as Italian folk medicine. Described in the lists below are the basic nature of the qualities, and how we can see them in relation to the body and plants. The reason this is so important to herbal medicine is that when we are choosing plants to apply to a specific condition or ailment, we need to know what type of energy they exert and then match that to the type of energy being exerted by the condition. In other words, a hot condition calls for a cooling plant and vice versa. If we apply a hot plant to a hot condition there is a potential to make the condition worse.

Hot

Nature: Active

Function: Disperses, separates, and divides

Appearance in the body: Inflammation, immune system activation, swelling, heart problems, digestion of food, detoxification, vitality

Related plant qualities: Hot plants are pungent, heating, and stimulating.

Cold

Nature: Active

Function: Gives form, pulls together, and when the degree of heat falls below that of our body, aggregates and condenses

Appearance in the body: Stagnation, lack of circulation, sluggishness, low immunity

Related plant qualities: Cooling plants depress function, cool, and calm.

Damp

Nature: Passive

Function: Allows pliancy, flexibility, and has no limit of its own

Appearance in the body: Edema, excessive urination, excessive sweating, and damp stagnation

Related plant quailities: Moistening plants increase secretions.

Dry

Nature: Passive

Function: Incoercible, creates structure, and limits

Appearance in the body: Nutrient deficiency due to lack of hydration or oils to deliver energy, toxic build up, and lack of elimination

Related plant qualities: Drying plants are diuretics, diaphoretics, and astringents.

The Degrees

When applying the four qualities to plants, we do so in degrees. Each quality has four possible degrees, or grades, that go from one to four with one being the lowest degree, and four being a highest, and each degree conducts a specific action or energy. The first degree is mild in effect, the second is mild to moderate, the third is moderate to strong, and the fourth is strong. A plant medicine that has an effect of the third degree or more can cause harm if overused and at the fourth degree can even be considered poisonous or low-dose medicines.

Assigning degrees to plants is how we identify the basic nature and characteristics of the plant. The degree of a quality in a plant tells us its scope or range of being and what it is related to. This is considered part of the "language" of the plants and is one of the ways they speak to us about themselves and how they can help.

The table at the top of page 119 shows the qualities and the effects they have depending on their degree. The table at the bottom of page 119 shows many of the plants used in herbal medicine and how they correspond to the qualities and degrees.

EFFECTS OF QUALITIES AT DIFFERENT DEGREES

Quality	First Degree Effects	Second Degree Effects	Third Degree Effects	Fourth Degree Effects
Hot	Opens pores; expands	Thins fluids; increases circulation	Warms, stimulates, and increases digestion and metabolism	Burns and penetrates
Cold	Refreshes	Cools and slows	Works as a sedative; contracts and condenses energy	Diminishes consciousness; stops pain; envelops
Damp	Moistens	Nourishes; thickens	Softens; smooths	Acts as a cathartic; flushes and purges bowels
Dry	Closes pores; strengthens constitution	Acts as an astringent; binds	Dries and stops discharge of fluids	Hardens tissues; draws; stops bleeding or the excessive loss of fluids

QUALITIES, DEGREES, AND CORRESPONDING PLANTS

Quality	Hot	Cold	Damp	Dry
First degree	Peppermint, Catnip, Calendula, Lobelia, Nettle	Fruits, Peach leaf, Elderberry, Lemon balm, Lettuce	Mallow, Violets, Comfrey	Witch hazel, Valerian, Onion, Nettle
Second degree	Elecampane, Fennel, Angelica, Mugwort	Elderflower, Yarrow, Wild cherry bark, Wild lettuce	Burdock, American ginseng, Slippery elm	Sumac, Yarrow, Red raspberry, Lady's mantle
Third degree	Cumin, Ginger, Hyssop, Black pepper	Wormwood, Juniper, Lavender	Mullein, Fenugreek	Nettle, Rue, Thyme, Lavender
Fourth degree	Garlic, Onion, Chelidonium	Opium, Hemlock, Henbane	Japanese knotweed, Poke root, Yellow dock	Garlic, Cayenne

Each plant will have a level of temperature and moisture. When we know which qualities are present at which degrees in a plant, we can match that plant to the person and the quality of their condition. For instance, if someone has a fever, they require a cooling plant. *Also important to note is that the energetics can change depending on the seasonal weather patterns and location of where the plant is grown.*

PLANTS AND THEIR DEGREE OF HEAT AND MOISTURE

Plant	Qualities and Degree
Angelica	Hot and dry in the third degree
Barberry	Cold and dry in the second degree
Borage	Cold and damp in the second degree
Cardamom	Hot and dry in the second degree
Chamomile	Hot and dry in the first degree
Cannabis	Cold and dry in the third degree
Chicory	Cold and damp in the first degree
Fennel	Hot and dry in the second degree
Garlic	Hot and dry in the fourth degree
Ginger	Hot and dry in the third degree
Hyssop	Cold and damp in the third degree
Licorice	Hot and dry in the second degree
Mallow	Cold and damp in the first degree
Mugwort	Hot and dry in the third degree
Nettle	Hot and dry in the third degree
Peppermint	Hot and dry in the second degree
Rose	Cold in the first degree, dry in the second degree

Another layer of these qualities can be created by combining herbs or substances to modulate the degree of heat or cold any given herb has. So for instance, if someone needs garlic for its antibacterial properties, but it's too hot in its raw form, it can be adjusted with another herb or substance. These "adjusters" are called corrigents. The table below provides examples of corrigents for yarrow, onion, and garlic.

QUALITIES AND CORRIGENTS OF YARROW, ONION, AND GARLIC

Plant	Qualities	Corrigent
Yarrow	Cold and dry in the second degree	Anise
Onion	Hot in fourth degree and dry in first degree	Vinegar, honey
Garlic	Hot and dry in fourth degree	Honey, lemon, butter

Excess and Deficiency

When we look at excess and deficiency as part of Traditional Western Herbalism, we see a strong similarity to the idea of sharing in Italian folk medicine. Identifying excess and deficiency is a way for us to begin to notice the way in which the four elements and four qualities are in relationship with each other in any given situation. Either excess or deficiency can occur in terms of an organ, a body system, the qualities, or elements, for example if there is too much heat or not enough moisture.

Excess is the overfunctioning of a tissue, organ, or system of the body, usually as a result of metabolic or neurological activity. This activity is always a response to some extreme influence, usually stress, illness, or a dysfunction of the inflammatory response. This response pumps more blood and other fluids to stimulate cellular function, which decreases blood supply and metabolism in another tissue, organ, or system.

Excess in one organ requires energy to be diverted from that organ to some other area of the body. Over time this leads to some type of deficiency in that organ. The idea is not to suppress excess, because the excess is the body's attempt to maintain dynamic equilibrium. Instead we want to determine why there is a need for excess function and then address that.

A physiological example of this is insulin resistance whereby the pancreas increases insulin secretion because not enough insulin is getting to the cells; the body "needs" more insulin. This eventually causes *deficiency* in the pancreas to the point where we can no longer make insulin and become dependent on prescription insulin. To address this we don't want to decrease insulin, we want to increase the capacity of the insulin receptors to uptake insulin.

When using herbs to treat some types of physiological deficiency, we often will choose an herb or herbal combination that is "stimulating," meaning that it will increase function or sensitivity in the area where that is needed. This can redirect energy away from the area of excess as well promote greater tone in the deficient area and make it stronger and more efficient. Or we might choose an herb that is "tonic" and will support the tone of the deficient area so that it becomes stronger and thereby functions more optimally.

The Four Vital Faculties

When viewed from the perspective of the human body, the four elements translate into the four vital faculties: radical moisture, vital force, innate heat, and thymos.

Radical Moisture

Radical moisture is the water of the body, which was thought to be the overall "life fluid" of the human body from which all of the humoral (humidities) fluids formed and emerged. Radical moisture is the fuel that feeds the "lamp of life," the nutritive, fluid fuel that provides the essential food that powers all other forces.

> The basic idea was that a human being was born with a finite amount of radical moisture—this derived from the sperm at conception— which was consumed during the span of life. The radical moisture could be replenished, but only to a certain extent and not indefinitely, since food, when it entered the human organism, was refined

so as to form a sequence of four "secondary humours"—often called "humidities" or "moistures" to distinguish them from the four constituent ("primary") humours—of which the fourth, and hence the most refined, was the radical moisture.[10]

Vital Force

The vital force is the fire of the body (described at length in chapter 5), the primal, evolutionary, kinetic force that inspirits nature and is sometimes considered the candle of god.

> *The Light of Nature . . . is the Secret Candle of God, which*
> *He hath tinned in the elements: it burns and is not seen, for*
> *it shines in a dark place.*
> THOMAS VAUGHAN, *LUMEN DE LUMINE*

The vital force, or vitalism, is the doctrine that an invisible power courses through all that is alive, animating matter with intelligence, energy, identity, and instinct. The vital force is self-organized, self-directed, and evolutionary. It quickens substance and animates matter in all of its manifestations and exists within all of the elements. Its doctrine has been entirely discredited by modern science, which is quite ironic because the very cornerstone of scientific theory and biomedicine was built on the work of vitalist philosophers, inventors, and theorists. Hippocrates credited the vital force as the natural, inherent healing quality of his patients and called it *physis*, a word that later evolved into *physician*.

The vital force was integrated into various philosophies and up until the past several decades, it informed all branches of scientific study including chemistry. Louis Pasteur himself conducted experiments regarding fermentation that led him to conclude that fermentation was a "vital action."

Innate Heat

Innate heat is the air of the body, the thermal, metabolic, and alchemical energy of the body and the body heat as a result of the breath and its circulation around the body via the cardiovascular system and the heart.

Thymos

Thymos, or Thumos, is the earth of the body and is often associated with "spiritedness."[11] In terms of herbal medicine it is the immune force generated by the distillation of the vital force and innate heat. The innate heat keeps the fire of the body stoked, and the vital force circulates it. This keeps outside pathogens from being able to settle anywhere for long. The concept of thymos can be thought of similarly as inflammation. Inflammation is how the body defends itself; it is our immune response that carries immune cells to wherever they're needed.

These four vital faculties are in continuous interaction and alchemy. Our innate heat is the spark that ignites the radical moisture, creating the vital force or flame of life. One common metaphor used to describe this is the burning oil lamp. The radical moisture of the body is robust during childhood but becomes more and more used up as we age. This is why babies, children, and pregnant and nursing people are viewed as "juicy" and "full of life." They are full of heat and moisture, or in humoral terms, are "moist" and "hot." From this view aging brings about coldness and dryness, which eventually leads to death.

The Four Humors and Temperaments

The four humors are the fluids of the body as they correspond to the four elements and the four qualities. The concept of the humors is accredited to the Hippocratics who developed them as a medical system around the third century BCE. Each humor is associated with a temperament, and each person has one that is dominant. A person's temperament is basically made up of their personality traits and underlying physical constitution that when in balance create a harmonious relationship between the humors and elements. When they're out of balance, however, illness will manifest. Each temperament has many associations and correspondences that hold the same energetic and elemental imprint as the temperament. These include organs, colors, tastes, and seasons.

The tables below show characteristics of and associations with the four humors and four temperaments.

THE FOUR HUMORS

Humor	Temperament	Qualities	Element	Organ(s)	Color	Taste	Season
Blood	Sanguine	Hot/moist	Air	Heart, but blood was believed to have originated from the liver	Red	Sweet	Builds in spring
Yellow bile	Choleric	Hot/dry	Fire	Liver/gallbladder	Yellow	Bitter	Builds in summer
Phlegm	Phlegmatic	Cold/damp	Water	Lungs, brain	White	Salty	Builds in winter
Black bile	Melancholic	Cold/dry	Earth	Spleen, any tissue that lacks oxidation or vitality	Bluish	Sour	Builds in autumn

THE FOUR TEMPERAMENTS

Temperament	Humor	Personality Traits	Physical Constitution	Useful Herb Types
Sanguine	Blood	Extraverted, cheerful, passionate, talkative, red complected or flush easily, clairvoyant	Prone to excess, inflammation, and hyperconditions, tend to overindulge and burn out	Nervines, cooling
Choleric	Yellow bile	Independent, ambitious, extraverted, confrontational, leaderlike, angry, perfectionistic, clairsensual (hearing, tasting, touching, etc.)	Tense, stressed, anxious or hypervigilant, prone to digestive issues, easily overstimulated	Relaxants, bitters, cooling, mucilagenous
Phlegmatic	Phlegm	Introverted, avoidant, sensitive, compassionate, empathic, humble, clairsentient	Tend toward mucus congestion, brain fog, fatigue, muscle-skeletal laxity/weakness, edema	Stimulants, astringents, expectorants, warming
Melancholic	Black bile	Sensitive, introverted, intellectual, perceptive, claircognizant	Depression, stagnation, lymph congestion, "hypo" conditions	Circulatory stimulants, lymphatics, warming, digestive

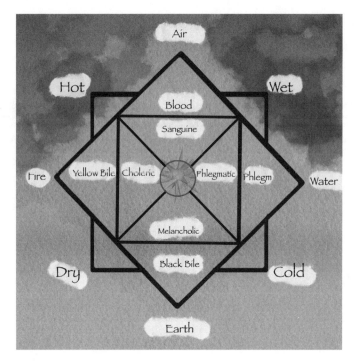

The four humors and temperaments

The Four Humors and Italian Folk Medicine

In Southern Italian folk medicine, the balance of humors, in particular the level of "humidity," is a major focus of health and medicinal or spiritual remedies. Many treatments are designed to revitalize the body and its vital fluids. It is thought that, through life from birth until old age, the bodily fluids are slowly consumed by living and that illness or disease is a result of dryness as is death.

A "good death" is one where the corpse is dry and even bathing the corpse was done with vinegar instead of water because any moisture could impede their smooth transition. In regions where water is given to the dead as a symbol of purification, it is customary to also give the dead a towel to dry themselves. In addition, dry leaves or straw might be added to the coffin. Newborn babies were thought to be in the most extreme state of radical moisture and in fact in places such as Abruzzo, the newborn child was placed for a while by the hearth in order to harden the bones. Small irregularities in the shape of the face and the body were corrected by strokes of the fingers, as the child's flesh was thought to be as soft and formable as wax. With increasing age, living organisms seem to become less humid, to become dryer, harder and wrinkled, and death implies an actual and radical loss of moisture, leaving behind dry material such as straw, shell or bone.[12]

It's important here to keep in mind that the context of the four humors as well as Italian folk medicine is a dry climate. Southern Italy, Greece, and the SWANA region of the world where the humors emerged has an arid climate. The importance of water and other liquids to health and well-being as well as even survival is an integral component of this tradition.

The Italian word for *dry* is *secco*, and there are several linguistic metaphors from the Italian language that show us how the drying of the body is perceived:

- Restarci secco ("to find one-self dry," "to be dry") = to die on the spot[13]
- *Fare secco* ("to make dry") = to kill him
- *Seccarsi* ("to dry up") = to suffer a loss of vitality and vigour
- *La morte secca*[14] or *mortesecca* ("the dry death") = death personified or simply death in general
- La commare secca ("the dry mistress") = the grim reaper

Ceneri, the Italian word for ashes—the ultimate dryness—refers to a human's remains even if they have not been cremated.

There are many ways to increase moisture and vitality, and the list below provides several examples.

Ways to Increase Moisture and Vitality
- Eating particular foods, such as meat and fat
- Drinking fresh blood
- Drinking mother's milk

❧ Calling on God or divine sources (grazia/grace) to give you vitality

❧ Bathing in an ocean or lake

❧ Soaking in dew

❧ Making talismans, charms, and other apotropaic tools using the color red to represent blood

In other geographical areas the humors and elements may be associated with different conditions. For instance, in a rainforest where mold is a major concern there might be more of an association between moisture and illness. In humoral terms when a person has an excess of moisture/humidity there are several remedies. Many of these make use of sympathetic magic, which employs objects and actions that correspond to or are antithetical to the quality of the condition. For example, contact with a corpse—touching the hands, feet, or head—could dry up excessive perspiration. An excess of humidity such as a swollen spleen or edema could be treated by taking a moist object, such as fresh leaf, a slug, or a juicy fruit to represent the area of the body and then drying it. Excessive drooling in a child could be remedied by touching its lips with a living frog, which then was hung up by the fireplace to dry. The cure started to work when the frog dried out completely and died. Vinegar and wine are both considered drying and wine is also considered hot, so either could be used to address coldness. And finally, *amaro* means "bitter," and a bitter taste is thought to counteract the excess humidity of malaria and other diseases that might cause a swollen liver or spleen.

Other conditions and illnesses associated directly with the humors, qualities, and elements include the following:

Poor blood: While strong blood provides good circulation, immunity, and health, "bound" or "poor" blood can lead to illness. A symptom of the malocchio is a "feeling of poor blood in one's head." A sign of being cursed is "that your blood is bound, it is encumbered with something dry, something tough."[15]

Mal vento[16] **(wind illness):** This is said to manifest as a form of dermatitis caused by either "poor blood" (sometimes called "weak blood") or from walking in the vicinity of where a murder occurred.

Mal aria (bad wind): As its name suggests, this is thought to cause malaria.

Phlegma: This is a state of weakness thought to be caused by witches.

Fuoco morto (dead fire): This illness causes dermatitis and is cured by lighting an oil lamp and saying the following:

> *Luce, luce della lontana via*
> *Guarisca 'stu fuchə murtə alla vita di [nome del paziente].*[17]
> Light, light of the faraway street
> Heal this dead fire illness in the life of [name of patient].

Italian folk medicine is a tradition set in a continuous timeline of history and connected to many other geographical locations, cultures, and peoples. Its basic tenets can be found in other iterations from ancient animism to modern medicine. Now we turn to astrology, a system that we don't necessarily see in day-to-day Italian folk medicine but more in relation to Traditional Western Herbalism. Folk medicine is embedded in astrology—in its symbolism, in the way that it expresses the relationship between energies and natural forces, and how it identifies the way the elements interact in relation to the cosmos.

Astrology

Astrology was one of the earliest codified explorations of consciousness and has always been an integral aspect of healing. The first plant-medicine people synthesized multiple methods of cultural and spiritual life into their healing systems and technologies. Indigenous and folk healers didn't fall into specialized categories such as "herbalist," "astrologer," "doctor," "bodyworker," and so on. Instead, they had a wide scope of skills that included attunement with the celestial forces.

Astrology can be used as a tool to discern the energetic background from which past, present, and future events may be made manifest but, in its essence, it is more of a symbolic language that describes and defines the holographic resonance that exists between the earthly and heavenly bodies. The concurrent motion of the planets and their influence on universal activities and functions have been studied, observed, and documented by some of human history's greatest scholars, philosophers, and scientists, with ongoing experiments being conducted based on numerous hypotheses regarding the reflection of astral light, electromagnetic resonance, and medical/physical correspondence.

Much of this information was categorized and thereby specified during the Renaissance when "scholarly" and mechanistic perspectives were valued over the more "primitive" folk traditions of the Mediterranean, Northern Europe, and Asia. Following the motion of the planets and the way they move with the fixed stars, the twelve signs and houses of the zodiac along with the luminaries (the Sun and the Moon) influence the agricultural cycle, crop outcomes, harvesting times, weather patterns, and all aspects of plant-based culture.

Each plant is thought to be "ruled" by a planet and zodiac sign that correspond to its elemental properties and the organ systems of the body that it affects. "Ruled" in this sense doesn't mean in a hierarchical manner but in resonance with each other. In other words, the plant is an earthly version of the same energetic imprint as is held in the planets, stars, and heavens.

Again we look at Dante and the way he described the understanding of the universe during this time period. The philosophers and astrologers of the Renaissance period had a fundamental understanding of the planets that was astronomically inaccurate but was still a valid framework for visualizing how the energetic dimensions of life were influencing and interacting with the Earth and its people.

Renaissance philosophy, which was an accumulation of the knowledge of the eons in that particular region of the world, envisioned the principles of descension and ascension or manifestation and liberation. The manifest world was created by the descension of the archetypal or preform, premateral, essence of the universe. These archetypal energies descended through the heavens via the magnetic orbits of the known planets. And in turn, for liberation or ascension to occur, the planets must be climbed in reverse.

The process or journey of the soul taken to either descend or ascend was considered a spiritual devotion and practice that required a level of skill and initiation to undergo. If the initiate was not prepared for the ordeal of traversing the universe, they would not be lucid or cognizant and therefore not "awake" to the journey and would miss the gates or thresholds to the planets that would lead them toward either liberation or manifestation. There were various practices and disciplines available to develop the necessary focus and skill for a successful journey, including meditation and prayer. Each planet was considered a threshold to another dimension or world in the progression of ascension or descension and as such were called gateways.*

The Gateway of the Moon

The Moon is the first gateway from Earth. It's the last gateway we pass through before birth and the first one we pass through after death on our way to the less-dense dimensions. We also move into the realm of the Moon during sleep, trance, and altered states of consciousness.

The Gateway of Mercury

The second gateway from Earth, Mercury, is associated with the god Hermes who enables divine communication. Mercury rules our ability to shapeshift and respond to changes with resilience and sensitivity. Hermes, considered to be androgynous (part of their shapeshifting capacity), is the god of healing and associated with Asclepius, technology, all forms of currency, and the state of semiconsciousness. When we pass through this gateway toward Earth, we begin to become self-aware or lucid, and our involuntary functions, such as breathing, begin.

The Gateway of Venus

The gateway of Venus is where our passion and creativity emerge. This is where we are in contact with the divine muses as well as unconditional love. It is also the realm of longing and Eros that provokes our desires, including our desire to follow the path of soul.

---

*The following sections on the planetary gateways was derived, in part, from Wolf-Dieter Storl's *The Herbal Lore of Wise Women and Wortcunners*.[18]

The Gateway of the Sun

The Sun is where we gain or lose our etheric body and vital force. The etheric body, or soul, is not the spirit but is an invisible, ethereal part of the physical body that is the container or mycelium of the material, visible, physical body. It is sometimes known as the "etheric double." Spirit and soul are different, although they are often used interchangeably. The spirit is the nonmaterial source of life, the body is the material, and the soul is the intermediary or synthesizer between them. The Sun is also the gateway from which all earthly rhythm emerges into day and night, the seasons, our heartbeat, circadian rhythms, and physical order. This gateway is midway between the planets and therefore is where the above and below energies are synthesized.

The Gateway of Mars

This gateway is pure heat and energy. Mars as the red planet is the force of discernment, differentiation, and defense. Mars is where our survival instinct emerges and animates the channels of the body and being through which the light of the Sun will flow. This realm is unconscious and forms our impulses and reflexes.

The Gateway of Jupiter

Jupiter is the gateway of wisdom, pure spirit, and clear perception of reality. Jupiter is where all that we have gained through our lifetimes culminates into joy and abundance. It is where the trials and tribulations of having a body become one with universal love and source. This is where we deepen into the inner (or upper) realms and become more universal and undifferentiated.

The Gateway of Saturn

This is the farthest gateway from the Earth and the threshold to primum mobile, or what we might call God. The realm of Saturn is where the first notions of form and reality emerge. This is a realm of complete unconsciousness except for the initiated who have mastered staying conscious through the realms of birth and death. The realm of Saturn is where the archetypes begin and where space, time, motion, concepts, and ideas are born.

After passing through all of the spherical realms there is the realm of the fixed stars and then the primum mobile. In Renaissance terms the primum mobile would be called the holy trinity.

Below is a list of the basic corresponding characteristics of each of the planets.

Basic Characteristics of the Planetary Spheres

Moon: Physicality and increase
Mercury: Thought, speech, and interpretation
Venus: Passion and longing
Sun: Sense perception and imagination
Mars: Bold spirit
Jupiter: Power to act
Saturn: Reason, understanding, and the contemplative state

The following list provides the symbolic glyph for each of the planets.

PLANETS AND SYMBOLS

Planet	Symbol
Moon	☽
Sun	☉
Mercury	☿
Venus	♀
Mars	♂
Jupiter	♃
Saturn	♄
Uranus	♅
Neptune	♆
Pluto	♇

Geocentric, Heliocentric, and Holographic Views

The astronomers of the Renaissance held a geocentric view of the universe, meaning that they believed the Earth was at the center of the universe.

The heliocentric view, or the theory that the Sun is at the center of the universe, was first written about by ancient Greek philosophers, but it didn't become the dominant cosmology of Western civilization until the sixteenth century when it was proposed by Nicolaus Copernicus. It was later discovered that the Sun is the center of our solar system and our galaxy but *not* the center of the universe and that the Sun itself is moving in orbit around the center of the Milky Way.

> Present estimates indicate that the sun is between 25,000 to 30,000 light years from the Milky Way's center. The sun revolves around this center with an orbital velocity of about 155 mi/sec (250 km/sec). One revolution around the Milky Way's center takes about 200,000,000 years. The sun is only one star among 100,000,000,000 or more other ordinary stars that revolve around the Milky Way's center.[19]

Although the planets and stars are located in the sky, they have corresponding placements on Earth based on the holographic view of the universe. This idea is also a form of collectivism whereby our basic nature is not separate from the basic nature of the universe. All of the elements that form the stars and planets are the same elements that have formed everything on Earth. As the saying goes, "There is nothing new under the sun."

The two charts on page 135 and 136 show how the characteristics of the human body and plants, respectively, echo the signs and planets and vice versa. Ultimately, we are not separate but are living from the same source from different realms and in different combinations.

The Signs and the Elements
Each of the twelve zodiac signs corresponds to one of the four elements, and each element has three corresponding signs that represent different phases or states of that element. These are illustrated in the lists on page 136.

The Zodiac Human

Aries-top of head, brain, face, muscles, carotid artery

Taurus-throat, neck, lower jaw

Gemini-lungs, shoulders, arms, hands, capillaries

Cancer-breasts, stomach, uterus

Leo-heart, back, spine

Virgo-intestines, liver, pancreas, assimilation, and absorption

Libra, kidneys, adrenals, lower back

Scorpio-genitals, colon, pelvis

Sagittarius-hips, thighs, buttocks, sciatic nerve,

Capricorn-knees, bones, joints, skin, nails, all mineralized structures of the body

Aquarius-legs, ankles, blood circulation, nervous system, spinal cord, electrical conduction of body

Pisces-feet, weaknesses anywhere in the body, lymph, fluids, immune system

Correlations between the zodiac signs and the body

Plant morphology and planets

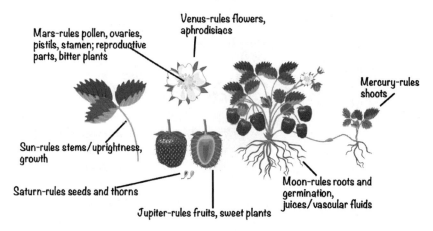

Mars-rules pollen, ovaries, pistils, stamen; reproductive parts, bitter plants

Venus-rules flowers, aphrodisiacs

Mercury-rules shoots

Sun-rules stems/uprightness, growth

Saturn-rules seeds and thorns

Jupiter-rules fruits, sweet plants

Moon-rules roots and germination, juices/vascular fluids

Correlations between the planets and the plants

Earth Signs

Taurus: Roots

Virgo: Soil, plants

Capricorn: Rocks

Water Signs

Cancer: Liquid, water

Scorpio: Ice

Pisces: Mist

Air Signs

Gemini: Wind

Libra: Equilibrium, aerodynamics

Aquarius: Compression, conductivity, electricity

Fire Sign

Aries: Ignition

Leo: Combustion

Sagittarius: Growth, expansion

Each of the zodiac signs also corresponds to one of three modes of action: fixed, mutable, and cardinal. Fixed signs are the most stable and least changeable. They are also the most dense and rigid. Mutable signs are the most changeable. They are shapeshifters and nonbinary. Cardinal signs are the most magnetic and initiatory. They start and attract movement in a forward direction. The three modes and their corresponding signs are listed on the following page.

Fixed Signs	Mutable Signs	Cardinal Signs
Leo	Virgo	Aries
Scorpio	Pisces	Cancer
Aquarius	Sagittarius	Libra
Taurus	Gemini	Capricorn

The list below provides the symbolic glyph for each of the astrological signs. This information will be helpful in understanding the wheel of the zodiac that follows.

ASTROLOGICAL SIGNS AND SYMBOLS

Sign	Symbol
Aries	♈
Taurus	♉
Gemini	♊
Cancer	♋
Leo	♌
Virgo	♍
Libra	♎
Scorpio	♏
Sagittarius	♐
Capricorn	♑
Aquarius	♒
Pisces	♓

The Wheel of the Zodiac

The wheel of the zodiac is the way in which ancient astrologers placed the location of the planets in space and where they are in relation to the zodiac signs. The wheel is, of course, two dimensional and representative of the multidimensional motion and position of the planets and signs. There are many methods of doing this from across the world, but in the ancient Mediterranean the primary method was "tropical" astrology.

Tropical astrology is based on the sacred geometry of where the Sun's ecliptic crosses the equatorial plane of the Earth. Basically it's a method that takes two cross-sections of the universe and measures time and space based on where they cross (see the image below).

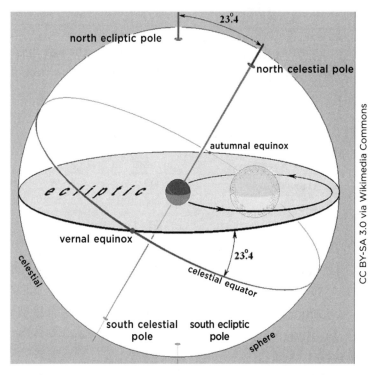

Sacred geometry of where the Sun's ecliptic crosses the Earth's equatorial plane

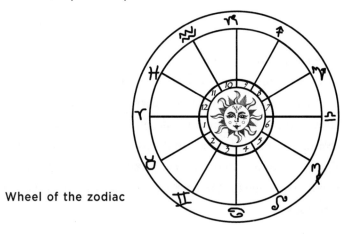

Wheel of the zodiac

Aries is the first sign in the zodiac and, in tropical astrology, begins on the spring equinox at the precise time that the ecliptic plane crosses the equatorial plane. This is 0 degrees of Aries. Each sign is then laid out on the wheel and given 30 degrees each.

Each person has an individual "birth chart" that is their own personalized version of the wheel of the zodiac. A birth chart shows us how the elements and basic qualities of the cosmos are arranged for us. Although a birth chart is considered to be personal, it is actually a map of how we are connected to and interdependent with the rest of nature and the universe. It is the way we are uniquely carrying or incarnating the basic energies of life.

As astrologer Dane Rudhyar says in his book The Astrologicial Houses,

Until the end of the "archaic" age in the sixth century BC . . . the consciousness of men . . . was fundamentally *locality-centered.* . . . The tribe constituted an organism; every member of it was totally integrated into this multi-cellular organism. Each member of the tribe was dominated psychically by the way of the culture, the beliefs, and the symbols of the group, whose taboos he or she could not disobey. There were no real "individuals" at this stage of human evolution; all the values upon which the culture and beliefs of the group were founded were expressions of particular geographical and climateric conditions, and of a particular racial type. The tribal community looked to the past for the symbol, if not the fact, of its unity; that is, to a common ancestor, or to some divine king who had brought it a revealed kind of knowledge and a special psychic cohesion.[20]

It is true, however, that in our current age, the idea of the individual has become more prominent and in fact is a strong value of the dominant paradigm. When we look at astrology from a more collectivist perspective we view the birth chart as a source of relational knowledge as well. Every person's chart is unique and begins with the rising sign. The rising sign is the sign that was on the horizon at the moment you were born.

Plants and Planets

Medical astrology, now seen as a specified branch of study, was at one time integrated into all medical doctrine and was long practiced by the physicians of antiquity that founded our current system of allopathic and technological medicine. Herbal medicine and astrology form a harmonious bond that offers a deeply coherent conception of physical, psychological, spiritual, and planetary resonance that was well defined and practiced by many Western herbalists of the past. The work of English herbalist Nicholas Culpeper (1616–1654), along with many other Renaissance scholars, provides us with one of the most extensively recorded treatises on planetary-plant-anatomical relationships that is still referred to today by Western herbalists.

The study of astrological herbalism is one of complex and interacting systems but a basic understanding can begin by learning the initial relationship of the plants to the planets, the planets to the human organ systems, and the planets to the signs of the zodiac. When we are working with the correspondence between plants and planets we are identifying the resonant and ultimately unified elements that define and link them together. These are called the sympathetic resonances. And in doing this, we gain a greater understanding of the plants and the energy and qualities that they have to offer as well as how those same patterns correspond to human life, behaviors, and conditions.

Sometimes, when we see plants and planets paired they are also antipathetic, which means they have opposing qualities. For instance, you might find a plant listed under "sun plants" that is not hot and dry but is cool and moist. This would be a plant that would balance the dry heat of sun-type conditions. This can make understanding plant/plant correspondences confusing at times.

The following subsections provide information on the qualities and types of plants that correspond to each of the planets as well as the plants that are ruled by them and the ways in which their energies affect humans.

MOON

Qualities: Cold and moist

Types of corresponding plants: Stomachics, demulcents, sedatives, galactagogues, hypnotics, calmatives, alteratives, cooling and mild vegetables

Plants ruled by the Moon: Mugwort, datura (moonflower), lotus, evening primrose, mariposa lily, pomegranate

One of the Moon's primary qualities is receptivity. The Moon has the capacity to receive and reflect the light of the Sun, and in doing so, has provided light in the darkness for all of the Earth's lifespan. It is well known that the Moon corresponds to emotions and our emotional relationships, but it also connects the emotions, feelings, and felt senses or sensory inputs to the nervous system. In this sense, as well as in other ways, the Moon is a bridge through the liminal places where the body and mind make contact and from where meaning emerges.

The Moon has often been perceived as diminutive compared to the Sun but in ancient times and in certain cultures, the Sun and the Moon are seen as equals and nonbinary. Seventeenth-century physician, botanist, and astrologer Nicholas Culpeper realized this during his own deep and devoted work with healing and the planetary influences: "Yet I can scarce be of that opinion, that the Microcosmical Sun and Moon, which reign like King and Queen of the body, should be confined to any particular place."[21]

Another quality of the Moon is moisture. The Moon is ruled by the water element in ancient alchemy, and this is a power that makes the Moon as formidable a force as the Sun. The Moon governs all of the waters on the Earth including those within plants and the human body.

SUN

Qualities: Hot and dry

Types of corresponding plants: Cardiacs, many brain herbs, tonics

Plants ruled by the Sun: Saint John's wort, calendula, goldenrod, angelica, sunflower, chamomile, hawthorne

The Sun has become associated with what are considered the "masculine" qualities of the universe. As patriarchy became more dominant, the Sun took a prevalent role in the applications and methods of astrology. Many of us think of our "Sun sign" as just "our sign." For example, if someone says they're a Libra they usually mean that their Sun is in Libra. This is an unbalanced perspective because the Sun's placement when we are born is only one of the significant aspects of our birth chart.

The most basic and essential energetic qualities of the Sun are the energies of heat, dryness, and radiance. The Sun is the fire at the center of the world and has been called the "divine light." Its radiance is expansive and mobile, and its rays move outward in all directions, carrying vital energy to the Earth. Alchemically, the Sun is the fire of transformation and has the power to create material changes and to shape which qualities are contained within all matter. We see how the Sun acts as an alchemist for the plants because it is the primary transformative agent in the process of photosynthesis. The Sun represents the vital force of the body.

MERCURY

Qualities: Cold and dry
Types of corresponding plants: Nervines, some antispasmodics
Plants ruled by Mercury: Parsley, skullcap, lavender

The planet Mercury represents all forms of communication, including messages from our unconscious or deep psyche. Mercury rules thought, speech, the nervous system, sensory gating, restlessness, and the processes of active perception. Mercury also causes us to become lost in details and miscommunication when channels of transmission are not clear. When Mercury is retrograde or poorly aspected in our chart, we can become oversensitive and overwhelmed by thoughts and ideas and may misinterpret information. Negative Mercury aspects can disrupt electrical signals causing the breakdown of technology and interfering with electronic messaging such as phone calls and emails.

VENUS

Qualities: Warm and moist

Types of corresponding plants: Anodynes, demulcents, some aphrodisiacs, sedatives, emollients, antispasmodics, calmatives, vulneraries, vasodilators, most sweet and juicy fruits, sweetly aromatic flowers

Plants ruled by Venus: Plantain, wild rose, pomegranate

In her planetary form, Venus, the Roman goddess of love and all things harmonious, brings peace, harmony, and resolution to all wounds and conflicts. Venus rules sexuality, art, poetry, and all forms of self-expression and relationships to others. It rules over all unions, contracts, and social endeavors. Where we find it in our astrological chart is where we best express our true beauty and gifts but also where we may have the greatest conflicts to resolve. However great the conflict, Venus has the capacity to bring resolution and further creation as a result of it. Venus is love medicine and at its worst can lead to vanity, laziness, overindulgence, and stagnation as it contacts our sense of contentment that, when in balance is a blessing but in excess can lead to negative consequences.

MARS

Qualities: Hot, dry

Types of corresponding plants: Stimulants, antibiotics, purgatives, male aphrodisiacs, diaphoretics, diuretics, all alliums, capsicums, rubefacients, emetics, anthelmintics, cholagogues, emmenagogues, carminatives, laxatives, some poisons, venoms

Plants ruled by Mars: Garlic, ginger, nettle

Mars is the Roman god of war and Earth and is symbolically similar to the Germanic god Thor and the famous Viking, Ragnar Lothbrok, as he is the warrior of the cosmos. Mars represents all things masculine, yang, and active. Mars is also a fertility god ruling virility, vitality, and energy. When Mars is in excess or poorly aspected in your astrological chart, you may find yourself in unnecessary arguments or feeling angry or aggressive. Mars must find an outlet for its forceful, swift, and highly charged energies or negative consequences can result. When thought, patience, and temperance are brought to Mars forces, great achievement, success, and strong work can be made manifest. Mars teaches us to set good, solid boundaries and to strengthen our egos to contain our vital, resilient energies.

JUPITER

Qualities: Hot and moist

Types of corresponding plants: Hepatic support, tonics, arterial herbs, galactagogues, alteratives, vasodilators

Plants ruled by Jupiter: White cedar, sage, dandelion

Jupiter is the Roman god of the sky and heavens and rules social justice, laws, light, and abundance of all kinds and is also a thunder god and the Roman equivalent of the Greek god Zeus. In astrology Jupiter is called the "greater benefic" and is usually considered the bringer of all that is good. Jupiter transits bring positive outcomes, ease of action, and expansion in any area of life that Jupiter aspects. The only downside to Jupiter is that it can cause a tendency toward overindulgence and a lack of moderation. Jupiter can be blocked if we are resistant to abundance or for some reason unable to receive it or recognize it.

SATURN

Qualities: Cold and dry

Types of corresponding plants: Astringents, nutritives, bone-building herbs, tonics, alteratives, ligament tightening herbs, vasoconstrictors, some poisons, drying herbs

Plants ruled by Saturn: Mullein, Solomon's seal, comfrey, hellebore, bleeding heart, echinacea, borage, bittersweet, nightshade

In our lives Saturn manifests as change and often the type of change we desperately need but are resistant to because of unconscious fears. This type of change can feel oppressive, as if it is happening whether we want it or not, and we usually don't, or so we think. As we experience the effects of Saturn we may feel depression, grief, and fear. Physically, Saturn is related to any condition of the bones and skeletal structure.

With the potential turmoil that can result from contact with Saturnian energy also comes enormous gifts as is often true when we are forced to look at aspects of ourselves that we are afraid of. Saturn helps us identify unconscious weaknesses that are the true obstacles to our destiny and our soul's purpose. Not only does Saturn shine light into the darkness, but it drags the darkness out into the light.

The "outer planets," Uranus, Neptune, and Pluto, cannot be seen with the naked eye. Therefore, they were not included in traditional Western astrology and herbalism. This was/is a complete system (without the outer planets) and was not lacking. Once the outer plantets were discovered, the characteristics already embedded in the qualities defined by the inner planets (Saturn, Jupiter, Mars, Venus, Mercury, Sun, and Moon) were further revealed and expressed at differing levels and/or octaves by the new planets. That said, there is less historical information to be found about them. And astrologers haven't had as many generations to gather insights about their effects, therefore they are not described in detail here. All of the outer planets are considered to be "impersonal" and have more collective and less individual impacts on life on Earth.

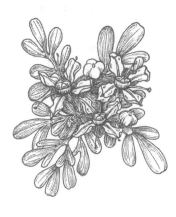

7

Stregoneria and Benedicaria

A Synthesis and Reclaiming of Italian Witchcraft and Magic

Come si divento guaritori? I modi sono fondamentalmente due: o per nascita o per "ereditarietà." Mi spiego subito: c'è chi nasce in circostanze tali per cui è subito chiaro che è destinato a curare certe malattie.

How do you become a healer? There are basically two ways: either by birth or by "inheritance." Let me explain immediately: there are those who are born in such circumstances that it is immediately clear that they are destined to cure certain diseases.

PAOLA GIOVETTI, *I GUARITORI DI CAMPAGNA*

FROM THE ANCIENT DOCTORS AND PHILOSOPHERS of the Mediterranean and the peasants of Southern Italy we have seen their unique version of folk medicine, spirituality, and culture become moveable as those that emigrated from Southern Italy settled in various diasporic locations. They brought their culture with them along with their pockets of seeds and stowed-away tomato plants. The Italian immigrants who came to the United States were largely agrarian peoples who had to adapt to living in urban areas. They often clustered in enclaves or neighborhoods where their diverse ways of life converged.

One of the dominant narratives that is now being pushed back on is the idea of the "melting pot" whereby diverse groups of people all acculturate into a homogeneous standard American, but that has proven not to be the case in all circumstances. Though many Italian immigrants came from diverse regions of Southern Italy and Sicily with different regional traditions and languages, they have maintained their distinctiveness as Italian American for quite some time. As M. Estellie Smith says in "Folk Medicine among the Sicilian-Americans of Buffalo, New York,"

> Despite—or perhaps because of—the more obvious assimilation process best illustrated by out-migration of the most "Americanized" enclave members, there continues to exist the Little Italies, Kaisertowns, Chinatowns, et al., which are perceived by their members to be "different" from other such units.[1]

Recently, Italian-American traditions have become increasingly popular, and many of those traditions have come under the title of witchcraft. This is partly associated with the stereotyping of Italian Americans as "superstitious," and many of their folk medicine practices are similar to those we see in various forms of modern witchcraft as well as historically in Italy and around the world.

Another reason for categorizing Italian-American folk medicine as witchcraft is that many of the newer generations have rejected the Catholic church and denounced the great harms it caused and continues to cause. Witchcraft is a heretical art that divests from religious hegemony and redirects our relationship with the divine back into the hands of the people, as does folk herbalism. Another component of this has been the popularity of modern Wicca and neo-paganism that converged with Italian folk medicine in the books of author Raven Grimassi. Grimassi based his writings on his Italian heritage, but he has been highly criticized for his inaccurate portrayal of Italian folk medicine as an intact, standardized tradition of witchcraft.

The modern and historical witchcraft practices of indigenous Europe have multiple variations, but all were at one time formed as place-based methods and systems used by folk healers to maintain a healthy and balanced relationship with the animate forces of nature for which we are inextricably linked. As for Italian witchcraft, the first question that arises, especially for those of us who are part of the Italian diaspora, is this: are witchcraft and the Catholic folk practices of the Southern Italian people two separate spiritual practices or are they one and the same? The answer is neither. They are both iterations of the folk magic of Southern Italy, and it is largely impossible to trace divergent paths back through time to determine succinct differences. It's absolutely true, however, that many ritual and healing practices of that region of the world were adapted to survive during major social and political changes over time.

There are three basic phases of cultural shifts in Southern Italy:

1. Prepagan animistic worship of Earth-based deities and spiritual matter
2. Pagan patriarchal Sun god worship
3. Christianity

We can only know so much about the transition from animist-based Earth worship to the pagan, patriarchal sky worship, but we do have a fair amount of information and documentation about the transition to Christianity. Much of what we have comes from testimonies during the trials of the Inquisition as well as from the writings of the poets, artists, and philosophers of the time. From this we know that folk medicine and magic became tools of the empire and a means of accumulating power over common people.

The Catholic church became a powerful force of government and was determined to be the sole purveyor of cultural magic. There is some controversy around what happened to the "old religion," or *La vecchia religione*, during this phase. Some say that it continued intact but was hidden; others say that it syncretized with Catholicism. I imagine that both are true, but it's definitely clear at this time that the folk medicine of Southern Italy and the Italian diaspora has been highly influenced by Catholicism to the point where the difference is largely indiscernible.

Regardless of the political and cultural narratives, the underlying themes remain the same; it is all folk magic, and many of those that practiced la vecchia religione during the times of the Inquisition did take refuge in Christian holy places such as monasteries. The prayers, chants, rituals, recipes, and initiatory rites as well as archetypal spirits and deities adapted to Christianity in a full range of variations. In Southern Italy today, these practices continue in their folk Catholic form mostly in the countryside and small villages. These people do not consider themselves to be witches or to be practicing witchcraft but instead identify as Catholics.

Witchcraft itself is not a centralized tradition and is instead full of diverse, local folk practices that are improvisational and syncretized to geographic and cultural imperatives that preserve the indigenous healing practices of the people through time. The rural village traditions in Southern Italy and the practices found in the Italian enclaves in North America may have been shaped around the dogma of the Catholic church, but they are still alive with the indigenous animism of the ancestors. I don't believe this is something that can be suppressed as the world of matter is alive, dynamic, and a force to be reckoned with. It always comes through as it is a natural part of being human. As Sabina Magliocco says in "Spells, Saints, and Streghe,"

Most peasants maintained a magical view of the world. Their universe was an interconnected whole, and tweaking one part of the fabric was likely to bring about changes in another. Rural people were thoroughly familiar with their environment; each feature of the landscape had its own name and legends. They knew well how to exploit it—where to cut wild beet greens in the spring before there were other vegetables to harvest, or where to find land snails to supplement their diet. They planted, harvested and butchered according to the phases of the moon and its position in the sky, believing that this affected the success of their enterprises, and therefore their ability to survive in harsh conditions (Cattabiani, 1988). The world was animated by a variety of local spirits, as well as by angels, demons and saints; these

beings could be invoked to aid survival, but could also be dangerous at times. Invoking or appeasing these beings was not considered
witchcraft, but common sense; it was not limited to a small group of
people in a village, but was widely practiced.[2]

Village and neighborhood healers can be found in many cultures
if not all. Even in our contemporary American/Western world, if you
think about it, I bet you know someone who fits the archetype of "village
witch" in some way or another. I'd venture a guess that village healers
can be found in apartment complexes, city neighborhoods, small towns
and villages, and all the places in between. It may not be someone that
has trained in a specific tradition (or it might be), but it could be someone with the desire or natural inclination to serve the community in
some way. We tend to believe that this type of medicine is in the past,
but the power of nature, the Earth, the soil, the seeds, and all the spirits
to emerge through us is implacable. It cannot be stopped.

Part of our ancestral remembering is learning that all of us originated from places where witchcraft and folk healing were practiced in
some way, and according to Francesco Scaroina in his article "Tra terra e
cielo: quando il popolo si faceva dottore" (Between earth and sky: when
the people became doctors),

> anthropologists steadily assert that people should become aware of
> their originality by studying their traditions and keeping alive the
> memory of what was born among the community. Medicine origi-
> nated from compassion toward human pain, thus seeking and experi-
> menting the most useful remedy in order to restore body health and
> soothe wounds.[3]

One of the most popular notions around Italian folk medicine in
the United States is the idea of the *strega*, or "witch." There is a widespread belief in the idea that Southern Italy hosts an ancient witchcraft tradition that is still practiced today. This is often coupled with
the image of a Strega Nona-type figure, an old grandmother who is

considered a witch and who works for her community as such. This is partly true in that there are still local village and neighborhood folks that practice folk medicine, but they generally consider themselves to be Catholic and use various elements of Catholicism in their practice; they do not go by the name of strega and, in fact, *strega* is considered a derogatory term in Italy.

The use of the word *strega*, however, has become reclaimed by the younger generations and is hopefully beginning to lose some of its negative stigma. And in the United States it has come to be used as a term of ethnic identity and style of practice in the witchcraft community. This is not to say that the practices of those who consider themselves Catholics and not witches could not be viewed as witchcraft depending on your definition of such. We can also view it as a form of magic:

> To approach the knowledge of folk medicine, we have to consider the possibility of a coexistence between rational and irrational elements, thus creating a modus operandi which is not always attributable to superstitions, but which derives from millenniums of experience, traditions and beliefs. The origin lies in a time when magic, religion and science were so related to look like an all-in-one reality.[4]

Healers of Many Names

One of the consistent elements of Italian folk medicine, both in the US and Italy and in traditional witchcraft practices is that it was transmitted orally. This means that categorizing any area of what remains is tricky, the variations of names and terminology are vast, and there is no way to know with any certainty how the language, practices, and rituals have changed or from where they originated.

As mentioned earlier, Italian witchcraft is not an organized tradition. It is naturally decentralized, local, and improvisational as a collection of folk healing practices that syncretized the animistic pre-Christian and pre-pagan indigenous spiritual traditions of Southern Italy with survival imperatives under harsh political and economic conditions. There has always been and, to an extent still are, village healers, and they go by many names in many dialects both in the United States and Southern Italy.

> At one time, many villages had a number of folk healers who could cure a variety of illnesses. They ranged from those who cured with herbs, magic formulas and prayers to professional sorcerers who were called in serious cases of magical attack. In practice, however, these practitioners overlapped, since almost any illness could be judged to be the result of a magical working. Folk healers seldom referred to themselves as streghe (although their neighbors might call them such), but as fattucchiere, "fixers," maghi (masculine plural; singular mago), maghe (feminine plural; sing. maga), "magic-workers." . . . In Sardinia they are simply known as praticos ("knowledgeable ones," akin to the English "cunning-folk"). Most inherit their craft from a relative, although occasionally a healer will acquire power directly from a saint.[5]

Often, folk healers are simply called *quelli che aiutano*,[6] or "those who help," and they were part of the natural healing function of the collective. Collectivism itself was part of community medicine. They also might have been called a *guaritori*, or "healers." This title was not a function of social status, and these people did not work alone and were not solely responsible for "healing" others but were part of larger communal networks—human, natural, and supernatural. Also, the "patient" had agency and was empowered by the reciprocal exchange between themselves and the healer.

The idea that there are networks that include unseen and spiritual forces is a common theme that we see across cultures, in particular in witchcraft testimonies whereby the "witch," a.k.a. community or village healer, "confessed" that they had help from a spirit of supernatural deity. Traditional healing presumes that there are elements of the universe and the biological field of life that we are not able to perceive just with our five senses.

The quelli che aiutano are in alliance with both sensory and extrasensory forces. In terms of the collective, the ailment or concern of the person they are helping is not the central focus of the relationship between them. The central focus is the relationship itself, which is usually long-term and often lasts throughout their entire life. Additionally, the person being helped is not alone in their ailment as they are also part of a greater community/collective that spans generations in all directions. This places the locus of disease or sickness beyond our fixed identity as individuals.

When a three-year study was done in the Lucania region of Southern Italy with Arbëreshë Albanian and Italian communities, it was found that the beneficial aspects of these practices "include prolonged personal contact between patient and healer and strong belief in the treatment regimen."[7] The individual being treated and the healer generate an emergent relationship that is part of the formula, and there is also a relationship between the healer and the entire social field:

> In part, healers gain authority by drawing on symbols and ideologies. Medicinal plants are often important in regional healing ceremonies, but the invocation of holy entities plays a central role. The helper alone is unable to heal the patient, even when botanicals or animal products are employed during the procedure. Often, saints and religious figures are invoked, though these entities may also be natural (e.g., light, water, or plants) rather than supernatural. As she bargains or pleads for help voicing oral formulas, the healer mediates between the perceived or mythic universe and the patient's experiential reality, helping her transition from illness to health.[8]

Below is a list of some of the titles or names that the local healers of Southern Italy and the Italian-American diaspora are known by, a few of which have been discussed earlier. There are certainly many more than are provided here as there are so many dialects and regional versions of the following. Some of the translations below are literal and others are not.*

---

*The Italian language as a standard national language has only been used since the risorgiemento (1860) and many regions still use their own dialect even today. In the United States we (Italian Americans) have our own dialect that is unique as well as a blend of many dialects as many of the immigrants that came didn't speak standard Italian. This gets confusing in terms of the plural/singular of words so for instance the word *practico* in Italian is masculine singular and to make it plural might be *practici*. There's no "s" on the end of words to make them plural, but in the United States we would say the "practicos." This is, of course, not proper Italian and I wouldn't use it in a book, but people could hear it and it's not necessarily *wrong*.

- ❦ Curatrice (curer)
- ❦ Fattucchiera (fixer/witch)—Standard Italian
- ❦ Guaritrice/guaritore (healer)—Standard Italian
- ❦ Janara (witch)—Beneventan dialect
- ❦ Le donne del segno (the women of the sign)—Standard Italian
- ❦ Magara (witch)—Calabrian dialect
- ❦ Mago (magician)—Standard Italian
- ❦ Masca (healer)—Piemonte dialect
- ❦ Masciara (witch)—Salento dialect
- ❦ Medicina contadina (peasant/farmer medicine practitioner)—Standard Italian
- ❦ Pratico (knowledgeable one)
- ❦ Sciamane (shaman)—Standard Italian
- ❦ Spilato (healer or witch)—Sicilian American dialect
- ❦ Strega (witch)—Standard Italian

Although there is no absolute or standardized way to categorize the various practices implemented by the above healers and no obvious division between witchcraft and folk Catholicism, there are three general terms in popular use that describe Italian folk medicine:

1. Stregoneria: "Witchcraft" in Italian
2. Benedicaria: "Blessing Way" in Italian-American
3. Stregheria: "Italian folk magic"

Stregheria is not an Italian word and is in no way historically accurate as it was invented by Raven Grimassi (an Italian American) and was never used before him. People make up words all the time and, in fact, that's how language emerges. However, it's important to note that there is no historical or cultural reference for this word.

Stregoneria and Benedicaria, again, can be perceived as one and the same with subtle differences and a lot of similarities making them often indistinguishable. The one precise commonality is that the individual practitioner comes to use their skill via the direct, oral transmission of knowledge combined with an innate capacity to do so. Traditionally the practitioner is chosen by an elder, usually the grandmother, who has determined that the person, usually a grandchild, has the inherited ability to heal. That inner ability is called "*la forza* (power), *la virtù* (virtue; also attribute), or *il segno* (the sign), and is believed to be inborn."[9] This method of transmission is based on communal, multigenerational living, which is becoming less and less common. In fact, it is becoming nonexistent. Therefore, the means of transmission are changing, as mentioned in the introduction to this book. That said, it is important to be aware of how it has traditionally been believed to operate as a lineage tradition that was often inherited.

Stregoneria

It is from Stregoneria that we get the word *strega*, and all of its associations with magic and the malevolent character of the witch and/or a longstanding pagan tradition that has remained underground through time. Although this idea has remained consistently in legends around Southern Italy, it has not been founded in any factual way except as syncretized with Catholicism.

Charles Leland, author of *Aradia, or the Gospel of the Witches*, did claim to have found a tradition in Southern Italy that was not syncretized with Catholicism, and he based his books on his supposed relationship with a genuine strega by the name of Maddalena. Leland wrote that "the witches even yet form a fragmentary secret society or sect, that they call it that of the Old Religion, and that there are in the Romagna region entire villages in which the people are completely heathen."[10] Though his claims are quite popular among neopagans, they have been largley disputed by ethnographers and scholars with the general consensus being that they are false.

Witches of Benevento

Another of the most famous and ongoing legends that does actually have substantive evidence is that of the witches of Benevento. Benevento, a region in the province of Campania that includes the city of Benevento, is so famous for its witchcraft tradition that it even has a museum dedicated to the history of its *janare*, or "witches." Benevento is often called *La città delle streghe*, or "the city of witches." *Janara* (singular form) is related to the Latin word *ianua*, or "door," or derived from *dianaria*, or "follower of Diana."

> The women seem like normal housewives until 11pm when they apply the olio stregato and fly out of the window to avenge some trespass by harming the babies of the family. They could fit through the keyhole in a door or any other crack in a door.[11]

The legend possibly originated from a sermon given by San Bernardino in 1427 who, going to Benevento at night, saw women, children, and young people dancing and was very afraid, yet curious enough that he eventually got up the courage to take part in what is described as a "witches' Sabbath." This is the first historical documentation of the dance of the witches in Benevento, but it is believed that these practitioners and their traditions have roots back to the ancient Samnite tribes, and they are sometimes referred to as the *le janare sannita* (the Samnite janare). The janare are often described as skilled herbalists and healers: "The Samnite Janare loved the mountains because their main task was to collect herbs, in fact, it is to try to heal both in a benevolent and malevolent sense."[12]

The witches' Sabbath at Benevento is said to have occurred around a walnut tree along the Sabato River. The Sabbath is conducted as a gathering as well as a ritual ceremony.

> It is told that, among their rites, the witches had the custom to meet, in the nights between Saturday and Sunday, around a big walnut tree to give birth to their demoniac Sabbath. The arrival to the place was rigorously flying on horseback of a broom after having spread themselves with a miraculous unguent that gave them not only the ability to fly, but also to become invisible to indiscreet eyes.[13]

The Sabbath at Benevento was well known and even documented in locations outside of the region. During the trial of Matteuccia de Francesco (died 1428), an alleged Italian witch from the province of Perugia who was burned at the stake, the testimony talks of the witches' Sabbath and says that witches flew to Benevento after rubbing their bodies with ointment and reciting a spell that made them able to reach Benevento by flying:

> *Unguento unguento portami al noce di Benevento, sopra l'acqua e sopra il vento sopra ogni altro maltempo.*
>
> *Ointment ointment take me to the Benevento walnut, over the water and over the wind over any other bad weather.*

This theme reoccurs through time as we see one hundred years later, in 1528, when Belleza Orsini, a skilled herbalist who could make medicines better than most *uomini medici ufficiale* ("official medical men," or doctors), refers to the walnut of Benevento and to these gatherings that took place precisely in this city.[14]

Accounts of similar Sabbats in Italy have been written about by Italian historian Carlo Ginzburg in his book *Ecstasies: Deciphering the Witches' Sabbath* and are based on testimonies from the European witch trials. As scholar Marguerite Rigoglioso notes:

> Testimonies indicate that men and women, but above all, women, would meet with her (Diana) in shamanic trance, usually at night. One group, the benandanti of the Friuli, fought during such episodes with malevolent "witches" who threatened the fertility of the fields. Sometimes shapeshifting into animals or insects, other times riding on animals' backs, they would end their journey by joining an otherworldly "procession of the dead." Various references to "toads" and ointments in the trial records, suggests Ginzburg, indicate that practitioners may have induced such trances by ingesting or topically applying hallucinogenic substances derived from toad's skin or psychoactive mushrooms.[15]

Witchcraft or Everyday Magic?

As we touched on earlier, the word *strega* and all of the negative connotations that have been associated with witchcraft and witches is a topic of

some confusion in terms of Italian folk medicine because of its syncretism with Catholicism. The village healers that identify as Catholics are
those that help the community and, from their view, witches are people
who are malevolent. But, when we look at the practical aspects of both
traditions we see uncanny similarities. This is likely due to the demoniza-
tion of women as well as the hegemony that the church had on the power
of healing. The local, vernacular methods of health care held by the common people, as well as their emotional and spiritual agency, were a threat
to the control that the church desired to have over the masses.

According to Angela Puca in her article "The Tradition of Segnature:
Underground Indigenous Practices in Italy," "The survival of vernacular magic among Italian people appears to be the product of history, fos-
tered by two endemic driving forces within the cultural fabric: tradition
(especially family tradition) and the rejection of authorities."[16]

Witchcraft in some of its forms, then, stems from tradition, meaning
it is a very ordinary, everyday, way of life. In terms of Italian witchcraft
or what might be called such, it has been a part of the cultural system; it
emerged from the people. It's natural magic. As Fabrizio Ferrari explains
in his book *Ernesto De Martino on Religion: The Crisis of Presence,*
"Magical practices are not extraordinary for those belonging to the cultural system that generates them. In fact, they are often not even considered magic at all."[17]

Origins of the Flying Witch

The word *strega* is derived from the Latin word strix, which means "a noc-
turnal bird," along with the ancient Greek *strix*, which means "screecher"
and also refers to the screech owl. This word led to the term *strĭga*, meaning "evil spirit, nightmare; vampire; witch." Interestingly the idea of a witch
or other supernatural being flying and/or having wings while at the same
time bringing healing to people, is based in both mythology and the Bible.

The origin of folk medicine is ascribed to the angels in the
Mediterranean region, particularly in Hebrew, Egyptian, and Greek
mythologies and cosmologies. Based on the documentation from
these traditions, the angels taught humans the ways of magic and folk

medicine. The Book of the Watchers in 1 Enoch (an ancient Hebrew text) describes how the fallen angels gave the following skills to human women in exchange for carnal/corporeal knowledge:

Shemihazah taught spells and the cutting of roots.
Hermani taught sorcery for the loosing of spells and magic and skill.
Baraqel taught the signs of the lightning flashes.
Kokabel taught the signs of the stars.
Ziqel taught the signs of the shooting stars.
Arteqoph taught the signs of the earth.
Shamsiel taught the signs of the sun.
Sahriel taught the signs of the moon. (I Enoch 8)

And the women also of the angels who went astray shall become sirens. (I Enoch 19:2)

Sirens in this sense are half bird, half human and are portrayed in a number of characters through time including the following:

Anat, the Canaanite goddess, is a vulture.
Ishtar, the Summerian goddess, is a hawk.
Babylon is equated with the gluten of the eagle.
Naples is a siren.[18]

The original mythological figures described here can be found across the world in many cosmologies such as the Germanic Norns, the Roman Fates, the Greek Moirae, and others. As Christianity took over, the powerful constellations of these figures became less universal and more localized within folklore and vernacular traditions and likely syncretized with the dominant religion. Eventually this idea of a female figure with healing powers and knowledge of herbs and spells became the target of the witch trials and anyone that displayed these talents was considered a "witch." However, as Jean de Blanchefort says in her book *Riti e magie delle campagne*,

It is useful to remember that with the term witchcraft I refer to a set of rites and practices that have nothing to do with black magic; these practices also included the use of herbs and vegetables, and sometimes even parts of animals aimed at procuring healing from certain diseases. Witches and Sorcerers often and willingly acted to help the inhabitants of the villages and the surrounding area where they lived; sometimes they also looked after the animals, tried with their rituals to interfere with the atmospheric conditions in case of drought and, last but not least, they practiced love spells for young women seeking husbands.[19]

Benedicaria

Benedicaria means "Blessing Way," or "Way of Blessing," and refers to a set of spiritual practices that are part of the folk Catholic traditions of Southern Italy and Sicily. By "folk Catholic" I am referring to the way Catholicism syncretized with the place-based indigenous healing methods and life ways of the peasants of Southern Italy. These same traditions are also known as Fa Lu Santuccio in the region of Campania, which literally means to "do a little holy thing." Many Benedicaria practitioners also simply refer to it as "the things we do."

The life ways of the peasants were based on village collectivism and small-scale sustainable farming, forestry, and land management that were inextricably linked to their relationships with the entire web of creation. These ways and traditions were manifested as rituals that strongly resemble the pre-Christian ancient Roman forms of animism, which are rooted in the pre-pagan cultures of Old Europe and the Mediterranean. The rituals include words—incantations, prayers, and blessings—often in an Italian dialect (the vernacular language of the various microregions of Italy), English, or both. Along with words, these rituals involve sacred or meaningful objects or materials that ranged from an altar to water, salt, candles, a rosary, and often sacred foods and recipes. They can also include home remedies, plant medicines, and fiber arts such as specific crochet patterns that have symbolic meaning and magical potency.

The word *Benedicaria* itself emerged from the Italian-American diaspora as a way to identify unique methods of cultural magic practiced by the Italian immigrants as well as their unique form of folk Catholicism. The Italian immigrants practiced Catholicism much differently than it was being administered by the churches in the United States. Most of the clergy in the United States during the initial immigration of Italians were of Irish or German descent, and Catholicism at that point had been somewhat Protestanized, or you could say, "Americanized."

As Frances M. Malpezzi and William M. Clements contend in their book *Italian-American Folklore*, when Southern Italians came to the United States the church saw them as a problem because they resisted the control it was forcing upon them, most likely because it felt like the same type of "oppressive forces which they had fled Italy to escape" and

> they found the tone of Catholicism much different from what they had previously known. Legalistic and formal, the Church focused on a patriarchal deity and opposed many of the practices which the Italian immigrants believed to be central to religious devotion. Consequently, Italian immigrants found the American Church to be "a cold and almost puritanical organization" that failed to meet their religious needs and in some cases overtly opposed their devotional activities.[20]

So because the Italian immigrants didn't like the clerical authority of the church in the United States, religion for the Southern Italians . . . "reflected the spirit of campanilismo, more devotion sometimes being offered to the patron saints of specific communities than to the Trinity."[21]

Benedicaria is a form of healing that is part of family and community life in Italian traditional culture and continues to be practiced today both in Southern Italy and in the Italian diaspora although it is becoming less and less common as the pull of modern Western life and global economics has left many of the "old ways" behind. Bendicaria, as it is called, is a word that emerged in the Italian Amerian diaspora though the practices that it includes are those that were brought with the Italian immigrants and adapted to life in the United States. In this sense it is more of an Italian American tradition, than an Italian one.

> *La peculiarità di questa Benedicaria è che in Italia non esiste. Almeno non in senso stretto. Gli unici a praticarla in verità sono gli Americani, spesso nipoti dei nipoti dei primi emigranti italiani. Facendo una breve ricerca fra i testi sulle tradizioni siciliane si evince che non c'è alcuna traccia di Benedicaria in Italia o di praticanti davvero italiani.*[22]

The peculiarity of this Benedicaria is that it does not exist in Italy. At least not strictly speaking. The only ones who actually practice it are the Americans, often grandchildren of the grandchildren of the first Italian emigrants. Making a brief search among the texts on Sicilian traditions it is clear that there is no trace of Benedicaria in Italy or of truly Italian practitioners.

In Southern Italy the methods and practices that are part of Benedicaria in the U.S. are not considered separate from the religious practices of Catholicism, nor are they considered separate from simple daily devotional means of navigating secular life. In other words, Benedicaria includes tools and practices that imbue mundane activities with blessings, spirit, and intent. It's not only a way of blessing daily life and activating the holy in the physical but also a practice of staying blessed and in alignment with spirit by reminding ourselves, our family, and our community that we are inherently holy, part of nature, and in continuous contact with the divine.

Practitioners of Benedicaria don't usually have a title or call themselves anything because Benedicaria is just a way of being in the world. However, a person might be called by the honorable name Benedetta or Benedetto (plural: Benedetti) when they become well known and trusted as someone who makes dependably successful cures or when a practitioner steps into the role of elder in a family or neighborhood, and people start coming to them regularly for help. Certain practitioners are known for the scope of their blessings and cures. For instance, some will be known for being good at curing the malocchio, and some may be known for other types of maladies or specific illnesses or conditions.

One becomes a Benedetta or Benedetto through lineage transmission. An elder practitioner will transmit the healing gifts to someone of a younger generation, usually a family member. Traditionally this transmission goes through the female line from grandmother to granddaughter, but this is not always so. While staying in a small village in the province of Salerno, I was told that the transmission must go from woman to man and then from man to woman and so on, changing genders each generation. Either way, at the end of their life, the elder person will pass down the prayers, rituals, and tools of healing and devotion to a younger family member who they have determined has a natural propensity for them or an interest in taking on the responsibility. In that sense, this is a lineage tradition, and the specific words and methods used are often familial or at least regional. *It is important to note here that our current cultural narratives and indoctrination around the ideas of "gender" belong to us and did not necessarily apply to our ancestors or our traditional cultures.*

The specific words and prayers used, the deities invoked or even the particular skills and ailments that the practitioner can cure are often familial, especially in the diaspora. Because people immigrated from all over Southern Italy where the traditions can vary greatly even from village to village, the diasporic communities that formed were a conglomeration of what would have otherwise been disparate groups of people with their own unique ways of practicing.

In my own community, there were several methods of curing the malocchio, each with different words, prayers, and phrases. The way my friend's nonna performed the malochhio cure was very different from the way mine did it, although to an outsider they might seem similar.

Italian immigrants brought their Blessing Way with them and carried it on in the New World as best they could, adapting it to life in a country where they were not immediately accepted and, in fact, experienced a great deal of alienation and discrimination. Benedicaria is an improvisational tradition that, because it makes use of the tools at hand, enabled the Italian diaspora to orient and ground with a familiar form of healing, worship, and faith. The peasants and contadini of Southern Italy were artists, as all peasant and indigenous peoples are, who knew how to identify and access the patterns of nature and the divine, or God, and channel them into generative forms of living and creativity.

Benedicaria is also a direct realization practice. This means that there is no intermediary needed for an individual to have contact with God. The Benedetta or Benedetto employs the aid of the Virgin Mary, Jesus, or other angels and saints via direct transmission during ritual and prayer. The healing that occurs is channeled directly without the need for a priest or other intercessor. The Virgin Mary and any of the Catholic deities are available to everyone at any time or place and therefore help and healing are also available.

It's no wonder that both Benedicaria and Catholicism in general have been often seen as forms of heresy and even witchcraft by Protestant and Evangelical denominations of Christianity. Often Italian Benedetti were called witches, and their practices called witchcraft.

Benedicaria does have links to Italian witchcraft, or Stregoneria, and many people consider Benedetti and streghe to be the same. But while they can be indistinguishable from each other in some practices, the Benedetti invoke Catholic deities, saints, and angels and use traditional Catholic prayers and practices, whereas the streghe work with pre-Christian and even pre-pagan elements, forces, and gods and goddesses. Both Benedicaria and witchcraft evolved from the ancient pagan cults and rites of Southern Italy as well as the animist pre-pagan forms of worship. Witchcraft, also called La vecchia religione (the old religion) as mentioned earlier, is a largely fluid definition of pre-Christian spiritual practices that did not merge with Catholicism but continued, often hidden and in secret or cloaked in Catholicism. Benedicaria can definitely be viewed as an iteration of La vecchia religione from this lens.

In his book *The Things We Do: Ways of the Holy Benedetta*, Agostino Taumaturgo says,

> What we can know with certainty about its history, is that in its origins, the practices of Benedicaria were thoroughly Pagan, and were most likely ties to the Domestic Cult (i.e., the practices of family and

household rituals) among the tribes of Southern Italy. Of note would be the Samnites, the Brundisii, the Calabri, and others whose names have passed into history. Whatever these original rites may have been, they would have been rites of home and hearth, centered on the individual's relationship with the gods or the family's spiritual well-being; perhaps the best modern parallel we could draw would be the praying of the Rosary in an individual or a family setting, or the practice of a family getting together to read a discuss a passage from the Bible.[23]

Practices and Rituals of Benedicaria

The healing blessings of Benedicaria are based on the Holy Trinity: the Father, the Son, and the Holy Spirit. To reframe this in pre-Christian terms, we might say body, mind, and spirit. The devotional practice of blessing works through the three realms of matter: solid (body), liquid (mind), and gas (spirit). The specific practices facilitate the awareness and distribution of these via ritual, contemplation, and connection with the divine. Combining these aspects of practice is intended to position us in a call-and-response engagement with creation whereby we both call and respond, act and listen, give and receive. We come into communication/communion with the sacred or holy through prayer, meditation, and ritual. We also enact our own agency, meaning we become agents of creation for the benefit of all beings.

The home is the center for the practice of Benedicaria, and described below are some of the most common elements of making a sacred household. Benedicaria is not an organized tradition with overarching rules, systems, or doctrine, beyond its adherence to Catholic precepts. Instead, it is improvisational and emergent, meaning that each practitioner will find their own style and methods based on experience and their personal connection with spirit.

Often a practitioner will include several consistent customs in their methods. These customs will often include building a home altar, making the sign of the cross, blessing with holy water, and reciting traditional prayers.

BUILDING A HOME ALTAR

A home altar, or several altars, is often the center of practice and the place where prayer and offerings are made, and building home altars and interacting with them regularly are primary practices of Benedicaria. It is important to keep your altars fresh and in motion, meaning to stay in relationship with them. You should clean them regularly, replace candles and other perishable items, remove items that are no longer relevant, and add seasonal or situational objects. An altar is a manifestation platform and a place where the material world represents the unseen. Home altars that we may pass by and/or sit with throughout the day represent the sacred and are a constant signal to our psyche to remember and shift our awareness from too much focus on the mundane.

It is important to carefully consider where to place your altar(s). Ancestral altars are sometimes erected in a main room or a place where they can be seen throughout the day and by other family members. It is generally recommended not to have ancestral altars in your bedroom or where you sleep. This is because having the image or a belonging of a dead ancestor or relative where you sleep can elicit disruptive energy while we're trying to sleep, particularly if it is an ancestor that we are working deeply with. This is even more pertinent if the ancestor is "unsettled," or not yet crossed-over in the otherworld.

Working with an ancestral altar is an active practice of presence and engagement, so it is often better suited for when we are fully awake. I like my bedroom altars to bring in peace and relaxation so a prayer altar or an altar devoted to protective spirits and forces might be more suitable here. Seasonal altars are also appropriate in a main living space. Ritual altars might be better in a less-active part of the house. Any flat surface can become an altar, indoors or out. The altar itself is blessed as is each item. A blessing usually involves sprinkling the altar with holy water and saying a prayer. A blessing can be any prayer that you prefer, but traditionally it would be an Our Father or Hail Mary.

Below are lists of traditional objects and more personal items that are often included in an altar:

Traditional Objects

- ❧ Altar cloth, typically white
- ❧ Statue of the Blessed Mother, Jesus, or a saint, or a crucifix
- ❧ At least one candle placed in front of an image of a saint or ancestor or a one on either side of the statue
- ❧ Rosary or scapular, often draped around the statue
- ❧ Small bowl of holy water
- ❧ Small bowl of salt
- ❧ Prayer book or Bible, usually familial
- ❧ Wine
- ❧ Incense and incense burner
- ❧ Photos of dead relatives/ancestors

Personal Items

- ❧ Flower essences or herbal remedies you are working with
- ❧ Live plants, seasonal objects gathered outdoors such as fresh flowers, seeds, pine cones, autumn leaves
- ❧ An item that represents all or any of the four elements: earth, air, fire, water
- ❧ Rocks or gems such as black onyx, amber, or any others that have meaning to you
- ❧ God/goddess/nature spirit statues or images
- ❧ Tarot cards (I often draw a new card and place it on my altar each time I cleanse it.)
- ❧ Any item you wish to "charge" such as a charm/amulet bag
- ❧ Prescription medications that you want to bless and hold sacred
- ❧ Sigils (symbols with magical power)
- ❧ An intention jar
- ❧ Empty space to see what comes up and wants to be on your altar

MAKING THE SIGN OF THE CROSS

The sign of the cross, symbolic of the cross that Jesus was crucified on, is a somatic sacramental movement or mudra, a bodily gesture that signals that sacred space is opening or closing. It is also an apotropaic ritual used to protect and bless people, objects, and places. The sign of the cross is made on the body of the person or over an object, a bowl of holy water, an altar, or any other place. It is at the very least a simple form of blessing and invoking presence in the moment. It can also be used at the beginning and ending of any prayer, when sitting before an altar, entering church or sacred space, or receiving communion, or at any moment during the day when one may need to center and focus or stabilize strong emotions.

The Blessing Hand: The blessing hand is the mudra used when blessing oneself. It's made by extending the thumb and index and middle fingers while folding in the ring and pinky finger. This may be different in other denominations of Christianity.

When blessing others or objects such as a bowl of holy water, you may see some or all fingers extended so the hand is flat but turned sideways.

The Motion: To make the sign of the cross, make a motion with your right hand starting at your forehead and then moving to your breast, to your left shoulder, and to your right shoulder while saying the following prayer:

> *Nel nome del Padre, e del Figlio, e dello Spirito Santo. Amen.*
> In the name of the Father, the Son, and the Holy Spirit. Amen.

Making Holy Water

Holy water is another often-used tool of healing in Benedicaria. It is used for blessings, for cleansing objects and spaces, and as a way to bring the water element to a living space or an altar. Holy water can be purchased at a Catholic store, but you can also make your own as described here.

You will need salt, water, and a large bowl or jar. Glass is preferable to plastic but in a pinch either will do.

Blessing the Salt: You can keep a separate container of Holy Salt that has been blessed and is ready to use, or you can bless the salt as you are making the holy water. Here is a traditional prayer to bless salt:

O salt, creature of God, I exorcise you by the living God, by the true
God, by the holy God, by the God who ordered you to be poured
into the water by Elijah the Prophet so that its life-giving powers
might be restored. I exorcise you so that you may become a means
of salvation for believers, that you may bring health of soul and body
to all who make use of you, and that you may put to flight and drive
away from the places where you are sprinkled; every apparition,
villainy, and turn of devilish deceit, and every unclean spirit;
adjured by Him who will come to judge the living and the
dead and the world by fire. Amen.

Exorcising the Water: Place the water in a large bowl or jar and place the
bowl on your working altar. Exorcise the water by either making the sign of
the cross and saying a Hail Mary or by saying this traditional prayer:

O water, creature of God, I exorcise you in the name of God the
Father Almighty, and in the name of Jesus Christ his Son, our Lord,
and in the power of the Holy Spirit. I exorcise you so that you may
put to flight all the power of the enemy, and be able to root out
and supplant that Enemy with his apostate angels: through the power
of our Lord Jesus Christ, Who will come to judge
the living and the dead and the world by fire. Amen.

Mixing the Salt and the Water: Place a handful (more or less depending on
how much water you have) of salt in the water and say the following:

May this salt and water be mixed together in the name of the Father,
and of the Son, and of the Holy Spirit. Amen.

You may also add this prayer:

God, source of irresistible might and king of an invincible realm, the
ever-glorious conqueror; who restrains the force of the adversary,
silencing the uproar of his rage, and valiantly subduing his wickedness;
in awe and humility we beg you, Lord, to regard with favor this
creature thing of salt and water, to let the light of your kindness

shine upon it, and to hallow it with the dew of your mercy; so that
wherever it is sprinkled and your holy name is invoked,
every assault of the unclean spirit may be baffled, and all dread
of the serpent's venom be cast out. To us who entreat your
mercy grant that the Holy Spirit may be with us wherever
we may be; through Christ our Lord. Amen.

Blessing the Water: Now bless the water:

Blessed are you, Lord, Almighty God, who deigned to bless us in
Christ, the living water of our salvation, and to reform us interiorly,
grant that we who are fortified by the sprinkling of or use of this
water, the youth of the spirit being renewed by the power of
the Holy Spirit, may walk always in newness of life.

RECITING PRAYERS

Traditional Catholic prayers are used during various rituals and blessings
or any time the practitioner seeks the intercession or guidance of God. The
prayers below are written traditionally but many modern Benedicaria practitioners alter them to align with our own personal faith, beliefs, and values.
In the more conservative sects of Catholicism, it is believed that traditional
prayers must be accurately recited in their original versions, but in my personal experience, using words and phrases that are incongruent to our inner
truths and values creates dissonance instead of blessing, or at least a disso-
nant blessing. When we fully resonate with the prayers we speak, they are
far more potent and healing; therefore altering a prayer to align with who
you are and what you believe can only be beneficial from this view.

Padre Nostro (Our Father)

Padre Nostro,
che sei nei cieli,
Sia santificato il tuo nome.
Venga il tuo regno,
Sia fatta la tua volontá,
Come in cielo, così in terra.

Dacci oggi il nostro pane quotidiano,
E rimetti a noi i nostri debiti
Come noi li rimettiamo ai nostri debitori.
E non ci indurre in tentazione,
Ma liberaci dal male.
Amen.

Our father
Who art in heaven,
Hallowed be thy name
Thy kingdom come
Thy will be done
On Earth as it is in heaven
Give us this day our daily bread
and forgive us our trespasses
as we forgive those who trespass against us
Lead us not into temptation
and deliver us from evil.
Amen

Ave Maria (Hail Mary)
Ave Maria, piena di grazia,
il Signore è con te.
Tu sei benedetta fra le donne
e benedetto è il frutto del tuo seno, Gesù.
Santa Maria, Madre di Dio,
prega per noi peccatori,
adesso e nell'ora della nostra morte.
Amen.

Hail Mary, full of grace
The Lord is with thee
Blessed art thou amongst women
And blessed is the fruit of thy womb, Jesus.
Holy Mary, Mother of God
Pray for us sinners

now and at the hour of our death.

Amen

Memorare (Remember)

Ricordati, o piissima Vergine Maria,
che non si è mai inteso al mondo
che qualcuno sia ricorso alla tua protezione,
abbia implorato il tuo aiuto,
chiesto il tuo patrocinio
e sia stato da te abbandonato.
Animato da tale confidenza,
a te ricorro, o Madre,
Vergine delle vergini,
a te vengo, e, peccatore come sono,
mi prostro ai tuoi piedi a domandare pietà.
Non volere, o Madre del divin Verbo,
disprezzare le mie preghiere,
ma benigna ascoltale ed esaudiscile.
Amen.

Remember, O most gracious Virgin Mary,
that never was it known
that anyone who fled to thy protection,
implored thy help,
or sought thy intercession,
was left unaided.
Inspired by this confidence
I fly unto thee,
O Virgin of virgins, my Mother.
To thee do I come,
before thee I stand,
sinful and sorrowful.
O Mother of the Word Incarnate,
despise not my petitions,
but in thy mercy hear and answer me.
Amen.

Gloria al Padre (Glory Be)

Gloria al Padre

e al Figlio

e allo Spirito Santo.

Come era nel principio,

ora e sempre

nei secoli dei secoli.

Amen.

Glory be to the Father,

and to the Son,

and to the Holy Spirit.

As it was in the beginning,

is now,

and ever shall be,

world without end.

Amen.

Benedicaria Sacramentals

A sacramental is any object, prayer, or practice that is used in an act of devotion. These are methods of channeling the healing power of the divine and facilitating grace or "grazia"(grazia is talked about in depth in chapter 9).

THE ROSARY

A rosary is a set of prayer beads strung together into specific sizes and sets. Rosaries were originally made from seeds or knotted fiber, thread, or rope and possibly even strings of flowers, or garlands. The name *rosary* stems from the Latin *rosarium*, which refers to a garland of roses or possibly a rose garden. According to legend, the first rosary was given to Saint Dominic, the twelfth-century Spanish saint and founder of the Dominican order, by the Virgin Mary during a vision. But we know that the history probably goes much further back than that to pre-Christian times.

The rosary is a tool to prompt and facilitate a state of prayer and meditation. The repetition of a series of prayers while using a tactile prompt, the beads, is not unique to Italians or Italian-Americans but is a cross-cultural form of meditation and prayer. For instance, we see the use of prayer beads in other religions such as mala beads used by Buddhists and Yogis.

The rosary consists of fifty-nine beads, and each bead corresponds to a specific prayer that is repeated. Each prayer is a mantra, and each bead is a place to say it. The beads provide something tangible, something physical to keep us present and grounded while we stay open and quiet as we pray.

While the prayers said on each bead can vary depending on the tradition, the following is a general standard:

1. Begin with the crucifix or whatever symbol is at the bottom of the rosary by saying a Memorare (a prayer to the Virgin Mary)
2. Say an Our Father at every large bead
3. Say a Hail Mary at every small bead
4. Say a Glory Be at the center

THE NOVENA

> *Of all the rites and "spells" performed by practitioners of Benedicaria, the most common component is the Novena. If fact, the Novena is so pervasive that one could say it is the heart and foundation of the Benedicaria tradition.*
>
> AGOSTINO TAUMATURGO, *THE THINGS WE DO:*
> *WAYS OF THE HOLY BENEDETTA*

Novena stems from a latin word *novem*, which simple means "nine" and refers to nine-day prayer cycles. Each day for nine consecutive days a series of prayers are said, usually in front of an altar with candles and sometimes an image or statue of a saint or deity. The rosary is usually incorporated into the novena and is prayed at least once on each of the nine days.

The novena is devoted or dedicated to some intention such as petitioning for healing, celebrating a feast or holy day, or commemorating a special event, or it can be a form of devotion to the Virgin Mary or a saint or a form of prayer to the Sacred or Immaculate Heart.

THE SACRED AND IMMACULATE HEARTS

The Sacred Heart is the symbol of the heart of Jesus, which is said to be the source of all love. It represents the center of the human body, the center of humanity as a whole, and the possibility of love suffusing the world as the heart suffuses the body with lifeblood.

The counterpart to the Sacred Heart is the Immaculate Heart, which is the symbol of the heart of the Virgin Mary. The Immaculate Heart is the vessel for the joys and sorrows of life. Both divine hearts are an important aspect of devotional contemplation and worship in Benedicaria. Prayers and novenas to the divine hearts invite and call on the energies they express to be remembered as part of our essential goodness and healing propensity.

Benedicaria Cures

Benedicaria is ritual and energetic medicine. It facilitates the flow and exchange of energy. The most popularly known rituals of Benedicaria are the ones that offer cures for ailments related to the malocchio discussed in earlier chapters.

The malocchio is often called the *maloik* in Italian-American vernacular, or sometimes the "overlook," but it has other names depending on the dialect. There is also a term used to describe the cure for the maloik, which is *fa maloik* or "make the maloik." So a malocchio cure or treatment would be referred to as fa maloik, and in Italian American we would say, "Can you do the fa maloik?" or "Does your nonna know the fa maloik?"

Malocchio is the seeking of equilibrium or homeostasis and is a natural part of being human. While living daily life, especially in a communal setting, it is natural to throw off overwhelming or uncomfortable energy onto others as well as take those energies on. This is largely autonomic/subliminal.

One form of malocchio is caused by envy or jealousy, whether it's unconscious or conscious. It is generally believed that it is not intentional but merely the result of someone looking at you or something you have and having a desire for it. This can include any item of clothing, jewelry, or any praise or acknowledgment, and even good luck that has been noticed by someone else. Because of this it is generally considered an act of malocchio to even compliment someone by saying something like "Your blouse is pretty." In this case, the person giving the compliment can prevent the evil eye from being cast in two ways:

1. By always ending any praise by saying "Benedica" or "Dio ti benedica," which means "God bless you"
2. By making a "spitting" sound three times: "Puh, puh, puh"

Whatever the cause or situation, when we have the malocchio, we have taken on the projection of someone else's unmanaged energy, and the Benedicaria cures for this disperse that energy. Many of the cures are done with olive oil, salt, and water—all simple and accessible items that are imbued with sacredness and magic through the ritual process and the experience and skill of the Benedetta. One such cure involves using scissors to "cut" the curse. This is done by pointing the scissors down into the water or above the bowl and making a "cutting" motion with them. Another cure involves dropping oil into a bowl of water and then observing how the oil behaves. Various oil globs and streams appear, and the way that oil moves around in the water will indicate whether the person has the evil eye and whether it was caused by a man or a woman. Then a special prayer is said to turn the evil eye away.

There are other cures that do not use either oil or water. Some use only prayers, gestures, or mudras and often incorporate the laying on of hands or herbs and other tools.

Malocchio cures are familial rituals as well as parochial (parochial here means that there are different methods in different parishes in Italy), and the knowledge of how to cure malocchio comes from direct transmission, usually from an elder family member. The elder teaches the younger how to perform the physical actions involved as well as what prayers and words to say. Often these prayers are only shared between the elder and the younger family member and are otherwise kept secret. The transmission is performed on specific nights of the year at midnight: Christmas Eve, Saint John's Eve (June 24), Good Friday, Easter, and Epiphany (January 6). This is thought to be the only time that this tradition can be passed on from one person to another:

> A cure was wrought by bringing in a woman who said an incantation learned on Christmas Eve. Anyone taught the incantation on the eve of Christ's birth has the power to cure "overlooked" persons; consequently, old wives knowing the charmed words are still much sought after, even in this country.[24]

The incantations vary far and wide and many practitioners choose not to share them too broadly because they are sacred and only meant to be handed down from elder to younger in a family lineage. That said, some people do share them, and here is an example from Taumaturgo's *The Things We Do*:

> *mmidia e malocchio*
> *curnucille all'occhio*
> *crepa l'ammidia e scoppia*
> *lu malocchio*
> *n' nome di Di e d' Santa Mari*
> *lu malocchio se n' pozza ye.*[25]
>
> *Envy and evil-eye*
> *little horns to the eyes*
> *Impolde the envy and*
> *explode the evil eye.*
> *In the name of God and of Holy Mary*
> *The Evil Eye must go.*

Both Stregoneria and Benedicaria, assuming they're separate practices, addressed specific types of psycho-somatic-spiritual ailments such as the malocchio. The prayers and rituals were performed at home in gardens and kitchens or anywhere that was necessary. The tools and objects were items that were available, and there was not a big fuss made around how they were used. Often a cure for malocchio or some other ailment would happen at the kitchen table or on the front porch with children running around, and other family members weaving in and out. In short, the above described practices, along with many others, were and are a way of daily living and part of the vernacular medicine of the peasants of Southern Italy.

Curses

One element in Italian folk magic that is often excluded from the discussion, or likely just forgotten, is the curse, which in general has come to be associated with malevolence and evil, or those who would cause harm. But that narrative emerges from our dualistic Abrahamic traditions that divided good and evil. From an animistic and what might be called an indigenous perspective, these so-called curses can also be intentional means of prevention and protection from pernicious external forces.

These rites and rituals come from a people who were under constant outside threat from foreign invasion, disease, and oppression by their own state. Examples of why a more severe and intentional curse would be used include finding thieves, protecting against marauders, stopping the spread of an epidemic, or any other manner of preventing or reducing harm. More serious spells and curses can be used to counter other spells and curses.

We discussed the most common ailment—the malocchio, or evil eye—in the previous section. Below are some other types of curses described by names that are often used interchangeably with *malocchio* and sometimes used to describe variations of the evil eye. Again, the term used depends on the region, family, or community in both Southern Italy and in the Italian-American enclaves. One important aspect to keep in mind about the malocchio as well as other curse-type spells is that not only humans are susceptible; all of life including horses, cows, crops, and even the elements can be subjects of curses.

JETTATURA

The word *jettatura* comes from *iettare* meaning "to jinx," "to throw," "to cast out," or "a spell." This curse is caused by someone with harmful intent who sends you bad luck. One such curse is the Sicilian u scantu, which is described as follows:

> *Una paura o un dolore improvviso, che spezza l'equilibrio della persona e consente la manifestazione di ogni tipo di malattia.*[26]

A sudden fear or pain, which breaks the balance of the person and allows the manifestation of any type of disease.

FATTURA

Fattura, or a "fixing," literally means "to invoice," as in "you owe me"; it's like getting tagged but not in a good way. This is a malevolent spell that often affects people in the solar plexus and affects their digestion and stomach. Sometimes a *fattura* is described as the way the evil eye attaches to a person. A local healer in the Campania region described fattura as a different type of affliction than the evil eye and according to Thomas Hauschild in *Power and Magic in Italy* a fattura is sent by raising the dead using dust or flour.[27] In these cases a fattura is a distinct, intentional ritual as opposed to the evil eye, which may simply be an unintentional energy exchange:

> *Si intende per fattura qualunque procedimento basato su concetti magici di simpatia, similarità e di contatto, diretto allo scopo di male contro una determinata persona, compiuto da persona adatta, con materiale particolare e particolari cerimonie più o meno complicate. Dicendo a scopo di male, non bisogna intendere pertanto che la fattura abbia sempre l'intento ai recare una vera e propria sciagura alla vittima. Sebbene questo sia lo scopo predominante, pure esistono fatti che hanno per fine costringere una determinata persona a compiere la volontà dell'operante, (come per esempio, nel caso di tiare innamorare un individuo restio), di ritrovare tesori nascosti, di ritrovare i ladri*

*ecc. questo secondo genere di fattura non ha, però, importanza nella
medicina e perciò basti soltanto l'averlo accennato. La fattura è il
grado maggiore di azione maligna.*[28]

By fattura we mean any procedure based on sympathetic magic, similarity and contact, aimed at the purpose of harm against a particular
person, performed by an appropriate person, with particular material
and specific, more or less complicated ceremonies. By saying for the
purpose of evil, it does not mean that the fattura always has the intent
to bring a real disaster to the victim. Although this is the predominant purpose, it is also done to force a certain person to fulfill the
will of the operator (as for example, in the case of falling in love with
a reluctant individual), of finding hidden treasures, of finding thieves
etc. however, this second kind of fattura has no importance in medicine and therefore it is enough to just mention it. Fattura is the major
degree of malignant action.

The idea of fattura is present in Italian-American neighborhoods as
well with the general understanding that it is a form of the malocchio but
with intent: "the only difference between the two being that an attitude
of deliberateness and malevolence surrounds the latter . . . one *gives* the
malocchio but *makes* a *fatura*."[29]

La Fascinazione or La Fascinatura

La fascinazione or *la fascinatura*, also *L'affascino*, is a type of curse caused
by a look, or someone with malintent looking at another, touching them
in some way such as with a caress, saying certain words (especially com-
pliments), and sometimes using specific gestures.[30] The consequences
of being the victim of la fascinatura can run from possession to being
the object of a love spell. Fascinazione is also sometimes interchangeable
with malocchio as it is considered to be an "influence [that has] darted
from the eyes of an envious or angry person, and so infected the air as to
penetrate and corrupt the bodies of both living creatures and inanimate
objects."[31]

ATTACCATURA

Attaccatura means an "attachment" or "binding" that attaches a hostile force to someone.

LEGATURA

As discussed in the beginning of this section, not all curses are used to harm. *Legatura* is another form of binding, but it is a means of reestablishing balance when it has been disrupted by an illness or curse, sometimes called a *narcatura* and associated with having *sangue guasto*, or "bad blood." Legatura is performed by "tying of a cord tightly around the ankle of a patient in order to obtain blood to counter the narcatura."[32]

SCIOGLIERE

Sciogliere, "untying," is the dissolving or melting of something, and in the case of folk magic, it is the resolution of or absolution from evil. It also refers to the untying or freeing of some type of obstruction or *nodi* (knots) in the spiritual or energetic sense and to "liberare da un impedimento" (free from an impediment).[33] So we can see here that "binding" can be both malevolent and benevolent depending on the circumstances: "Fatture indicates the creation of powerful magic, generally magia nera 'black magic,' although one who possesses the power of fatture also has the ability to create sciogliere 'absolution from evil.'"[34]

Sympathetic Magic

The manifestations of so-called curses and conditions discussed above can be treated in a number of ways. So far we have discussed the basic foundations of Italian folk medicine from ancient history to modern herbal medicine and other forms of folk healing. The vital force and the four elements are at the core of how illness or imbalance expresses itself in both the human body and the social field that includes other species and the ecology. We also discussed the concept of "sharing" that helps us to understand how various healing practices were designed to keep the flow and circulation of the vital force in balance between people and their environment. We now move on to another core aspect of this tradition and its variations along the spectrum of folk Catholicism and witchcraft: a technique called sympathetic magic.

The word *magic* comes from the Proto-Indo-European root *magh-*, which means "to be able" or "to have power." Magic is the practice of bringing our awareness to our relationship with more than our three-dimensional space-time as full participants in the forces of nature, the imaginal realm, and the vital force of healing not to manipulate them but to serve and interact with the sacred in ourselves and all of life. Magic allows us to embody the mythic and archetypal elements of the divine or multidimensional reality that guides our earthly human work to the benefit of creation.

Sympathetic basically means "alike" or refers to "mutual association" or "affinity." Sympathetic magic, then, is a magical technique that uses practices, objects, and rituals that resemble or are symbolically associated with whoever or whatever one wishes to influence. This idea goes back to our discussion of the holographic universe and an understanding of nature as being a continuous field of experience whereby the entire wisdom of the "whole" is contained in every molecule. Sympathetic magic uses this understanding to recognize and connect patterns and then merge their properties, usually via some ritual or formulation, to elicit a rebalancing or elemental exchange between entities that creates healing. Sympathetic magic also employs the practice of imitation, or mimesis, whereby "any effect may be produced by imitating it"[35] and *antithetical* practices, or practices that are "not like" or contrary to what is being influenced; for example, using a moistening herb to counteract dryness.

Much of what has been deemed "superstition" in Italian and other forms of folk medicine is based in sympathetic magic, and this technology can actually be seen in both Catholicism and witchcraft practices. As author Frederick Thomas Elworthy says in *The Evil Eye*, "Surely in the act of baptism we hope for the spiritual effect we imitate or typify by the actual use of water. So in the highest of our sacraments we spiritually eat and drink, by the actual consumption of the elements."[36]

The following are examples of sympathetic magic taken from Gabriel Peroni's *Le nostre nonne si curavano così* and Paola Giovetti's *I guaritori di campagna*.

Ad Arcisate (Va), si consigliava alle persone affette da pertosse (detta tosse asinina) di bere l'acqua da un recipiente in cui aveva bevuto un somaro.[37]

In Arcisate (Varese), people with whooping cough (known as donkey cough) were advised to drink water from a container in which a donkey had drunk.

Nel Salernitano l'anziana guaritrice Maria Servita per curare la milza ingrossata stacca da un albero di noce un pezzo di corteccia corrispondente alla forma della pianta del piede dell'ammalato, e la mette poi a seccare sul fuoco dopo aver recitato certe preghiere e dopo averla segnata, compie senza saperlo un tipico rituale di "magia simpatica," o "magia per analogia": ella ritiene infatti che via via che la corteccia si secca e raggrinzisce, anche la milza ingrossata si riduca di proporzioni, tornando a poco poco alla normalità.[38]

In the Salerno area the elderly healer Maria Servita to cure the enlarged spleen removes a piece of bark from a walnut tree corresponding to the shape of the sole of the patient's foot, and then puts it to dry on the fire after having recited certain prayers and after having signed it, she performs without knowing it a typical ritual of "sympathetic magic," or "magic by analogy": in fact, she believes that as the bark dries up and shrivels, so does the englarged spleen shrink in proportion, gradually returning to normal.

Oppure prendiamo le numerosissime cure contro i porri che ho trovato un po' dappertutto: un guaritore sardo, zio Palmerio, prende un giunco, gli fa tanti nodi quanti sono i porri da curare, lo segna, recita le sue formule e poi lo seppellisce oppure lo getta in un fossato: ed è convinto, e i suoi malati con lui, che via via che il giunco si consuma e marcisce, debbano sparire anche i porri. L'operazione infatti richiede una quarantina di giorni.

Lo stesso principio è alla base di interventi che ho trovato in Emilia: qui si prende del grasso di maiale maschio, lo si strofina sui porri e lo si seppellisce in una concimaia. E mentre il grasso si sfalda, spariscono anche i porri. Ancora una volta, magia per analogia.[39]

Or let's take the numerous cures against warts that I have found almost everywhere: a Sardinian healer, Uncle Palmerio, takes a rush, makes it as many knots as there are warts to be treated, marks it, recites his formulas and then buries it, or he throws it into a ditch: and he is convinced, and his patients with him, that as the rush wears out and rots, the warts must also disappear. The operation in fact requires about forty days. The same principle is the basis of interventions that I have found in Emilia: here male pork fat is taken, rubbed on worts and buried in a manure pit. And as the fat flakes off, the warts disappear too. Again, magic by analogy.

Di tipo magico sono anche altri riti tesi a trasmettere a un oggetto il male che affligge la persona: zia Angelina, in Sardegna, trasmette ai rami di fico, che poi brucia, la sciatica che tormenta i suoi "clienti." Per la cura dei vermi ho trovato in più parti la consuetudine di ricorrere a fili di cotone che alla fine del rito vengono anch'essi bruciati a indicare l'eliminazione degli sgraditi ospiti.[40]

Other rites aimed at transmitting to an object the evil that afflicts a person are also magical in nature: Aunt Angelina, in Sardinia, transmits to the branches of a fig tree, which she then burns, the sciatica that torments her "clients." For the cure of worms I have found in many places the custom of resorting to cotton threads which at the end of the rite are also burned to indicate the elimination of unwelcome guests.

Reclaiming the Magico-Religious Tradition

As we have seen, Italian folk medicine and indigenous healing are sourced in a magico-religious history that combines local healing practices with vernacular or folk magic and the regional spiritual practices of the people. Since the time that Christianity took over Europe, these healing practices have been transformed from their pagan character and qualities and intertwined with Italian Catholicism.

As many of the modern generations of Italian Americans have sought to reclaim and remember their cultural history and resist further assimilation, these traditions have been resurging in the context of an era where witchcraft, as a healing art, is also resurging, and although the term *strega* may have negative connotations in some contexts, it has been reasserted as a valuable and explicit word to describe the full spectrum of inherited and reclaimed practices of Italian folk magic as they have been adapted in the Italian diaspora.

Though we may not know much about how the world was for our ancestors we do know that they were tasked, like us, with being the living generation that would lead the way for the next. And we, the streghe in North America right now, are future ancestors and as such our task is to begin.

The word *return* is from the Latin *tornare*, which means "to turn." With the prefix *re*, it means "to turn back." And although we can't go back in time, we can turn back to what we know while standing in the here and now. When we seek to fully live and feel and connect to the place and the "who" that we returned to, we turn back to the raw elements of creation and culture. We turn back to what is before us, and we make that holy and sacred as our ancestors did and discover the sentient presence in every atomic, electric, heated cell on Earth.

Because of this, I believe that the reclamation and reappropriation of the word strega in the context of Italian-American folk magic is both authentic and accurate even though it may have negative connotations in Southern Italy. It is also a word that is continually being defined, as are all words, and it is our willingness to dialogue about who we are, where we are, and what our context of relationship is that is the guiding principle.

The Old Gods still speak, but they must do so with young voices. Every age needs the Devil reborn, not complacency or nostalgia, but paradoxically the experience of this truth can transport vertiginously back to a confrontation with the origins of who we once were and who we can truly become.

PETER GREY
IN *APOCALYPTIC WITCHCRAFT*

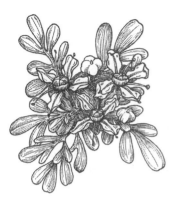

8
Segnatura

The History and Practices of the Language of the Soul

Il linguaggio dell'anima

The language of the soul

ALICE IMBALZANO

SEGNATURA (PLURAL: SEGNATURE) is "the language of the soul" as described by Alice Imbalzano in her master's thesis "Segnare la malattia."[1] *Segnatura*, or *segnare*, doesn't directly translate to English. *Segnare* literally means "score," "mark," or "sign," and *segnatura* translates as "signature," but in this healing practice it refers to a specific set of practices that involve formulas and techniques applied to relieve and resolve certain ailments, both physical and spiritual.

The segni (signs) are specific hand gestures and movements that resonate and conduct "healing" energy. These segni are combined with other techniques to make formulas that are then applied by the practitioner to those who need it. Segnatura is a technology, a system, and process used by the village healers of Southern Italy and the Italian diaspora, and in fact, it is at the core of these traditions.

The word segnatura has become popular in recent years as a way to describe this phenomenon and can be found in various iterations all over Italy, as well as in the enclaves of the Italian diaspora. The Italian immigrants brought this practice with them and have continued to pass it down through the generations in America.

The origin of the word used in this context and the techniques that it refers to often have no name; they are not "called" anything, and they are not standardized or systematized in any way. The practices involved vary from region to region and are performed by certain individuals who have been transmitted the healing gift via oral transmission. In the United States and other diasporic places, there has been a convergence of regional practices even within families because although Italians often married other Italians, the regional lines were blurred.

These practices were not written down or codified in any way until recently. The use of the word *segnatura* to describe these practices can be found in historical use in several regions especially Emilia-Romagna and Garfagnana (Lucca). I have found its use in writings from many regions all over Italy, although just as often those that performed these rites had no name for it or used other names or phrases in their specific dialect.*

In her thesis on the topic, Alice Imbalzano says, "One aspect that struck me during the research is the fact that the segnitori do not identify themselves with a precise word: there is talk of "having the sign" ("avere il segno"), or "knowing how to score" ("saper segnare")."[2]

More recently the word *segnatura* has been popularized by Italian religious studies professor Dr. Angela Puca, who conducted research and writing on her findings in the various regions of Italy and the similarities found in the diversity of practices. The use of the word has also become popular among younger generations of practitioners.

Originally, folk healing practices were much less mobile and communication was slower. With the increase in technology and social media, as well as the increased incidence of people relocating and moving about the world more quickly than our ancestors, the spread of knowledge has taken on different forms. Groups of practitioners have even formed on social media and other communication platforms where people have come to use segnatura as a generally agreed upon term to define their knowledge base.

---

*Note here that the nation-state of Italy includes multiple regions that have and to some extent still have their own language. Standard Italian is the language/dialect of Florence. When doing research about Italy, descriptive words can vary greatly.

I do not know of a word in modern American English that can convey the full meaning of segnatura as it is a pluralistic practice of relational knowledge. Folk medicine is difficult to package or brand under one umbrella as it is intrinsically mutable as well as rhizomatic. It can't be "mass distributed" in any way that keeps its integrity because it is a living force of moving, dynamic presence in the full spectrum of creation at any given moment.

Transmission

Segnatura is relational, meaning that it can't be taught or learned from books. The tools, techniques, and instructions can be taught, but those are only part of the magic. The Segnatrice, or a practitioner of Segnatura, has embodied knowledge that they received from living and being in communication with their place, community, ancestors, and the divine. The specific physical and material technologies are transmitted based on social contracts and long-term, multigenerational relationships. Segnatura becomes the form these combined healing treatments and formulas take when the Segnatrice conducts these emergent properties.

Il potere, or the power, to practice Segnatura can only be transmitted on Christmas Eve, Epiphany, Saint John's eve (June 24), and, in some lineages, Pasqua (Easter). The knowledge and healing power, as well as the specific formulas, are traditionally passed from one generation to the other within families; usually from grandmother to granddaughter. Once passed, the receiver of the knowledge has to keep it secret and can't pass it on until the right time and only to the right person, or it is said that they will lose their abilities. The secret words, prayers, and gestures are handed down orally and if perchance they are written on paper, they must be burned.[3]

Basic Tenets of Segnatura

The basic tenets of Segnatura are prayers, hand gestures, and the use of certain objects, plants, and other substances such as oil and salt to resolve some physical or psychic ailment. These techniques of Segnatura must be applied and practiced in relationship and reciprocity with life and presence.

Scongiuri (Conjuring)

The prayers or words used in Segnatura are sometimes called *scongiuri* (conjuring) and involve a "magic formula" of words in the form of a prayer or rhythmic poetic phrases that are repeated several times out loud but under the breath so that only the practitioner knows what they are as they are considered *la segreta* or secret. Scongiuri does two things:

1. Invokes a deity or divine power
2. Requests the help needed for the person with the ailment

The reason for *la segretezza* or the secrecy of the words whereby the practitioner speaks them so that they can't be understood is an ancient practice of word magic. Words are another form of pattern recognition and expression as the vocal symbolic forms that emerge from natural patterns, particularly when these words are spoken in vibrational languages. Even in modern English, however, spoken words are expressed by vibrational resonance and pulsation that channel sound frequencies. These same frequencies that originated in an ancient language have evolved (or devolved) from those primordial sounds.[4]

La storia della magia della parola è assai lunga. Per conoscere le sue origini potremmo partire dall'area mediorientale, dove scorgiamo i primi esempi di scongiuri e di esorcismi. Se però la parola è il fulcro della magia, il vero potere è serbato nel nome, come descritto dal mito egizio del dio Ra, che dopo aver creato il mondo gli diede vita attraverso il suo nome, che era tenuto da lui segreto. Anche nelle religioni monoteiste troviamo la stessa convinzione. Si narra infatti che Dio si rivelò a Mosè con il nome di "Yhwh," ovvero "io sono colui che sono," e gli affidò il compito di liberare gli israeliti dalla schiavitù egiziana. Ebbene, come pare evidente, la divinità insegna il suo appellativo ma non il suo vero nome. Anche le quattro lettere del tetragramma ebraico . . . che costituiscono il nome di Dio, la cui traslitterazione più comune è YHWH, sono, nella tradizione, impronunciabili, in quanto si scatenerebbero tutti i poteri in loro racchiusi.[5]

The history of word *magic* is very long. To know its origins we could start from the Middle Eastern area, where we see the first examples of conjuring and exorcisms. However, if the word is the fulcrum of magic, the true power is kept in the name, as described by the Egyptian myth of the god Ra, who after creating the world gave life through his name, which was kept secret by him. Even in monotheistic religions we find the same conviction. In fact, it is said that God revealed himself to Moses with the name of "Yhwh," or "I am who I am," and entrusted him with the task of freeing the Israelites from Egyptian slavery. Well, as seems evident, the divinity teaches his appellative but not his real name. Even the four letters of the Hebrew tetragrammaton . . . which make up the name of God, whose most common transliteration is YHWH, are, in tradition, unpronounceable, as all the powers contained within them would be unleashed.

Gesti Rituali (Ritual Gestures)

Gesti rituali, or ritual gestures, are another major element of Segnatura. These segni, or signs, are movements of the hands in certain formations such as the sign of the cross. They can include what might be called mudras, such as *il mano cornuto*, or the horned hand. This element is the signing or marking part of the practice for which the word segnatura is derived. The gestures are often made on the area of the body where the healing needs to occur or can be made over the healing medium or menstruum. The healer often will make a gesture, again usually it's the sign of the cross, at the beginning and end of the ritual and will "bless" themselves as well.

Some practitioners have their own unique signs. These personal gestures can be for specific ailments or general blessing or healing. One practitioner who treated me gave me her sign at the end of the session for continued general health and protection after I left.

Gestures of both body and hand are our most primitive forms of nonverbal communication, and in Italian culture they have remained strongly linked to language and self-expression. Many of the apotropaic (able to ward off evil) gestures known in Italian folk medicine originated with the ancient Etruscans and were used as tools of exorcism.

Objects and Substances

Sacred objects and substances make up the third element of Segnatura but are not always present in the process. I've received both treatments and transmissions that use only words and gestures. This is partly a regional and familial feature whereby some lineages use objects and some don't. It is also dependent on what is called for and what is available in any given situation. For instance, if we require an action when we're not home or are in public, we may use more subtle formulas that only require a quick gesture or a word or two under the breath.

In other instances, we might use common substances such as oil, water, and salt. Sometimes herbs may be added or included in the rite in some way. Other possible objects include scissors, gold rings, saint medals, keys, nails, candles, and knives. These objects will generally be included as part of the gesture and are symbolic as well as physical containers or vessels for the patterns of consciousness we want to conduct and therefore introduce specific resonances into the field of experience.

One example is with the popular *riti di malocchio* (rites of the evil eye). This is probably the most well-known of all the rites. As described in chapter 7, it is sometimes done with just gesture and prayer but often includes the use of oil, water, and salt whereby olive oil is dropped in water to divine if someone has the evil eye, and salt is used to dispel it. In more serious cases scissors may be used to break up the "eye." I have heard of one practitioner that uses a knife combined with a gesture to remove the malocchio.

Types of Ailments Treated

Other ailments commonly treated by Segnatura are sciatica, lower back pain, Saint Anthony's fire (usually refered to as shingles), warts, parasites, and more. The practitioner is only able to treat the maladies that they have been transmitted the "signs" for. Because these are traditionally shared through lineage, individual practitioners will be known for treating different conditions. For instance, if you have Saint Anthony's fire you have to find the healer that knows how to treat that. Or you just go to the healer that knows the malocchio signs and hope that getting rid of the evil eye will cure your Saint Anthony's fire. This is changing now, however, in that "signs" are being shared between practitioners offering each one a broader scope of practice.

Syncretism with Christianity and Catholocism

One of the central aspects of Segnatura is its syncretism with Christianity and Catholicism. All of the *Segnatori* I have ever known use Christian prayers and invoke Christian deities in their practice. They also consider themselves Catholic, not witches or even pagans. However, these practices have been picked up by modern witchcraft and pagan practitioners, and they have been deemed Stregoneria, or witchcraft, by some. Others have attempted to separate the two, but the differences don't seem obvious. Ultimately, this is a practice of folk Catholicism or what might be called Catholic witchcraft or *magia Cristiana*[6] (Christian magic). It is also sometimes referred to as a practice of Benedicaria.

This has presented some confusion about the context and origins of these practices, and it can be triggering because the Catholic church has been responsible for so much harm. Yet the reality is that our traditional folk healers from Southern Italy consider themselves Catholic and use Catholic signs and prayers. One way to look at this that might bring some clarity is from the perspective of how these formulas syncretized from their pagan and animistic roots.

It's also important to recognize that, as my friend Marybeth Bonfiglio says, "Being anti-church doesn't mean we're anti-Catholic". The words and gestures of Segnatura are in essence ancient magic formulas, and the saints and Catholic divinities invoked can all be linked to ancient deities and animistic beings. As Andrea Romanazzi maintains in his book *Stregoneria popolare italiana*,

> *Lo scongiuro popolare non è, dunque, molto differente dalle formule magiche dell'antichità. Per il popolo, infatti, i santi sono divinità, risultato di una vera e propria coinonia tra un politeismo antico e le nuove religioni monoteiste, forse troppo lontane dai bisogni e dalle necessità dell'uomo. Non è dunque solo la fede a promettere guarigione al credente, ma anche l'inconscio background magico che si cela tra storie, leggende e tradizioni.[7]*

Folk conjuration is not, therefore, very different from the magic formulas of antiquity. For the people, in fact, the saints are divinities, the result of a real coexistence/communion between an ancient polytheism and the new monotheistic religions, perhaps too far from the needs and necessities of man. Therefore, it is not only faith that promises healing to the believer, but also the unconscious magical background that is hidden among stories, legends and traditions.

> *Tutto ciò non ha nulla a che vedere con le preghiere cristiane con le quali, a causa della similitudine di figure, il magismo può essere confuso. Se infatti la preghiera è un muovere a pietà il divino, chiunque esso sia, lo scongiuro ha in sé il potere della forza magico-evocativa. E' la bassa orazione che contiene quella scintilla divina alla quale la divinità non può sottrarsi. È quindi espressione di quel mondo numinoso che non ha mai abbandonato i suoi figli. È per esempio lo stesso Leland a smentire l'idea secondo cui, quando una magara si rivolge a un santo dei Cristiani, o quando proferisce il Pater Nostro, si sta rivolgendo direttamente a loro: "Dire il Paternoster così è della stregheria, e non della vera religione cattolica."[8]*

All this has nothing to do with Christian prayers with which, due to the similarity of figures, magic can be confused. In fact, if prayer is a move to petition the divine, whoever it is, the conjuration has within itself the power of the magical-evocative force. It is a short prayer that contains this divine spark from which the divinity cannot escape. It is therefore an expression of that numinous world which has never abandoned its children. For example, it is Leland himself who disproves the idea that, when a magara addresses a saint of Christians, or when she utters the Our Father, she is addressing them directly: "To say the Paternoster (Our Father) in this way is of witchcraft, and not of the true Catholic religion."

Segnatura and all of the elements of Italian folk medicine that are merged with Catholicism contain, at their origins, the roots of a life and a world much more primordial. That said, I totally understand the resistance some have around using Christian language and do believe that adaptations can be made as long as the cultural context is kept conscious. However, in my own practice I continue to use the Catholic language and symbolism that I was taught.

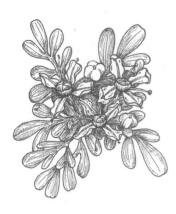

9

Grazia and the Holy Wonderworkers

The Magic of Grace of the Saints

GRAZIA *MEANS "GRACE,"* and the idea of obtaining grazia was directly linked to Italian-American folk Catholicism and what has been called the "cults of the saints." This idea of receiving grazia is not considered "magic" in the sense that an individual is no longer subject to the consequences of their actions and habits. Grazia is given to make us aware of how we ended up needing it in the first place and to support our capacity to change what is changeable about our circumstances and to notice if there are ways in which we are contributing to our own negative conditions. Certainly, grazia can be miraculous at any given moment, but it will not stop us from repeating negative habit patterns in the future unless we choose to stop doing so ourselves.

As mentioned in the previous chapter, Italian Americans did not align well with American-style Catholicism because it sterilized their *paese*, or village, form of devotional practice. Devotion to the saints was a major component of adaptation for the immigrants as the saints and their corresponding *feste* (feasts) linked them to their homeland villages and neighborhoods as each town and village in Italy has its own specific patron saint. "On a day-to-day basis, Italian Americans continued to cultivate affective relationships with supernatural figures 'who seem[ed] so human to them,' entities such as the Virgin Mary, the patron saint of the paese, and other saints as needed."[1]

Along with the saints, Italian Americans were also devoted to various angels and even a system of "demonology" that included regular ritual and practices to counter the influence of malevolent spirits. These devotional systems were often admonished by the American Catholic Church and even considered part of the "Italian problem" because "many of these ostensible Catholics did not attend or support the Church, preferring to devote themselves to what one observer called "a hideous web of superstition."[2]

These "superstitions" were also a source of social discrimination for Italian Americans, causing many immigrants to keep their devotional practices hidden. This also served to slow down the assimilation process as it kept Italians separated from other ethnic groups and kept them holding close to their own social networks. Benedicaria, as discussed in chapter 7, is included in this style of Catholicism as are some of the same facets of spiritual practice that are called "witchcraft." We can see here why it is difficult to make a clear division between the two, particularly when taken out of the context of Southern Italy. In Southern Italy these practices were not witchcraft but a longstanding devotional system of Catholicism. In the United States they were either diminished to "superstition" or considered to be witchcraft or magic of some sort.

Thaumaturgic Saints

One of the principles of a saint's cult and devotional practices is the thaumaturgic, or magical, capacity of a saint to perform specific types of miracles. Also important to this concept is the idea of what a "cult" is. The use of the word *cult* in the context of folk medicine and magic is not the same as our current application of the word to mean a "nefarious mind control predatory group, guru, or organization that brainwashes and steals people's autonomy." The definition of *cult* in folk medicine is "a system of worship," and it derives from the Latin word *cultus*, which means to care, tend, or cultivate. The original use of the word *cult* was to identify certain forms of devotion and spiritual practice.

According to Robin Clark, a linguistics professor in the School of Arts and Sciences at the University of Pennsylvania,

> The word "cult" originally designates a practice of religious veneration and the religious system based around such veneration—for example, the cult of Our Lady of Guadalupe. . . . However, the word was co-opted in the first half of the 20th century by sociology, and has come to denote a social group with "socially deviant" beliefs and practices, like a UFO cult.[3]

The ancient mystery cults and the cult of saints are systems of veneration that emerged in the context of collectivist style social life. They are place based and decentralized so, although they often center around a specific deity or ideology, they are not part of the dominant paradigm. Our cults today, although seemingly unorthodox, are exploitative and therefore very much in alignment with the dominant culture:

> In recent years the term cult has become a widely used popular term, connoting some group that is at least unfamiliar and perhaps even disliked or feared . . . . This popular use of the term has such credence and momentum that it has virtually swallowed up the more neutral historical meaning of the term from the sociology of religion.[4]

Keeping the original understanding of a "cult" in mind, the cult of saints can be understood as a devotional practice that is central to Catholic culture and Italian folk medicine. The saints are venerated and thought to be thaumaturgic, which means they are believed to be "miracle workers" or "wonderworkers." The thaumaturgic saints are humans who died and became divine beings who are still able to intercede in the lives of humans. Specific saints are thought to perform certain functions and to heal, resolve, and aid in various categories of needs and illnesses. For instance, one prays to San Giuseppe (Saint Joseph) for help in finding a home, to Santa Lucia for healing eye ailments, and to San Giovanni Battista (Saint John the Baptist) for protection.

Ne consegue che non tutte le parole sono gradite alla divinità, e che non tutte le divinità sono adatte alla risoluzione dei problemi. Si genera così l'idea dell'esistenza di una caratteristica intrinseca alle divinità, che si rispecchierà nella tradizione popolare quando, agli antichi dèi pagani, si sostituiranno i santi cristiani. Le varie "specializzazioni" di quelli che potremmo chiamare "Santi-Taumaturghi," non sono però casuali, e scaturiscono da loro episodi di vita. Ritroviamo la stessa dinamica pagano, dove le opere di un dio sono la base del potere al quale si appellano i fedeli sul principio del "come-così." Il legame tra santi e stregoneria è un elemento peculiare italiano. Per il popolo i Santi Taumaturghi diventano vere e proprie divinità di un politeismo eretico di cui è intrisa la tradizione popolare. Il Santo taumaturgo esula, dunque, da ogni canone di fede o dogma religioso.[5]

It follows that not all words are pleasing to the deity, and that not all deities are suitable for solving problems. Thus the idea of the existence of a characteristic is generated intrinsic to the deities, which is reflected in folk traditions when the ancient pagan gods were replaced by Christian saints. The various "specializations" of those we could call "Thaumaturgic Saints," however, are not casual, and derive from their life stories. We find the same pagan dynamic, where the works of a god are the basis of the power to which the faithful appeal on the principle of "come-cosi" ("as so" or the result leads us to the cause).

The link between saints and witchcraft is a peculiar Italian element. For the people, the Holy Wonderworkers become real divinities of a heretical polytheism of which popular tradition is imbued. The holy thaumaturge therefore goes beyond any canon of faith or religious dogma.[6]

Grazia

The saints act on the human realm via grazia, which they can convey to humans through a variety of practices. These practices are relational, which means that the practitioner must form a reciprocal relationship with the saint or deity. This relationship is somewhat of a sacred contract that includes devotion, discipline, and commitment to reverence and veneration. The simplest method of eliciting grazia from a saint is via prayer. Prayer is both an act of devotion and a request.

Other methods of obtaining grazia are through devotional practices. These are rituals and technologies that are meant to bring an individual into contact with the divine. Because the saints were once considered to be human, or at least semihuman, they are understood to inhabit the human realm even after death. The saints in Italian folk Catholicism are perceived as a direct all-powerful link to God and are even considered superior to the Holy Trinity, which is partly why Italian immigrants had a challenging time adapting to the American Catholic Church that places "God the Father " above all. In both Italy and the Italian enclaves around the world, the saints did not rank any lower in the divine hierarchy than did God, and, in fact, the patron village or neighborhood saint or Madonna was often considered superior to all and any other divine figures. In *Bodies of Vital Matter*, Per Binde describes how the saints are viewed in Sicily:

> Christ is counted higher than the Eternal Father and the Holy Spirit, who is lesser than all. Mary is regarded as superior to her Son and, between one Mary and another, adored in different churches and villages, and under different titles, there are differences, and one is counted as superior to the other, all according to the faithful who are under the direct patronage of one or the other of them. Saint Joseph, the universal father, is regarded as higher than the Eternal Father, Christ and the Madonna together; but then, immensely superior to each and all of the saints of Paradise is for a village the saint who is its patron. . . . [A]ll legends, all traditions, all past and present facts and acts show clearly as daylight that the Patron Saint has no superiors, that he can do everything and that he has absolute rule over everything and everyone. The superior position of the village patron in relation to other divine beings derive from his position as protector of the community. The patron saint belongs to the community; he is one of its members. The relics or image of the patron are kept in the community's principal church, and can be easily visited and addressed directly.[7]

Sanctuaries

The saints and their relics, including statues, are often held in the local church or sanctuary. A sanctuary can be anything from a simple roadside shrine to a chapel or even a cathedral that is dedicated to the veneration of a specific saint or deity. A sanctuary can also be a cave or a holy well or sometimes the top of a mountain. Wherever it is located, a sanctuary is sacred ground, and any object in or around it, including the ground itself, is imbued with grazia. Touching any part of the sanctuary can be a method of obtaining grazia and even just being in such a place is thought to invoke the healing powers of the saint or deity.

A pilgrimage to a sanctuary or sacred place is a major component of folk Catholicism and is done not only to request healing but as a rite of passage and a form of devotion. We see this practice across religious traditions and even in secular culture; for instance, the at least once-in-a-lifetime or even yearly pilgrimage Americans make to Disney World.

It seems that humans have an innate desire to go to a geographical location where they can meet with something beyond their daily encounters. The journey itself becomes part of the process and is a method of somatically shifting consciousness. As we travel—whether by foot or mechanical means—with the intent to meet with the divine, our scenery changes, and our body, mind, and psyche shift states, making us more aware and receptive to divine contact and intercession.

Once at the pilgrimage site there are a few basic practices that are performed. Often shoes are removed not only as a way to show respect for "hallowed" ground but also because of the belief that chthonic power from the Earth could be absorbed through the bottoms of the feet or anywhere that the body was touching the ground. Other practices of pilgrimage include bringing offerings to the pilgrimage location, bringing or saying prayers at the location, being immersed in the landscape and culture of the place, and participating in ceremonies such as in a pilgrimage to a church or a cathedral. Immersion type pilgrimages involve participation in cultural events, festivals, and perhaps learning from locals either by formally taking a class or just by engaging in local activities and meeting people.

Relics and Statues

Relics are associated with a specific sanctuary in the form of local mythology. Many sanctuaries are built around the exact location where a relic was supposed to have been found and/or where an apparition of the deity was experienced. There are many examples of the Virgin Mary appearing to people in specific locations, and often a sanctuary will be built to venerate her there. Sometimes a sanctuary is built where a relic was unburied from the ground, found in a cave or near a large tree, or floating on the water of a stream, river, or inlet. There is usually some legend that surrounds how the relic was found that involves supernatural experiences and the sense that the person who found it was being "guided."

Reciprocity and Votive Offerings

Because the relationship between the saints and humans is just that, a relationship, reciprocity is of utmost importance. This type of reciprocity is based on being in a conversation or a call-and-response type of relationship with nature and the divine. This is itself a cyclical practice whereby we open and listen during one phase, and then we focus and respond in the other. In between is a phase of alchemy or digesting when we metabolize and synergize the exchange of energy between ourselves and the universe. Our relationship with this medicine is emergent, which means that our experience with saints, grazia, and folk medicine is indeterminate and always unfolding depending on the context and conditions of the here and now.

Votive literally means "vow" or "offering," and it is often associated with sacrifice. A votive is basically a method of honoring an agreement between the petitioner and the saint from whom they are asking a blessing or miracle. Offerings can also be made as simply a form of love or devotion and as a way of giving thanks. When we make offerings of thanks we call them *ex-votos*. *Ex-voto* comes from Latin *ex voto suscepto*, which means "from the vow made" or "fulfillment of a vow."

An ex-voto can be any gift made in thanks for healing or the fulfillment of a prayer. An ex-voto is often a replica of the body part that was healed and is left at the altar or statue of a saint or deity.

Plants and Grazia

Plants are almost always a part of any devotion or healing ritual that invokes a saint or deity. And most saints and deities have specific plants or plant preparations associated with them. Plants are often used in formulas along with prayers and gestures and as herbal preparations. The plant used depends on the condition of the person and what they are requesting and/or which saint or deity they are requesting help from. A plant that is associated with a saint is considered to be an extension of that saint and their unique healing propensity. As we look at some of the most revered saints, we will see which plants they are each associated with. Plants are also central to specific rituals and celebrations as we discussed in chapter 4.

One poignant example is the use of palm leaves during Pasqua (Easter) and how they are made into palm crosses, representing Jesus. These crosses are made from palms given by the church on Palm Sunday and are considered blessed. The crosses are hung as talismans and for protection for the entire year and then burned just before the subsequent Palm Sunday when they are remade again.

Sometimes the saints are directly associated with a plant, such as La Madonna della Melagrana, or Our Lady of the Pomegranate, most notably depicted by fifth-century Italian artist Sandro Botticelli. The pomegranate is associated with Our Lady as a symbol of fertility but also is said to correlate with the chambers of the heart as the pomegranate, when ripe and sliced open, looks like the anatomical heart.

Dream Incubation

Dream incubation, first discussed in chapter 2, is another practice of the cult of saints. Dream incubation began long before Christianity with the cult of Asclepius and the dream temples erected at healing sanctuaries across the Mediterranean. Once Christianity took hold, the practice shifted to a component of pilgrimages whereby devotees would travel to a sanctuary and spend the night there, usually on the bare ground or on the floor of the shrine. The purpose of Christian dream incubation was basically the same as the pre-Christian type: to be healed or given grazia during a dream. During ancient times, it was in hopes that the god Asclepius would appear during sleep and heal the petitioner. During Christian times it was in hopes that the patron saint would come.

> The practice of incubation fuses several significances. First, to sleep outdoors or on the hard floor of a sanctuary is an act of penitence, equivalent to fasting, flagellation and other forms of self-mortification. Second, as in numerous other practices, described above, that aimed at obtaining grazia through physical contact with stones and earth, there is a notion that the direct contact between body and earth during sleep had as an effect an absorption into the body of vitalizing forces from earth. Third, the emphasis on sleeping and dreaming—states in which revelations were received and healing took place—can be construed as another expression of the momentary creation of a different kind of existence during pilgrimages and at the feasts of saints.[8]

Holy Manna

Manna means "windfall" and is considered to be a gift from heaven or a form of grazia. Manna is mentioned in the Bible as a superfood elixir given to the Israelites by God when they were starving in the desert. Manna is also mentioned in the Quran and is considered something that actually exudes from the Catholic saints. In terms of the cult of saints, manna is usually considered to be some type of liquid—particularly a bodily fluid such as blood or tears—that emanates from the saint's image, burial site, or site of death or any object or place associated with them. In ancient Greek and Roman times manna was referred to as "perspiration from the sky" and "saliva of the stars."[9]

Manna also refers to the sweet syrup that drips from the ash tree in Sicily and dries into solid sweet chunks that people eat as it begins as a liquid, solidifies, and then provides moist nourishment. Manna is generally associated with the vital force as it is liquid and humoral, or associated with humors of the body, which are the biological expression of the vital force. Manna is thought to be exuded by the saints from their statues or even sanctuary walls and is the material form taken by grazia that could be consumed by eating or drinking blessed food. The holy manna of a saint is an expression of their physicality, for although they are perhaps ascended or enlightened, they are still carnal beings and that carnality is a source of grazia. Manna is believed to bring about miraculous healing when eaten or applied to the body. Touching a statue or relic of a saint and/or wiping it with a cloth is considered a way to collect manna directly from the saint.

There are many patron saints known to offer holy manna, one of which is San Biagio, an Armenian saint, whose sanctuary is in the village of Maratea, Basilicata. San Biagio's relics are held there, and his statue is said to exude liquid manna. The manna is collected by his devotees and used to cure illness. San Biagio's feast day is February 3, and he is also celebrated during the second week of May.

Feste

Feste, or feasts, are held around the saint both within the sanctuary and in the homes or communities of devotees. A *festa* is traditionally held in the village where the patron saint and their relics abide, but the Italian immigrants carried their patron feasts with them to the New World. The immigrants have often recreated sanctuaries and devoted churches to their collective patron saints and madonnas. A festa includes a procession where the saint statue is decorated and carried through the street, a mass, music and dancing, and eating celebratory foods.

From New York City during the 1930s, an account of the many festas reads,

[H]ardly a day passes without some sort of festa in one or more of the half hundred churches of the city's several little Italys. Most are purely logical, given in honor of some patron saint of some city in Sicily, Calabria, or Campania (Naples) from which most of the worshippers originally came. These local celebrations are on a small scale and far from elaborate. In fact, one may see similar celebrations in almost any small city in the United States that has an Italian colony.[10]

In the city of Utica, New York, where I grew up, the Italian-American community hosts an annual festa for Saints Cosmas and Damian. Also called *i santi medici* ("healing saints"), Cosmas and Damian were Arab physicians and twin brothers born in a place called Aegeae between Turkey and Syria. They have been venerated all over the world starting in the Mediterranean and SWANA region in the fourth century CE. A major shrine to them was built in Bari, Italy, and it was some immigrants from Bari that started the festa in Utica. They are called on for healing of any kind but specifically for physical illness. Multiple miracles are attributed to them in legends.

Universal Saints and Madonnas

As mentioned, every city and village has their own specific patron saint or Madonna, but some saints, such as those listed below, are more universally celebrated for their healing and protective qualities, as Angela Puca describes in "The Tradition of Segnature":

The saint is believed to possess powers that affect the natural order; a saint can calm a storm at sea and help stricken ships. He or she can induce or dissipate rain if needed and foretell the future. But what all saints are best known for and are most worshiped for is their ability to heal illnesses, to the point where their importance is proportional to the efficacy shown on such matters (Sallmann 1979, 593). Since saints operate within a Catholic theoretical framework and still perform "magic" in the form of miracles, they represent the best role models for vernacular healers, who believe that by using Catholic symbols (the cross) and prayers while performing their rituals, they are doing nothing that would be considered in opposition to their identity as Catholics.[11]

Santa Agata (Saint Agatha)

Birth date or origin: Catania, Sicily, 251 CE
Feast day: February 5
Plant correspondences: Olive and primrose

Santa Agata is known for healing conditions of the breasts and issues around breastfeeding. She is known also to protect against volcanic eruptions as per her legend where she caused Mt. Etna to erupt and/or caused an earthquake as a result of being tortured.[12]

Santa Rosalia, a.k.a. La Santuzza (the Little Saint)

Birth date or origin: 1130 CE, Palermo, Sicily
Feast day: July 14 along with a pilgrimage on September 4 where devotees walk barefoot up Mount Pellegrino in Sicily to where her sanctuary is located
Plant correspondences: Rose and lily

Santa Rosalia is known to perform miracles of any kind, and she can be asked for anything.

Santa Lucia (Lucia of Syracuse)

Birth date or origin: 283 CE, Sicily
Feast day: December 13
Plant correspondence: Golden trumpet tree, a.k.a. Saint Lucy's Eyes

Santa Lucia is said to have gouged out her own eyes to avoid marriage and/or her eyes were gouged out by Roman authorities for refusing to marry, but her sight was restored by God or a miracle. Thus, she is known to imbue her devotees with clairvoyance and heal conditions of the eyes. She is also known as the matron saint of witches and folk magic. In a similar vein, her amulet is a pair of eyes that can ward off evil. Santa Lucia is also associated with the pagan goddesses, Juno Lucina, Freya, and Hulda.[13]

San Antonio (Saint Anthony of Padua)
Birth date or origin: 1195, Lisbon, Portugal
Feast day: June 13
Plant correspondence: Lily

San Antonio is considered a wonderworker, or miracle worker, and the patron saint of lost things. Pray to him when you have lost something. He is also associated with the pagan god, Mercury.

Padre Pio (Father Pio)
Birth date or origin: 1887, Pietrelcina (Campania)
Feast day: September 23
Plant correspondence: Violet

Padre Pio another wonderworker who can heal any and all ailments. He is said to have received the stigmata, or the wounds of Christ, on his own body. This is a sign that he has been embraced by and united with Jesus.

San Giuseppe (Saint Joseph)
Birth date or origin: 30 BCE, Bethlehem
Feast day: March 19
Plant correspondence: Saint Joseph's Lily

San Giuseppe is the patron saint of workers, peasants, and common people. Pray to him for finding or selling a home and if your request is granted, be sure to donate to the poor. Also Saint Joseph's oil, a holy oil made at the shrine of St. Joseph or with St. Joseph's Lily, can be used for healing.

*La Madonna di Montevergine, a.k.a. Mamma Schiavona (Madonna of Montevergine)**
Birth date or origin: She is an iteration of the Virgin Mary, and her sanctuary was built in Avellino, Italy during the twelfth century.
Feast day: May 22, yearly pilgrimage to her sanctuary on February 2

---

*This is a Black Madonna

Plant correspondences: All roses and all plants associated with La
Madonna/the Virgin Mary

Mamma Schiavona is the patron saint and protector of the LGBTQ community and the *femminielli*, or queer, third-gender people of the region.
The Wikipeida definition of femminielli is "a term used to refer to a
population of homosexual males with markedly feminine gender expression in traditional Neapolitan culture." Mamma Schiavona is also the
"slave mamma" who protects the poor and marginalized. La Madonna of
Montevergine is the Christian version of the pagan goddess Cybele, and
her sanctuary is built on what once was Cybele's temple.

Our Lady of Mount Carmel

Birth date or origin: She is the patroness of the Carmelite order who
was called the Lady of the Place by the hermits who lived and prayed
on Mount Carmel in Northwest Palestine.

Feast day: July 16

Plant correspondence: Roses and lilies; Our Lady is considered the Flos
Carmeli, or the Flower of Carmel (see the prayer on page 210)

Mount Carmel was the first church dedicated to the Virgin Mary, and
there is a basilica to her at the port of Naples where most of the Italian
immigrants to the United States left from. Our Lady was a prominent
figure in Southern Italian Catholicism and devotion to her was carried
over by the immigrants; therefore many churches established in Italian
enclaves are dedicated to her. In fact she became a beacon for Italian
Americans as they didn't fit in well with American-style Catholicism:

> The Irish Catholic hierarchy did not know how to respond to Italian
> expressions of faith, practices that seemed almost pagan. This, com-
> bined with the society's general anti-Italian bigotry, manifested itself
> in the church's open hostility to Italian immigrants. It is little wonder
> then that the Italian community did not feel welcome in Manhattan's
> great Saint Patrick's Cathedral. They want a church of their own, a
> church that would reflect their culture. So, they set to the task of

building it. Each evening, after a day of hard physical labor, the Italian community of East Harlem came together to build their church with their own hands. Despite this effort, when the building was complete, the Catholic Church could not see past their bias, relegating the Italians to worship in the basement. When it came time to name the church, however, the Italian community stood strong, insisting that it be called Our Lady of Mount Carmel.[14]

Our Lady of Mount Carmel is known as a miracle worker, particularly for her miracle in Palmi, Calabria, which was recognized by the church. For seventeen days before a major earthquake whose epicenter was in the middle of the city of Palmi, it is said that the statue of Our Lady moved its eyes and that its skin turned color. This prompted the congregation to hold a procession whereby they carried the statue to the outside of the city center. Once they were at the border of the city, the earthquake shook and destroyed most of the homes there. Because most of the population was not in the city due to the procession, only a few people were harmed.

The following is a prayer to Our Lady the Flos Carmeli:

Flos Carmeli Prayer (Flower of Carmel Prayer)
O beautiful Flower of Carmel, most fruitful vine,
Splendor of Heaven, holy and singular,
who brought forth the Son of God,
still ever remaining a Pure Virgin,
assist me in this necessity.
O Star of the sea, help and protect me!
Show me that Thou art my Mother.
O Mary, conceived without sin,
pray for us who have recourse to Thee!
Mother and Beauty of Carmel, Pray for us!
Virgin, Flower of Carmel, Pray for us!
Patroness of all who wear the Scapular, Pray for us!
Hope of all who die wearing the Scapular, Pray for us!
St. Joseph, Friend of the Sacred Heart, Pray for us!

St. Joseph, Chaste Spouse of Mary, Pray for us!

St. Joseph, Our Patron, Pray for us!

O sweet Heart of Mary, Be our salvation!

Amen.[15]

San Gennaro (Saint Januarius)

Birth date or origin: Third century in Benevento

Feast day: September 19

Plant correspondences: Olive and walnut trees

San Gennaro/Saint Januarius is the patron saint of Little Italy in New York City and Naples. He is associated with the miracle of blood liquefaction and three times each year his devotees gather in Naples to witness his blood, preserved in glass vials, liquefy at the masses held in his honor. The blood liquefies in response to the prayers and faith of his followers. He is petitioned for the healing of any blood disease as well as for protection from the evil eye.[16]

The name Januarius is derived from the Latin Ianuarius meaning "consecrated to the god Janus,"[17] who is the god of doors, portals, and transitions. Also the masculine form of Diana/Ianara and, of course, Diana is associated with the Janare.

San Michele (Saint or Archangel Michael)

Birth date or origin: The archangels are beings that emerged from the Abrahamic religions, but their archetype goes much further back to ancient Sumeria.

Feast day: September 29 (Michaelmas)

Plant correspondences: Garlic, Michaelmas daisy (aster), *Angelica archangelica*

The word *angel* means "messenger" and *arch* means "chief," so together you have chief angel or angel of the highest order. The list of archangels varies by tradition, but the Catholic church acknowledges seven archangels but only three by name: Michael ("one who is like god"), Gabriel ("god is my strength"), and Raphael ("god is my health").

Saint Michael is probably the most well-known of the archangels and is the one to pray to for protection. He is also known as the leader of the "army of God" and is often depicted slaying Lucifer. He is also petitioned to bless amulets and *brevi/abitini*, which are worn to keep the evil eye away.

Demons

Italian folk medicine and magic, as well as Italian Catholicism, also acknowledge other beings that might be called demons. These are often similar to our idea of fairies from the Celtic culture. It is important to acknowledge the "demons" in this tradition because they are the expressions of the fullness of the universe and on the spectrum of dark and light. Generally, demons or other malevolent spirits are only problematic when they are ignored or forgotten about. When we make continual effort to be in relationship with them, they can even become helpful. They are also sometimes thought to be similar to the Latin concept of the genius loci, or the "spirit of place."

Munacielli (Little Monks)

Munacielli, a.k.a. little monks, are supernatural beings that can cause minor mischief and annoyances. They have many names throughout Italy and in Italian America. In New York City it is believed that they live in the subways and alleys.

> They are tiny little creatures—merry, airy creatures running here and there. They delight themselves with procuring all sorts of annoyances to Christians: they tickle sleeping men under their feet, lift the blankets from the beds, throw sand grains in the eyes, upturn wine glasses, disguise themselves in the air currents to better shuffle all the papers; they drag laundered suits to the ground and filth them, pull the chairs from beneath women's bottoms, hide things in the most unpredictable places, make milk curdle, they pinch you and pull your hairs, buzzing and hissing like mosquitoes, and by night entangle the horses' hair and tail.[18]

Munaciello is the name for them in Naples, and it is connected to a legend about a poor dwarf man with supernatural powers who fell in love with a woman from the upper class. He always wore monk's clothes as his family had to move into the monastery because they had no money. It was not uncommon at one time for children of poor families to be abandoned at monasteries and convents, becoming forgotten and pitied members of society and therefore attributed to be malevolent or, at the least, an aspect of community that was relegated to the shadows.

Le Donne di Fuori (Women of the Outside) or Le Donne di Foresta (Women of the Forest)

Le Donne di Fuori or Le Donne di Foresta refers to a specific type of streghe from Sicily who are *a metà tra fattucchiere ed esseri fatati*,[19] or "halfway between witches and fairy beings." These beings have a direct relationship with the forces of nature, and it is believed that humans can attract them and receive their blessings by having their house in order and burning incense specifically made with rosemary and alloro (bay leaf).

Festivals on the Religious Calendar*

The festivals that celebrate patron saints and madonnas are held within the annual religious calendar. This provides a framework for cycling around the wheel of the year and is aligned with natural cycles as well as significant pagan holy days. These sacred celebrations mark different points during the year, and each offers its own specific type of healing qualities as well as rites and rituals that promote healing only on those days. Below are the basic holy days for the Catholic religious calendar and their associated magic and medicine.

Natale (Christmas)
Date: December 25
Deity: Jesus

---

*Note that I have taken liberties here with the calendar including some of the major holy days recognized by the church as well as some that are significant to Italian folk Catholicism.

Pagan correspondences: Winter solstice and Yule

Agricultural correspondence: The seeds are planted (buried) during this dark phase of the year.

Natale, or Christmas, might be the most sacred holy day of the year as it marks the birth of Jesus Christ. This is one of the only times during the year that the healing methods of the malocchio and other formulaic cures are transmitted. Christmas is also known as the night when diving into the sea can cure illnesses, water collected from a public fountain is used to cure "milk crust," and salves made from oil, lard, or butter are imbued with the ability to heal arthritis.[20]

L'Epifania (Epiphany)

Date: January 6

Deities: The Magi and La Befana

Pagan correspondences: Purification and death practice. La Befana is a pagan figure.

Agricultural correspondence: Time when the seed drops its skin into the earth, giving itself up to be renewed

L'Epifania, or Epiphany, is sometimes known as Three Kings Day when the Magi arrived to meet the baby Jesus. In Italian culture La Befana, a witch, rides her broom on Ephiphany Eve (January 5) leaving treats for children in exchange for a special cake. This is part of death practice and ancestor veneration whereby the dead leave their vital energy to new life. And in completion of this cycle the living feed the dead with ritual cakes. It's also about liberation of the past and the integration of grief to be purified or alchemized into a more expansive entity. By "purified" I don't mean puritanical. It means the essential vital force is released and recombined. This is also another time when malocchio cures can be transmitted, although this is not particularly common.

L'Annunciazione (The Annunciation)

Date: March 25

Deities: Archangel Gabriel, Artemis as Virgin (parthenogenetic) Goddess

Pagan Correspondence: The Spring equinox
Agricultural cycle: Rebirth, the beginning of growing season

L'Annunciazione, or The Annunciation, celebrates the incarnation of Christ when the Archangel Gabriel visits the Virgin Mary to tell her, "Do not be afraid, Mary, for you have found favor with God. And now, you will conceive in your womb and bear a son, and you will name him Jesus. He will be great, and will be called the Son of the Most High, and the Lord God will give to him the throne of his ancestor David. He will reign over the house of Jacob forever, and of his kingdom there will be no end (Luke 1:26–38). This is also the time when hernias in children heal by "passing the sufferer three times across a split tree or in a circle created by a branch split in two for the occasion."[21]

Pasqua (Easter)
Date: Sunday following the first full Moon after the equinox
Deities: Jesus, Persephone
Pagan correspondence: Ostara celebration
Agricultural correspondence: Blessing the field and gardens, planting seeds

In Italian and Italian-American culture Easter is called Pasqua and is celebrated throughout "holy week" with processions, church services, and family feasts. It is a time of resurrection and the rising of Jesus Christ from the underworld, three days after his crucifixion. Resurrection is a symbolic theme that spring festivals and rituals have been associated with in cultures throughout history. From Greek and Roman culture we have the myth of Persephone's resurrection from the underworld.

The iteration of spring resurrection in Christian cosmology is the ritual sacrifice and resurrection of Jesus Christ known as the celebration of Easter, which is also connected to the Jewish celebration of Passover. Jesus was crucified during Passover, and Easter, or Pasqua, and Passover share the same ancient name of Pascha, which is Greek for Passover and derived from the Hebrew word Pesach, which also means Passover and commemorates the exodus and liberation of the Jews from

Egyptian slavery. In fact, the Last Supper was a Passover seder (ceremonial dinner).

The word Easter was first added to the King James Bible in place of the word Pascha. It's an Old English word thought to have derived from the word Ostara, or Eastra, that referred to the pagan spring festival that celebrated the rising of the Germanic spring goddess, Eostre. Easter is also another traditional day to transmit the rites of malocchio.

La Festa di San Giovanni Battista (Saint John's Day)

Date: June 24

Deities: John the Baptist, the Green Man

Pagan correspondences: Summer solstice, Roman celebration of the sun gods and goddesses, e.g., the Roman sun god Sol Invictus (Unconquered Sun)

Agricultural correspondence: Harvest of sacred plants for use throughout the year; St. Johnswort in particular

La festa di San Giovanni Battista, or Saint John's Day, in Southern Italy is celebrated with processions and community gatherings. Bonfires are often lit at crossroads, particularly in front of or near churches where the celebrations are focused. Saint John's Day or Eve is the best time to gather the Saint John's wort plant for use in medicine and protective amulets and devices and to make *l'acqua di San Giovanni* during this celebration. The rites of malocchio can also be transmitted on this eve.

Assunzione (Assumption)

Date: August 15

Deities: The Virgin Mary, Diana, Artemis

Pagan correspondences: Ferragosto, or Feriae Augusti (festival of the Emperor Augustus), originally a Roman holiday that gave the agricultural workers time off from their labor in the fields. Also Nemoralia, the festival of Diana, which is on August 13.

Agricultural correspondences: Ripening fruits, the beginning of the harvest

Assunzione, or Assumption, is the day that celebrates the Blessed Mother's ascension to heaven. The dominant narrative tells us that this is when Mary, the mother of Jesus, left Earth behind and went to some paradise in the sky that was beyond or "above" the paradox of birth and death we live with here. But I prefer the idea that she was *subsumed*, or taken in by the earth as she was buried. The word *assumption* comes from the Latin *assumere*, which means to "take up, take to oneself." This is also a day of protecting the harvest and blessing of the fruits.

Ognissanti (All Saints Day) and Giorno dei Morti (Day of the Dead)

Date: November 1 and November 2, respectively
Deities: All saints, ancestors
Pagan correspondence: Samhain (Halloween)
Agricultural correspondences: Reaping harvest, preparing for winter

Ognissanti, or All Saints Day, and Giorno dei Morti ("Day of the Dead") or All Souls Day, are holy days that honor the ancestors, the saints, and the beloved dead. They are days for contacting the ancestors and releasing souls from purgatory. All Souls Day, also sometimes called the Feast of All Souls, is celebrated by going to mass and eating traditional foods such as ossi dei morti, or "bones of the dead," which are hard, crusty biscotti (see recipe below).

Bones of the Dead

As mentioned above, ossi dei morti, or "bones of the dead," are hard, crusty biscotti that are shaped to look like bones. They are eaten as part of the overall festa/celebration and can be used as an offering to the dead by placing them on an ancestor altar or offered to the grave of a loved one.

The tradition of making sweet treats, cakes, or other grain-based offerings to the dead and the spirits of the otherworld goes back to ancient times. One example is a *mola salsa*–literally, *mola* meaning "milled" and *salsa* meaning "salted"—which is a flat cake made from salted grains (usually some type of emmer grain). We also have the Greek cakes called *popanon* that were made to be left as offerings on the altars of the gods.

These cookies have other purposes as well. A little family story about them that I recently heard from my cousin is that her nonna makes them as teething biscuits for her kids. They are meant to be hard and dipped in espresso or coffee, so they're not as chewy as typical biscotti.

🌿 Ossi dei Morti Biscotti (Bones of the Dead Cookies)

This is a recipe that I improvised from several as I usually don't have all of the specific ingredients, and since I practice the art of substitution, I never make these the same way twice. Therefore, I recommend using this as a starting point and then experimenting with your own ingredients.

> 1 cup of almond meal/flour
> 1½ cups of granulated sugar
> 1 teaspoon of baking powder
> ½ teaspoon of salt
> ¼ teaspoon of cinnamon
> 3 tablespoons of softened butter
> 2 eggs
> 1 teaspoon of white wine
> ½ teaspoon of orange blossom extract
> ½ teaspoon of almond extract
> 1½ cups of all-purpose flour

1. Preheat oven to 300ºF.
2. Mix sugar, baking powder, salt, and cinnamon, then add softened butter and cream together.
3. Add eggs, wine, and extracts and mix well.
4. Add flours (both almond and all-purpose) and beat until a sticky dough forms.
5. Form dough into a ball, adding flour if it's too sticky. Then take small amounts of dough and roll them into 1-inch thick logs about 2 to 3 inches long. Shape as desired to look like bones.

6. Place on a parchment-lined baking sheet about 2 inches apart and bake for 20 minutes.

7. Enjoy by dipping in espresso or coffee!

Note: This makes about 3 dozen cookies depending on how big you shape them. They can be made smaller or larger.

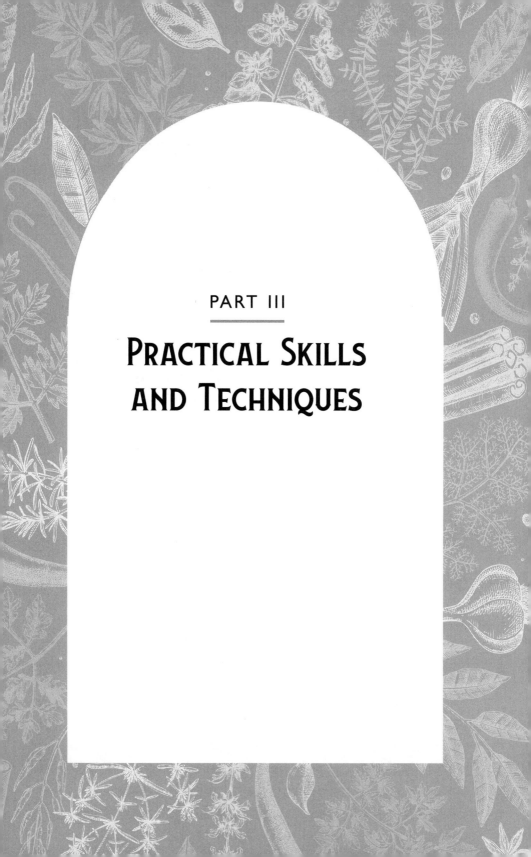

PART III

PRACTICAL SKILLS
AND TECHNIQUES

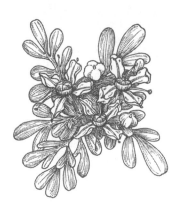

10
Preparations and Treatments
Basic Herbal Medicine and Kitchen Magic

Il materiale che viene usato è quello che si trova a portata di mano; fiori, steli di grano, rami di fico, grani d'orzo o di frumento, corteccia d'albero, acqua e sale, qualche goccia d'olio per diffusissimo rito contro il malocchio, lievito di pane, un po' di vino e così via: semplici ingredienti quotidiani che usati in un certo modo, all'interno dei riti, acquistano un significato speciale.

The material that is used is that which is found at your fingertips: flowers, wheat stalks, fig branches, barley or wheat grains, tree bark, water and salt, a few drops of oil for the widespread rite against the evil eye, yeast of bread, a little wine and so on: simple everyday ingredients that used in a certain way, within the rites, acquire a special meaning.

PAOLA GIOVETTI, *I GUARITORI DI CAMPAGNA*

ALONG WITH THE CULTURAL and spiritual devotion to practice, folk medicine includes the basic methods of preparation. The way a medicinal food, object, or herbal medicine is formulated is the container for the healing energy to be imbibed by those who need it. Italian folk medicine includes the making of many types of herbal preparations along with the magical, religious, and energetic relationships that practitioners cultivate with plant allies.

Most of the plants used in folk herbalism in general are traditionally bioregional. This means that herbal preparations are made from locally harvested plants. Of course, with modern commerce this is no longer the case exclusively. We sometimes have access to plants from all over the world that have traditional uses in many cultures and medicine practices. In terms of what it means to practice folk medicine, it's not so much that we have a dogmatic idea about where we get our ingredients from but more that we use what is available to us and that it is the best quality that we can find from the most ethical source we can find. Folk medicine isn't elitist in any way. Our ancestors had to make due with the ingredients that were available to them when they immigrated even if they weren't used to them, or they weren't exactly what was called for in a recipe.

Folk medicine preparations are adaptable, and part of the practice is improvisation. We try our best to use what's right around us and if we need to source from outside of our bioregion we try to find the best quality products that we can. It's also very important that those of us who are living on colonized land are in tune with the endangered status of native plants, avoid harvesting any endangered native plants, and do not plant or transport seeds from plants that are potentially invasive. For some good information and resources on this check out United Plant Savers.

The use of plant medicines and preparations is traditionally a form of common knowledge. That means it is not a specialized practice and requires no formal training or certification. Herbalism and the idea of an "herbalist" in the modern world is a fairly new concept. Our village healers weren't "herbalists," although they may have done some of the same things that current herbalists do. Their treatments could range from a simple remedy to more complicated energetic, spiritual, and medicinal techniques. Plant medicine was not used exclusively by herbalists; it was a part of daily life in every household, particularly when it came to minor ailments. For more complex issues a healer with greater skill would be sought out.

Paolo Luzzi, head of the Botanical Garden of Florence, describes three degrees of knowledge of herbal medicine[1]:

1. A first level regards general knowledge and species known by the whole community, plants that are often harvested and consumed such as chamomile, catmint, etc.

2. A second level involves specialists with knowledge passed down from family, often only oral, sometimes secret, sometimes sold (and thus easier to trace).

3. A third level is magical knowledge held by rare specialists and handled with strict secrecy. Often these specialists do not even pass the knowledge on, as they believe they are the elected bearers of the powers of the direct and essential effect of the healing capacity of a single plant or single best preparation. Very often, these practices also have religious values that interact with and complicate the rituals of preparation and their detection in the folk tradition.

Basically, there is a range of skill and practice from the household vernacular use of herbs to the skilled practitioner's use. In a traditional village or neighborhood, the skilled practitioner would be in service to everyone in the community and often for free. In fact, in terms of Segnatura and particularly the rites of malocchio, it is consistently stated in books and by practitioners themselves that they cannot accept money for their services. They will often accept trade and, in modern times, it is not unheard of for some practitioners to accept money, but it's generally rare. This does not mean that no one should charge for their services, especially in a capitalist economic complex where there are no communal or collective support systems. Just be aware that traditional health care in the form of folk medicine was accessible to everyone and that the practitioner did not need to charge to meet their own basic needs.

Using Ancestral Plants for Ancestral Revival

Plants have coevolved with human community and continue to do so. As we have discussed throughout this book, cultural ritual and tradition almost always include some plant preparation or other association with the spiritual/energetic qualities of plants. Many of those that have emigrated from their original homelands did so because of some plant-based oppression that made life difficult or even impossible. For the Italian immigrants it was the lack of access to fertile farmland. For the Irish it was the potato famine, during which it is estimated that one million people died and around six million people were forced to emigrate.[2]

We also know that plants and humans growing in the same location are nourished by the same ratio of basic elements. Forensic chemists are able to trace the location of where illegal drugs were grown based on their isotope ratios because their constitution of elements such as carbon and nitrogen is exactly the same as the ratios in the soils, water, and air where they are grown.[3]

This is also the case with the human body. Criminal investigators can now use isotope forensics to determine the trajectory of a corpse preceeding a death. According to Sarah Everts in "Isotopes Mark the Spot," "Checking these elements' isotope ratios against databases that contain global isotope abundances can provide investigators with the victim's probable trajectory during his or her last weeks, months, and years."[4]

Plants are also capable of changing their chemical compostion in response to human and animal behavior. I learned this one year when I put my horses out to pasture in the spring and noticed that they all started foaming at the mouth profusely. I called the vet who asked me if the pasture had been overgrazed the previous season, and I said that yes, it had been. She then informed me that when this happens plants, in this particular case it was red clover, will increase a specific chemical that causes grazing animals to foam at the mouth to make it harder for them to eat as quickly and efficiently, thereby protecting the plant from further assault.

My own venture into ancestral work began when I started intently sitting with plants and listening to them, observing them, and just being with them. This became a practice that sometimes included smelling and tasting plants. One day in my teacher Pam Montgomery's garden, I was sitting with a plant I had never known before, and yet I had the experience of deep familiarity. I didn't know the name of the plant but I "knew" it in a way I couldn't explain. I went to Pam and asked her about it, and she told me that it was probably an ancestral plant. I subsequently identitfied the plant and found that it was, in fact, a species of *Veronica* that grows in Ireland, one of my ancestral homelands. This obvsiously led me to where I am now with plants becoming the beacons of my ancestors and doorways into my own intrinsic ancestral memories.

While the following sections list various traditional herbal preparations that can be used as medicines and as mediums for our connection with our ancestral relationships with both humans and the greater ecoscape of our genetic origins, preparations are not required to elicit these types of connections. Any kind of plant contact is an option, even if it's just researching or reading about a plant and calling it into consciousness. Plants are always accessible. Ideally, however, sitting with a live plant in its natural environoment or in a garden is optimal. I often suggest to students that they do not try to identify or look up the "uses" of plant before they begin to work with them. This is to avoid internalizing any expectations that might interfere with authenthic communication. I also suggest working with one plant at a time and doing so for at least one week up to one month or even longer.

This usually involves having some type of contact and exchange with the plant on a daily basis and can be in any form but should at least include opportunities to taste and smell it. (Note: Do not taste any plant that you have not positively identified). Taste and smell are keys to our ancestral memories as our olfactory receptors on our tongue and in our nasal passages go right to our limbic brain: "Odors take a direct route to the limbic system, including the amygdala and the hippocampus, the regions related to emotion and memory."[5] Along with this are recent genetic studies that show how taste and smell change DNA. One study showed how the grandchildren of mice that were trained to have an aversion to the scent of cherry blossom also had an aversion although they had no previous exposure to that smell.[6]

Our relationship with plants as food, medicine, and cultural allies continues to shape and evolve through time but will always be at the center of human survival and adaptation to life on Earth. We cannot live here without them. The medicines and foods we make using plant ingredients have served as both health care and tools of the magical and divinatory arts.

Basic Herbal Medicine Terms

Below is a list of some basic terms and possible preparations that are used both in Italian folk medicine and basic herbalism. There are many variations and formulas. In a place-based culture, whether a neighborhood or village, adaptations are always part of the process and there is always some trial and error involved. Medicine making is one of the best ways to get to the plants and see how their medicinal qualities operate in different mediums.

Estrazione (Extraction)

Estrazione, or extraction, is the core activity of creating herbal preparations. This means extracting the medicinal compounds of a plant into a form that makes them bioavailable to humans as well as animals (pets and farm animals) by basically separating medicinal constituents by dissolving or suspending them in a suitable solvent.

Il solvente, or *menstruum*, is a solvent (e.g., water, oil, alcohol, vinegar, food, glycerine, honey). Water is the universal solvent as it extracts a wide range of plant constituents. Other popular solvents are wine, honey, and especially food. Food is not specifically a "menstruum" but the recipe or meal can be seen as one.

La Raccolta (Harvesting)

La raccolta, or the harvesting, of plants in the wild or from cultivated gardens is another central component of Italian folk medicine and includes the drying, garbling, storing, and grinding of plants. Harvesting is often a seasonal practice that aligns with the agricultural cycle.

Plant Preparations in Italian Folk Medicine

Below are the descriptions of some of the most common preparations in Italian folk medicine.

Tinture (Tinctures)

Alcohol *tinture*, or tinctures, are not commonly used in Italian folk medicine. There are several alcohol-based preparations, but they are generally liquors, wines, and *amari* (bitters) made with herbs. In terms of modern Traditional Western Herbalism, tinctures are probably the most commercially available and well-known form of herbal medicine. These are usually an alcohol extract but are sometimes made with vegetable glycerine as well. Basically the chosen fresh or dried herb is steeped in 100 proof alcohol for 4 to 6 weeks then strained and taken in drop doses.

Infusi e Tisane (Infusions and Teas)

Infusi e tisane, or infusions and teas, are two of the most ancient and simple methods of taking herbal medicine. They are made with the universal solvent, water, by boiling 1 cup of water and pouring it over 1 to 3 teaspoons of dried or fresh herb. The difference between a tea and an infusion is the amount of time it is steeped. A tea is steeped for 10 to 15 minutes, and an infusion is steeped for longer than 15 minutes and up to several hours.

Decotti (Decoctions)

A *decotto*, or decoction, is another water-based herbal preparation and is probably the most popular and commonly made in Italian folk medicine. In general, herbalists often make a decotto with seeds, berries, roots, and barks as opposed to leaves and flowers. This is because it is harder to extract medicinal compounds from seeds and such as they have harder cell walls. The longer heating time enables appropriate extraction.

To make a decotto, place 1 to 3 teaspoons of dried or fresh herbs in a pan with 1 cup of water, bring to a boil, then turn down heat, cover, and simmer for 20 to 30 minutes. Turn off heat, let cool, and strain. Drink like you would a tea.

Sciroppi (Syrups)

An herbal *sciroppo*, or syrup, is a great way to extract nutrients, concentrate them, and add to the shelf life of a decotto without using alcohol. We add sugar or some other sweetener to a syrup, which makes them quite agreeable and tasty to take. They make excellent tonics for children and, because honey or molasses can be added, they can carry additional medicine.

🌿 Herbal Syrup

1. Gather your chosen herbs. This can be seasonally based depending on what's in bloom or ready to harvest. Roots are generally harvested in the fall or spring, and aerial plant parts are picked at their peak of bloom.
2. Chop and measure the herbs. If using fresh herbs use 3 ounces of chopped herb mixture to 1 pint of water. If using dried, use 1 ounce of chopped herb mixture to 1 pint of water.
3. Combine the herbs and water in a pan.
4. Bring to a boil then turn heat down, cover, and simmer for 20–30 minutes.
5. Strain the herbs out of the liquid.
6. Reheat the liquid and simmer uncovered until the liquid is reduced down to half.
7. Add a sweetener such as sugar, honey, maple syrup, molasses, or vegetable glycerine. The ratio is 1 cup of sweetener to 1 cup of liquid, but I think that is way too sweet, so add liquid to suit your taste.

Note: Syrups will keep at room temperature for several months but refrigeration will ensure quality and increase shelf life. Any amount of brandy or other alcohol will also increase shelf life as well and can be added at the end of the process. Once the heat is off you can stir the alcohol into the pan or add it to the jar along with the syrup.

Oleoliti (Infused Oil)

Oleolito is an infused oil and another ancient method of imbibing herbs. Oils are made by infusing the chosen plant in either vegetable oil or animal fat. Most commonly these days folks use olive oil, coconut oil, or some other vegetable oil. To make an oleolito requires a heat source. This can simply be the Sun if you live in a warm climate.

❧ Simple Infused Oil

1. Choose a clean completely dry glass jar with lid.
2. If using a fresh plant, cut it into very small pieces and fill the jar to capacity. If using dried herbs, only fill jar 1/2 to 3/4 full.
3. Add enough oil to the reach the top of the jar and cover. The herbs will expand as they absorb the oil.
4. Place the jar in a cool, dark place for 4 to 6 weeks.
5. Strain the mixture through cheesecloth and store the oil in a cool, dark place.

Tips: Some oils infuse better dry than fresh. In fact, some herbalists prefer to infuse most of their herbs dry. This is because fresh herbs can become moldy when they are left in oil. To avoid this I will sometimes place cheesecloth over the jar instead of a lid. I also wipe any excess moisture that accumulates on the lid or the rim of the jar. Allow fresh herbs (except for Saint John's wort) to wilt before putting them in the oil.

You can also use an oven, double boiler, Crock-Pot, or even a woodstove as your heat source for infusing oil. Recipes for each method can be found below.

❧ Oven-Extracted Oil

1. Preheat oven to around 200ºF.
2. Place 2 to 3 ounces of herbs in an oven proof dish and cover them with oil.
3. Cover the dish with a lid and place it in the oven.
4. Allow oil to infuse for 2 to 3 hours. Be careful not to heat it too much, or you will deep fry your herbs. You may also use just the pilot but if you do, increase heating time to 2 to 3 days.
5. Strain the mixture through cheesecloth and store the oil in a bottle.

❧ Double-Boiler Oil

1. Place 2 to 3 ounces of herbs in the top of a double boiler and cover them with oil. If you don't have a double boiler you can use a glass measuring cup in a pan of water or a heat diffuser.

2. Cook over boiling water for 20 to 45 minutes.

3. Strain the mixture through cheesecloth and store the oil in a cool, dark place.

🌿 Crock-Pot Oil

1. Place 2 to 3 ounces of herbs in a Crock-Pot and cover them with oil.

2. Heat at the lowest temperature setting for 2 to 3 days. You may have to turn the Crock-Pot on and off to make sure it doesn't get too hot.

3. Strain the mixture through cheesecloth and store the oil in a cool, dark place.

🌿 Woodstove Oil

1. Place your herbs in a glass canning jar and cover them with oil.

2. Place the jar near the woodstove for 2 weeks.

3. Strain the mixture through cheesecloth and store the oil in a cool, dark place.

Oli Benedetto (Blessed Oils)

Oli benedetto, or blessed oils, are made with specific plants associated with a saint or angel whose medicine you want to imbibe in the oil. These are commonly made with essential oils but can also be made using infused oils. I recommend infused oils as much as possible because essential oils have become so commercialized that the plants used to make them are becoming overharvested and even endangered, and it requires a large amount of plant material to make a small amount of essential oil. Essential oils are also extremely potent; in fact, they have to be diluted, whereas infused oils are already diluted and thus more simple to use.

A blessed oil can include certain herbs or be any oil that has been consecrated or blessed. Blessed oils are used to anoint the body during rites and sacraments as well as during illness. They are also applied for spiritual protection and to consecrate sacred objects. Chrism oil is used by the Catholic church to anoint and bless those going through the various sacraments.

Blessed oils include the following:

Oil of the catechumens: Sometimes called "the oil of exorcism," this is a
pure olive oil used in baptism and anointing.

Chrism oil: Used during rites of passage and the sacraments, this is usually olive oil with balsam resin but may include myrrh essential oil.[7]

Oil of the sick: This is pure olive oil applied to the sick during the "laying on of hands" by a priest. The oil is applied by making the sign of
the cross on the forehead and hands of the person.[8]

Oils devoted to angels or saints include olio di San Michele, or Saint
Michael's oil. This is usually made with frankincense and olive oil, but I
like to make it with my local variety of angelica (*Angelica atropurpurea*).
This type of blessed oil is made to imbue the healing power of the saint
by pouring the determined oil or mixture into a bowl and reciting a
prayer asking the saint to bless the oil. Sometimes this is done in the
presence of said saint or the saint's relics or images or by touching a relic
or image to the oil or the bowl. When the oil is applied it is done while
also reciting a prayer to the saint or deity and usually while making the
sign of the cross or other segna. A blessed oil devoted to a saint can usually be obtained at a sanctuary dedicated to them or at the celebration of
their feast day.

One very special oil is offered for free at the Sanctuary of La
Madonna of Montevergine in Campania. The following suggestions for
the oil's use are printed on the package it comes in:

> *Ungere con l'olio benedetto la parte malata pregando con fede Maria
> Santissima di Montevergine. Si può recitare la preghiera qui riportata,
> tratta dal rituale della benedizione dell'olio o qualche altra preghiera
> spontanea e personale.*

> Anoint the sick part with blessed oil praying with faith to Maria
> Santissima di Montevergine. You can recite the prayer shown here,
> taken from the ritual of blessing the oil or some other spontaneous
> and personal prayer.

Pregheria O Signore che hai insegnato agli apostoli ad ungere i corpi infermi con l'olio tratta dal succo delle olive, concedi a noi che ti sup-plichiamo con fede, ungendo questo corpo malato, di ottenere la tua Grazia e la guarigione che fiduciosamente imploriamo dal tuo divino Figlio Gesù per intercessione di Maria Santissima nostra Madre e nostra Regina. Salve Regina.

Prayer O Lord who taught the apostles to anoint sick bodies with oil taken from the juice of olives, grant us who beg you with faith, anointing this sick body, to obtain your grace and the healing that we confidently implore from your divine Son Jesus through the interces-sion of Mary Most Holy our Mother and our Queen. Hail Queen.

Unguenti (Salve)

Unguenti, or salves, are made using beeswax or animal fat. Salves are applied locally to heal wounds and to relieve pain. They have also been used and continue to be used in traditional witchcraft as ointments that are applied to the skin so the medicinal qualities will be absorbed sys-temically into the bloodstream.

🌿 Herbal Salve

1. Start by making an herb-infused oil using one of the recipes above.
2. In a pan, add 2 ounces of beeswax to each cup of herbal oil. (Note that in the summer you may want more beeswax, in the winter you may want less because the temperature will change the consistency. More beeswax will make it more solid and vice versa.)
3. Melt the beeswax and oil mixture on the stove on low heat. (If beeswax is not "clean," heat it separately and strain it through cheesecloth, then add it to the oil and heat them together.)
4. Once melted, remove the mixture from heat and immediately add to jars.
5. If adding essential oils do it after the heat has been turned off and the salve has cooled slighthly, cover immediately or the oil may dissipate with the heat.

Flying Ointment

The flying ointment is one of the most well-known remedies related to Italian witchcraft as well as many other witch traditions. It is both a historical and mythical symbol of witchcraft and plays a role in many legends about witches and their ability to "fly." The exact formula of this sacred preparation is one of mystery, and it is quite likely that there are many variations using plants and substances that will elicit a trance allowing the witch to "fly." It is not clear what the legends mean by "fly." It is often literally translated to mean actual flying, and specifically, flying to the walnut tree of Benevento for the witches' Sabbath. Another interpretation is that it means to take a "trip" like the type associated with the use of psychedelics.

The few things that we know for sure about flying ointments is that they are based on a simple salve recipe but usually use some type of animal fat/lard. Traditional salves were often made this way. Many of the legends accuse "witches" of making this ointment using the fat of babies or young children, but I believe we can rule that out as a patriarchal narrative demonizing community healers.

We also have several possible entheogenic plants that may have been added to these ointments. Eyewitness accounts from Inquisition records describe that people who have applied the ointment to themselves fall into a deep slumber where they appear almost dead but when they wake up they insist that they had been bodily transported to the Sabbath. The following is from Giovanni Francesco Pico della Mirandola's dialogue *Strix* (1523), published in the aftermath of a series of witch trials he had participated in:

Apistio: You believe then that the witches are always brought to the game [of Diana] in the flesh?

Dicasto [the Inquisitor]: I do not deem that they are always brought bodily to this game, because at times they have been found holding to a wooden beam, in such a profound slumber that they could not feel anything, even when strongly beaten. Afterward, they were convinced that they had been carried to the game but in fact they never moved.[9]

Some of the possible plants and other entheogens that were included are as follows:

- ❦ Belladonna/*Atropa belladonna*
- ❦ Aconite (monkshood)/*Aconitum napellus*
- ❦ Mandrake/*Mandragora officinarum*
- ❦ Thorn apple/*Datura stramonium*
- ❦ Opium poppy/*Papaver somniferum*
- ❦ Ergot/*Claviceps purpurea*
- ❦ Mugwort/*Aremisia vulgaris* and other various species of *Artemisia*
- ❦ Amanita/*Amanita muscaria*
- ❦ Psilocybin mushroom/*Psilocybe* spp.

Un Miele Alle Erbe (Herbal Honey)

Un miele alle erbe, or herbal honey, is another popular Italian folk medicine. Honey is an ancient ancestral elixir, and honey bees were a collective deity that inspired many cults around the Mediterranean.

Honey bees are believed to have originated in South Asia and spread to the Mediterranean from there. Honey was a food staple in ancient Rome, and both honey and the bee became a part of Roman and Greek mythology. Both Zeus and Dionysus are said to have been raised on the honey of sacred bees.

The uses of honey are well documented. Cato the Elder, the ancient Roman who wrote *De agri cultura* (*On Farming and Agriculture*) said that honey "was used as a sweetener, a preservative and an ingredient of marinating. Besides, it was also a very important ingredient in healing. It was used in ointments to treat ulcers, as a remedy for coughing and internal organs. In addition, it was used for the expulsion of tapeworms."

In his work, *Gynaecology*, Soranus refers to honey as a type of contraceptive: "It is also aids in preventing conception to smear the orifice of the uterus all over before with old olive oil or honey or cedar resin or juice of the balsam tree, alone or together with white lead."[10]

🌿 Un Miele Alle Erbe (Herbal Honey)

Herbal honey is used both internally and externally. It can be made with fresh or dried herbs, but traditionally it is made with fresh herbs that have been left to wilt for several hours to reduce excess water content.

1. Put the herbs in a glass jar until it's about half full and fill the rest of the jar with honey.
2. Let the mixture steep for 4 weeks, then strain it through a fine mesh sieve into a new jar. Note that the honey may have to be heated until it's a smooth, liquid consistency before it will easily strain.

Suffumigi (Herbal Steam)
A simple *suffumigi*, or herbal steam, can be made by placing aromatic herbs in a pan of steamy water and breathing in the released medicinal compounds.

Pulizia (Energetic Cleansing)
Pulizia, or energetic cleansing, is part of regular daily health care and is also used during times of illness. Types of pulizie include *fumigazione, incenso,* and *sciumiento.*

FUMIGAZIONE (SMOKE)
Fumigazione, also called *pulizia del fumo,* or purification by smoke, is the Italian word for *fumigation,* or the burning of plants to purify, to protect, and to consecrate rituals and sacred space. It's a practice that can be found in many forms all over the world and comes from ancient times in the Mediterranean. Southern Italians and Italian Americans, as well as other European-descended peoples, often think of fumigation as we were taught in folk Catholicism. This is where a thurible, or incense burner, is filled with ritual herbs and swung during ceremonies, masses, and sacramental rites.

INCENSO (INCENSE)
Incenso, or incense, is made from a blend of herbs, resins, and sometimes honeys, meads, and other natural substances, but single herbs can be burned alone or together.

Sciumiento (no translation)

Sciumiento is burning herbs on coals from the fireplace and breathing them in or letting the smoke waft around the room.

Uovo (Egg) Pulizia

The quote from ancient Roman culture, *omne vivum ex ovo*, means "all life comes from the egg." Eggs are seen as an important symbolic and energetic medicine often used for cleansing and purification. Many folk practitioners will use an egg in various methods to cure or heal a physical ailment or psychic distress:

> In pagan times, eggs were part of the Bacchic or Dionysian myster-
> ies, possibly a symbol of the underworld; they could be used to cast
> spells and, conversely, to offer protection. A fortified castle built in
> the 15th century in the Bay of Naples has a connection to this ancient
> Roman practice, as legend has it the poet Vergil (1st c BC) buried an
> egg on the site for protection, hence the modern name of the struc-
> ture: Castel dell'Ovo.[11]

In Italian folk medicine we have an egg healing or "cleansing" prac-
tice called an egg pulizia. Eggs can be used externally and internally. It is sometimes recommended to drink a raw egg on specific holy days to elicit healing for certain ailments. For instance, it is recommended to "drink an egg produced on Good Friday"[12] for a headache.

Externally a whole egg can be placed near or on an area of the body in need of healing as it is believed to be a drawing agent that can pull out and absorb negative influences. There is a full ritual that can be per-formed for the all-over healing of physical or spiritual conditions that goes as follows:

Take a raw fresh whole washed egg and pray the Apostle's Creed, an Our Father, and a Hail Mary over the egg. Next anoint the egg with holy water. Then run the egg over the entire body either actually rubbing/rolling it directly on or almost touching the body. Go from the head down as if tracing a line around the outline of the person. Then run the egg up and down the center line, including the neck and give special attention to any area of the body that is particularly affected. Once the ritual is complete throw the egg out by either breaking it and flushing it down the toilet or breaking it and throwing it into a compost being sure to bury it under debris.[13]

Bagno alle Erbe (Herbal Bath)

Bathing as both a healing and sacred ritual incorporates the use of both plants and blessings. In terms of folk Catholicism we have the sacrament of baptism and the use of holy water (discussed in chapter 7) as wells as the other water preparations described in the following sections.

Guazza (Healing Water)

One of the most well-known herbal bath preparations is L'acqua di San Giovanni, or the "Water of Saint John," which is made from both plants and *guazza*, or dew collected on Saint John's eve. *Guazza* refers to both the healing water and the dew that it holds. Plants to make the guazza are gathered the morning of June 24 when they are considered magically potent for protection via the blessing of Saint John. Water is placed in a sacred bowl and several aromatic leaves and flowers are added to it. It is left outside overnight in the moonlight while the dew collects and combines in the bowl with the water and flowers.

Other holy days to gather guazza are Easter Eve, the two equinoxes, saint days, full Moons, and new Moons. Note that each day will imbue the water with its own energies.

L'Acqua di Medaglia (Medal Water)

L'acqua di medaglia, or medal water, has several purposes and there are different methods for making it, but basically a sacred medal, usually Saint Benedict, is used to sanctify and bless water. The water is then either drunk or used externally in a bath or applied directly to an area of the body.

There is also a L'acqua di medaglia practice used as part of *il rito del malocchio* (rite of the evil eye) where a sacred medal is used to break up the evil eye.

🌿L'Acqua di Medaglia

1. In the evening, fill a glass of water.
2. Using a saint medal that has been consecrated, make the sign of the cross over the glass three times.
3. Say three Hail Marys.
4. Make the sign of the cross with the medal three more times.
5. Say three Our Fathers.
6. Make the sign of the cross three more times.
7. Say three Glory Bes.
8. Place the medal in the water and leave overnight.
9. In the morning the water is ready to be used like holy water for blessing, prayer, and anointing for protection of objects, home, or self.

🌿To Make an Herbal Baths

An herbal bath is another form of pulizia. It involves using one of the above preparations and fully submersing the body in it, pouring it over the whole body at the end of a bath or shower, or washing, rinsing, or soaking a specific area of the body.

Almost any medicinal herb can be used, but here are some suggestions, depending on the effect you wish to achieve:

Artemisia (Mugwort): Clearing, pulizia, protection
Rosmarino (Rosemary): Protection, pulizia, stimulating hair growth, controlling dandruff and itchy scalp
Rosa (Rose): Calming, clearing, soothing the skin, acting as an anti-inflammatory, reducing redness
Calendula (Calendula): Soothing the skin, reducing redness and irritation, acting as an antifungal
Malva (Mallow flower): Soothing and cooling the skin

A handful of herbs of your choice (see list above for ideas)
1 cup to 1 quart of water
Bathtub or basin

1. Bring water to a boil in a pan on the stove.
2. Add the herbs and turn off the heat.
3. Cover and let the herbs infuse for 1 hour or more.
4. Strain the liquid, add the infusion to the bath or basin, and soak for at least 20 minutes.

Optional: Add salt or apple cider vinegar to bath
Alternative method: Simply add herbs directly to the water in a bath or basin and steep yourself in them. (Just be careful not to clog your drain if using a bathtub.)

Cucina (Kitchen) Medicine

One of the primary modes of imbibing the medicine of herbs in Italian culture and all traditional cultures is through food and cooking. Herbs are used directly in recipes or made into vinegars, wines, and oils that are added to recipes or used as condiments. The kitchen, in the life of common people, is the anchor of the soul. Transformation occurs there on many levels from physical digestion to relationships, magic, and spiritual alchemy.

Our societal move toward "laboratories" and pharmacies has bypassed an important grounding center of cultural life that is accessible to everyone. As Jungian analyst Marion Woodman describes in her interpretation of the Grimm's fairytale "Allerleirauh":

> Culturally, the kitchen work is still not being done. . . . Without the diligence to bite off, chew, swallow, digest, and assimilate the new energy available in the kitchen, the ego is often too weak to take time to evacuate. Certainly, it is too lethargic to build a fire. Without fire, no transformation can take place. No passion ignites matter. No phoenix can rise from no ashes.[14]

The kitchen is where a great deal of Italian folk medicine happens. It happens amidst pots of sauce, dishes, and ongoing conversations. In this sense, folk medicine is an ordinary part of life and a way to be continually engaged with the presence of the moment.

The kitchen is often thought to have its own guardian spirit who protects and guides whoever is doing the cooking and healing work, and in Italian folk medicine that is often the kitchen witch. My nonna and zie (aunts) all had their own kitchen witch. I inherited my nonna's! Sometimes there might be a statue of the Blessed Mother instead or there might be both. Either way the kitchen is honored as a sacred place with its own animating spirit and energy. In my family, and in many immigrant households, the kitchen was kept clean and tidy. The care and cleaning of a home and kitchen is a form of devotion and a meditation that keeps the hearth fire burning. The kitchen can be thought of as the heart of the home where there is always a flame kept going for family members and friends to gather around.

The Roman goddess Vesta (Greek goddess Hestia) is the goddess of the hearth and household, and all household events and ceremonies would begin by invoking her. Vesta keeps the flame of the hearth from ever going out. Her temple in Rome was where the Vestal Virgins tended her sacred fire. The temple of Vesta is the hearth of the city, and its flame has to burn perpetually as a symbol of the city's life force.

Tools for Kitchen Magic

Kitchen magic can happen anywhere: at a campsite, in an RV, under a bridge in a big city, off-grid, or in any place that is home for a moment or a lifetime. The basic tools are fire, which can be anything from a stove to a hot plate or a simple open fire, a vessel, cooking implements, and ingredients. Other basic tools include the following:

- Recipe box/spell book
- Mortar and pestle, or in the modern world, a blender, food processor, or herb grinder
- Measuring cups
- Cauldron (i.e., pots and pans)
- Jars and bottles for storage
- Labels for jars and bottles
- Strainer and cheesecloth
- Broom for sweeping both the floor and unwanted energy

Ritual Ingredients

The ingredients below are often considered sacred and hold both nutrient and medicinal power as well as magical power. They are also simple household substances that are easy to find in any store.

SALT

Salt is a foundational ingredient in pretty much every recipe on Earth and is used for making holy water, performing malocchio cures, clearing energy in a room, and casting spells. Salt absorbs and neutralizes, cleans and purifies. I recommend using either Mediterranean or Celtic sea salt. I don't recommend using dead sea salt because it's my understanding that it's being overharvested. A pinch of salt can be added to a bucket of water for cleaning or placed in bowls on a shelf or windowsill to purify and protect a room as well as absorb negativity.

VINEGAR

Vinegar is nutritional and healing, is an excellent preservative, and has extractive abilities, so it can be used as a menstruum for making herbal preparations. One of the most common preparations made from vinegar for herbal medicine is an oxymel.

Oxymel is the combination of two Greek words, *oxy* and *meli*, which mean "acid" and "honey." Cato the Elder described an oxymel as a wine made from vinegar and honey. Oxymels were common herbal remedies in ancient Greece that were often stored in amphoras, or vases, that depicted four male figures, all nude and bearded, being stung by bees. The figures are Laios, Keleos, Kerberos, and Aigolios, who plundered from the hives the honey on which the infant Zeus was nourished.

🌿 Simple Oxymel

1. Fill a jar with fresh plant material (any of the herbs you might use for a tincture, infusion, tea, etc.). If using dried, fill the jar half way.
2. Cover the herbs with vinegar. I prefer apple cider vinegar.
3. Let sit for 2 to 6 weeks, then strain.

4. Add honey to taste. Some recipes call for 1 part honey to 1 part vinegar but that is too sweet for me.

Note: Some recipes call for the honey and vinegar to be added at the same time, and some use heat to mix them.

WINE

After tea, wine is probably the second oldest method of herbal preparation. Like beer, it is one of many fermented traditional beverages. The fermentation process itself provides a healing liquid and herbs are added for further medicinal and nutritional benefit.

Parsley-Elderberry Honey Wine

Parsley-elderberry honey wine is a recipe from the ancient mystic and healer Hildegard von Bingen. This recipe is made after the wine has already been cured, so it's a secondary process to fermentation. The fermentation process itself provides a healing liquid, and herbs are added for further medicinal and nutritional benefit. Wine, particularly red wine, is a healing beverage even without the added herbs because grape skins contain resveratrol, which is an antioxidant and, of course, wine is full of beneficial enzymes and yeasts when made without added preservatives.

2 tablespoons of wine vinegar

1 quart of red wine

1 cup of fresh elderberries or 1/2 cup of dried

10 fresh parsley leaves and stems

1 cup of raw honey

1. Place vinegar, wine, and elderberries in a pot and, if using fresh elderberries, mash them a bit with a potato masher to release the juices.
2. Add parsley and bring to a slight boil. Then turn down heat and simmer for 5 to 8 minutes.
3. Let cool until warm but no longer hot.
4. Strain and add honey while it's still warm. I sometimes strain it and put it back on the stove on low for a minute to make sure the honey

is blended. I don't like to heat the honey too much because that destroys its vital enzymes.

5. Next, bottle it. I usually pour it right back into the wine bottle. It will store well in a cool place for about 1 year, but it doesn't last that long around my house!

6. Take one shot glass of wine up to 3 times per day.

Optional: Adjust the amount of honey to your taste. One cup is too much for me, so I use about half a cup.

AMARO

Amaro, which means "bitter" in Italian, is a traditional Italian herbal remedy or digestif. It is usually made with bitter herbs and taken after meals to aid the digestion of food. In Italy, these herbal remedies were made in every village and each village had their own recipes based on the plants that grew around them locally and the yearly health needs of the community. The formula was intended for the whole community and was made collectively in the piazza or center of town, according to ethnobotanists and historians.

I learned about the historical process of making amaro from Paolo Luzzi, the head of the Botanical Garden of Florence. He explained that every village made a collective seasonal medicine that everyone in the community would take to ward off illness throughout the year. Each community had their own special recipe and ritual-making process that was performed in public with group participation. Once Christianity became predominant, the church took over the distribution of health care.

The medical and pharmaceutical practice in Tuscany is linked from the beginning to a strong and widespread religious spirit closely linked to the assistance to the sick and practiced in many monastic orders, since 1000 A.D. in the wake of compliance with the Rule of St. Benedict, as stated in chapter 36: "First of all we must take care of the sick brothers really served as Christ himself because he says, 'I was sick and you visited me' and 'what you did for one of these my smaller brothers, you did for me,' confirming the close relationship between love for God and love for our neighbor, especially the last, selected from the suffering people, elderly or sick. God and man closely linked by bond assistance.[15]

These formulas were primarily bitters/amari that addressed digestion on a multisystemic level. Even today in Southern Italy, many localities have their own recipe for bitters. Local bitters formulas were often considered to be elixirs of life/health, and the formulas and herbal knowledge held within them were a part of cultural and spiritual relationships.

Kitchen Spells

The traditional Italian American or Italian kitchen is not only a place where meals are prepared but it also the center of the home, where healing remedies are prepared, and where magic spells are cast using household ingredients and recipes.

BREAD SPELL

A bread spell can be a prayer, an intention, or an incantation, and there are a variety of ways to make one. Some involve carving symbols into the bread after it's baked. Some involve speaking spells into the bread. And some are written onto paper and cooked in the bread (this should be done with food grade ink or food coloring).

Simple Bread Spell

1. Use any bread recipe that you like; usually it's a yeast bread but it could be sourdough.
2. Place bread dough in a loaf pan. You may want to make small loaves because you will be burying the bread. If you want one to eat, you may want to divide the dough in half or quarters.
3. Write a spell on a small piece of paper and place in the center of the bread or speak a spell into the center of the bread. Other options are to write the spell on the bread with milk or butter.
4. Bake bread per recipe.

5. When the bread is done and has cooled, bury it outside.
6. Sprinkle salt or protective herbs over the area where the bread is buried.
7. Say this prayer:

May this bread be taken by the earth.
May this bread be taken by the soils.
May this bread be eaten by the spirits underground.
So that my prayer (wish, spell) is turned into the flesh of the earth
and made real.

Freezing

This is a protection spell specifically for when you are in a human-to-human conflict with someone, and you think they may be causing you harm whether psychically, emotionally, or physically. It requires that you have a freezer.

Note that I do not recommend this spell for conflicts involving primary relationships. This is more for work or social conflicts.

🌿Freezing Spell

Piece of paper
Something to write with
Small container such as a flat metal tin or a small plastic box
Freezer

1. Write down the name of the person whose energy you do not want affecting you any longer.
2. Fold the paper and place it in the container.
3. Say this: "May this person no longer impose on my energy field. I pray that no harm comes to them but that they will no longer be in my life."
4. Place the container in the freezer.

The Kitchen Garden

Having herbs and fresh veggies right outside the kitchen door, if possible, is the ultimate boon to kitchen healing. This can even be pots of herbs grown inside. I had a friend who lived in a renovated warehouse apartment in Brooklyn who built large indoor raised beds inside next to a large window.

Traditional Italian gardens include some or all of the following:

- Tomatoes
- Peppers
- Basil
- Parsley
- Oregano
- Eggplant
- Figs
- Lemons
- Lettuce
- Legumes/some type of beans

Traditional Foods

Although there are many plants that have become synonymous with Italian culture, and we certainly do love them, it's important to know their historical context. Take tomatoes, for instance. They are a major staple in Italian cuisine, but they are not native to Italy and in fact were brought to Europe as a result of Spanish colonization of South America. At first it was actually thought to be poisonous because of its resemblance to poisonous nightshades. The same goes for hot peppers/pepperoncini. Even our beloved eggplant, *melanzana*, is not from Italy but originated in Southeast Asia.

There are many dimensions to our relationship with cultural plants and foods that include our relations with other peoples, white supremacy, European supremacy, and colonization. Another dimension is the agency of the plants themselves and how intentional they are about traveling and seed spreading. This touches upon human supremacy whereby we believe that it is solely our choices that lead to the movement of various plants across the globe. I find this to be an extremely narrow view. Plants do have agency, and they in fact can move at will and make themselves desirable in a way that will enable them to proliferate. For humans to think that it is purely our conquests that have broadened the range of plants is inaccurate based on my understanding and experience.

Traditional foods of every culture become deeply entwined with humans and even provide the essential materials for the replication of our DNA. In this way we coevolve. Plants also adapt to landscape and weather variations, so the coevolution is a network between people, pollinators, other species, and the land as well as the social, political, and economic climate where they are grown and harvested or where they grow wild.

Before tomatoes became so prevalent in Italian cooking, our food included olives, beans, and traditional grains. In fact, many of our traditional feasts and rituals involve recipes made from legumes and beans. Below is a family recipe from my Calabrian side. Note that this has been Americanized to adapt to available ingredients.

🌿 Pasta e Fagioli (Pasta and Beans)*

2 pounds of ground beef (optional: I prefer mine without beef but most recipes include it)

1 tablespoon of olive oil

1 cup of onion, diced

2–3 large carrots, chopped or shredded

3 large garlic cloves, minced

2–3 stalks of celery, diced

1 48-ounce can diced tomatoes

2 cups of canellini or white kidney beans

2 cups of red kidney beans

2 quarts of chicken or beef broth

2 quarts of tomato sauce

1 tablespoon of oregano

5 teaspoons of chopped fresh basil or 3 teaspoons of dried

2½ teaspoons of ground black pepper

---

*This recipe is adapted from a family recipe that my cousin Renee Ward included in a recipe book she curated.

8 ounces of ditalini pasta

5 teaspoons of chopped fresh parsley or 3 teaspoons of dried

Extra water as needed if it's too thick (it should be somewhere between a soup and a stew)

1. In large Dutch oven, brown the beef in the olive oil until it is no longer pink and is starting to brown.
2. Add onions, carrots, garlic, and celery and cook until translucent, about 5 minutes.
3. Add tomatoes, beans, broth, tomato sauce, oregano, basil, and pepper to the pot.
4. Bring to a boil, then simmer on low for about 45 minutes.
5. Add pasta and simmer until pasta is fully cooked. I sometimes cook the pasta separately and then add it to the rest, so it doesn't become too mushy.
6. Stir in parsley just before serving.

Note: This recipe makes a lot, so you might want to cut it in half.

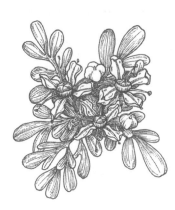

11

Protezione

Tools, Charms, and Practices for Averting Harm

PROTEZIONE, OR PROTECTION MAGIC and medicine, can be found in all cultures all over the world and are a major focus in Italian folk medicine. The idea of protection, or of needing protection, is often misunderstood as defensiveness and/or being in a state of hypervigilance when, usually, it is not. Though there are certainly times in life when we need to be in "'fight or flight" mode, the idea of protection in Italian folk medicine has a much wider scope than that.

The etymology of the word *protection* comes from the Latin *pretegere*, which means "cover in front," from pro-, meaning "before," and tegere, meaning "to cover," but it also means "keeping, guardianship, [and] act or state of protecting."[1] From this we often think of shielding or defense but also an act of agency where we keep or steward our energy as well as define its boundaries and limitations. When we understand the concept of "sharing" in Italian folk medicine, we can think of protection as a form of discernment and justice as well as a framework or container for relaxation. In terms of our daily and cultural magic, it is more a method of maintaining dynamic equilibrium in body, mind, and spirit.

Apotropaic Medicine

The techniques we use to invoke protection are called "apotropaic." Apotropaic is the power to avert harm or "evil" and comes from the

Greek word *apotropaios*, which means to "turn away, avert" or "turn from."[2] From this definition we can also interpret apotropaic magic to be a form of discernment where we choose to turn something away or turn ourselves away from something.

Ernesto de Martino who wrote *Sud e magia* (*Magic: A Theory from the South*), a book about Southern Italian folk magic, describes protection magic as a method of reinstating the centered presence of the individual in the body and mind. It can be thought of as a way to counter, neutralize, and/or integrate the negative aspects of life as a form of self and community care. Martino describes it as "the risk that the individual presence itself gets lost as a center for decision and choice." Basically, protection magic reembodies us from dissociation and reinstates our agency to face daily and lifelong challenges from our natural center.

> Being in the world—maintaining oneself as an individual presence in society and history—means acting [agire] as a power of decision and choice according to values; it means always performing anew the never-definitive detachment from the immediacy of mere natural vitality and rising to cultural life. The loss of this power and even the spiritual possibility of exercising it, represents a radical risk for a presence unsuccessfully engaged in resisting an attack in the form of the experience of being-acted-upon, where being-acted involves the personality as a whole and the operative powers grounding and supporting it.[3]

Protection magic is what gives us the "will to reply," and thereby we become engaged in the world and present. It is also a practice of taking up space in our bodies and lives, of being fully present and being who we are, knowing our existence is valid and that in that existence we become part of the universe that is essentially interactive. When we live in an interactive, call-and-response universe, we naturally have agency and choices that will unequivocally influence the web of connections.

The tools of protection accomplish this in many ways. They evoke awareness and can shift our focus from being acted upon to being agential (having agency) or being the actor, the person doing the acting. When protection medicine is embedded in culture and thereby repeated throughout life, it becomes an inherent access point to presence. This type of presence can be thought of similarly to the way people are taught to respond to conflict using martial arts. When we are facing confrontations—physical, spiritual, or otherwise—the art of protection puts us in the flow of consciousness of the moment so that we can act skillfully to avoid harm and diffuse the situation, turn it away, or turn ourselves away from it.

Overall, protection magic is, in this sense, a form of nourishment. If you remember our discussion on the four humors in chapter 6, we talked about dryness and how we use up our radical moisture as we go through life. Protection magic is one of the ways we can preserve our radical moisture, as it provides us and others with a sense of center and presence that prevents the unnecessary expenditure of our life source while maintaining a "stable sense of being."[4]

Protective Devices

Protective devices include many cultural practices that are inherent in daily life and those that are performed with various degrees of intention. The purpose is to relieve the individual or group that is experiencing distress or, as mentioned above, a loss of presence, using apotropaic tools that bring them back to their fullness of being. According to Ernesto de Martino these techniques are fundamentally provided by the culture, yet adaptive and improvisational. However, if the culture is not intact, for instance due to the process of alienation and assimilation, these tools will not be as effective. Just knowing the steps or formula will not necessarily lead to healing. Ernesto concluded that "when the crisis of presence is not overcome, it means that culture has been absent or so underdeveloped as to be useless at channeling the emotions' overwhelming power."[5]

When we are living in diaspora, this is one of the areas of ancestral work that requires our deep devotion. Of course, we can't go back in time or recreate an Italian village culture, but we can develop a relationship with our apotropaic magic that places us on the continuous motion of history whereby we take our place in it as we are. This is why knowing our ancestral past is essential to revitalizing our traditions and bringing them to life in the here and now. The process is different depending on the individual, their community, and the circumstances, but we can always regenerate these techniques by practicing them, listening to how they speak to us, being honest with ourselves about our loss of connection, and continuing to devote ourselves to rebuilding it.

Another aspect of protection is how we protect others. As mentioned in the section about the evil eye, we can unintentionally throw bad vibes toward others when we feel a sense of loss or a lack of presence. From this perspective, apotropaic magic is about self-care and nourishment.

Charms

Apotropaic charms are a primary means of protection in Italian folk medicine. Charms are often made from metal or some type of stone or gem and hung on a necklace or bracelet. Part of what activates the magic of a charm is that it is given to you by someone else. The rule is that you can't buy your own charms, but I do believe that there are exceptions to this as we do have to improvise and sometimes we have to buy ourselves a charm. If this is the case I suggest creating a small ritual of giving the charm to yourself. Another option is to ask someone to give you a charm. Recently a friend and I were shopping for charms together and agreed to pick out the ones we liked and have the other purchase it and then exchange.

Giving charms to others is a very common practice in Italian-American communities so, usually, charms are regularly provided to a person by others. Charms are often given at birthdays and other rites of passage such as first communion. It is customary to have charms available to give to others if the need arises. Other times that charms may be given are before travel or during a difficult or challenging time. My practice is to always have charms ready to go if someone needs them and in that way no one ever has to buy their own.

One of the most famous charms from Italian folk medicine is the *cimaruta* (chee-mah-roo-tah) or "charm of rue." The cimaruta is a metal charm made to look like a sprig of rue with specific apotropaic symbols attached to it. Different regions of Italy had different symbols but here are some possibilities:

- Fish
- Key—represents Hecate and gates/portals
- Flower
- Bird
- Dagger
- Rooster—symbolizes guardian energy
- Snake—represents Proserpina/Persephone
- Crescent Moon—for the goddess Diana

Each of these has its own apotropaic magic.

Another popular charm is the *cornicello* or "little horn," known in the Italian-American diaspora as the "Italian horn." This is usually made from red coral or gold and worn on a gold chain around the neck. Both coral and the symbol of the horn are considered to have protective powers. It's also common to hang a cornicello from the rear-view mirror of a car. The horn is associated with the horn of a bull and represents strength and virility. It also looks a lot like a chili pepper, and sometimes the horn and chili pepper are used interchangeably. The chili pepper also looks like a horn, so as a symbol it represents the same fertile energy, especially since chili peppers are used as an aphrodisiac.

The Color Red

Anything red is considered apotropaic, partly because red is the color of precious coral, which is considered protective as well as lucky. Coral is actually a type of limestone that was used as a protective shield by marine creatures called polyps.[6] Red is also associated with blood and the blood mysteries. Menstrual blood was considered extremely powerful and magical to the Romans and many other ancient cultures, and it is associated with the Blessed Mother. It was thought to contain unlimited powers that could drive away natural catastrophes and cure many illnesses, and it was symbolic of fertility and life itself.[7]

In Italian culture red clothing is often worn and, in my family, we use red ribbons. A red ribbon is always tied somewhere in a new car that has just been bought. Red ribbons can be tied anywhere around anything to invoke the color red and its apotropaic qualities.

Nazar (Glance)

> There is a mystery called the glance, the gift, nazar.
> COLEMAN BARKS

Another popular charm is the *nazar*, or "glance," which looks like an eye and is believed to have originated in ancient Turkey and then spread all over the Mediterranean and SWANA regions of the world. The nazar is known to ward off the evil eye, or malocchio, and is often incorporated in protection charms with other symbols such as the cornicello. The nazar, also called the "evil eye stone," is made from glass into a flat circle bead that looks like an open eye. It has sometimes been considered the eye of God. Rumi, for instance, spoke of the power of the divine "glance" of truth and enlightenment.

Hand Gestures and Mudras

These hand gestures are used as a way to prevent or block unwanted negative energy, usually against the malocchio, but for protection in general.

MANO CORNUTO (HORNED HAND)

The *mano cornuto*, or horned hand, is a gesture to protect and ward off the malocchio. The mano cornuto is thrown or cast in the direction of the threat and is often worn as a charm. It's made by folding the middle and ring fingers and thumb into the palm and extending the pinky and index fingers, like horns. When throwing the mano cornuto, it is sometimes customary to say, *Tiè, tiè*! which means "Take that!"

Mano Fico or Figa (Fig Hand)

Mano fico or *figa*, meaning "fig hand," is another gesture of protection against the malocchio and can also be worn as a charm. It's made by making a fist and sticking the thumb through the index and middle fingers. It is sometimes considered an obscene gesture because *figa* is slang for female genitalia, and the fingers represent a vulva and vagina, and the thumb a phallus; so basically, sexual intercourse.

This hand gesture can be worn as a charm but is also "thrown" or gestured toward someone or something.

Brevi and Abitini (Amulet Bags)

Italian amulet bags are most generally referred to as *brevi* bags, but they are also called *abitini*. *Brevi* literally means "short" or "brief" because they are small bags, but also because a brevi is usually made for acute needs at any time during life. *Abitini* is used interchangeably with *brevi*, but it also can refer to a specific type of amulet bag made for rites of passage such as a baptism. A brevi bag, then, is used in the moment for a specific purpose such as curing an illness, and an abitini is kept throughout life or at least through childhood or through a certain phase of life as a memento of protection and support.

> *Chiamati anche devozionali o devozioni, abitini o abbatini, i brevi sono piccoli sacchetti di stoffa cuciti a mano e recanti all'interno oggetti apotropaici per proteggere dal male come erbe, piccole frasi scritte, pietre, peli di animale, cera di candele benedette e via dicendo.[8]*

> Also called devotionals or devotions, abitini or abbatini, brevi are small hand-sewn fabric bags containing apotropaic objects to protect against evil such as herbs, small written sentences, stones, animal hair, wax from blessed candles, and so on.

Brevi and abitini are made from pieces of cloth and are worn similarly as charms. The folk Catholic version of these are scapulars. A scapular has two small pieces of cloth, usually wool, that are hung on ribbons or some type of cord. One piece hangs from the front, and one from the back. Usually the scapular has an image on it of a saint or other deity and sometimes other ornamentation such as embroidery.

Amulet bags have ancient roots in many cultures. In ancient Rome it was customary for boys to be given a *bulla*, and girls to be given a *lunula*. These were usually made from gold, were similar to lockets, and would contain a charm or coin.[9]

Make a Brevi

Making your own brevi can be a simple or extravagant process. Below are some basic instructions on which you can elaborate. It is customary to say a prayer before and after making one. This can be a Hail Mary or a prayer to Saint Michael.

1. Cut out a 4″ x 4″ piece of cloth. Red cloth is traditional, but any material can be used, including old towels or T-shirts.
2. Lay the cloth on a flat surface and place the apotropaic items in the center of it. These items can be charms, saint cards, herbs, or written words or prayers.
3. Fold the four corners of the bag together and tie with a ribbon or string.
4. These bags can be worn inside of a coat, tied to a baby's crib, worn on a string around the neck, or carried in any other possible way that works for you. Often Italian women place them inside their bra.

Note: You may want to add a small safety pin to the outside of the bag so that the person you are making it for can pin it to their clothing.

Sale (Salt)

As discussed in earlier chapters, salt is a potent and universal cleanser, protector, and neutralizing agent. It can be sprinkled around the perimeter of your home, your property, or a room. Bowls of salt can also be placed in a room to keep it clear and protected.

In the tradition of Benedicaria and other folk Catholic practices ritual and protective salt must be blessed before it is used. You can find instructions for doing so in chapter 7.

One traditional practice from the Benevento region of Italy is to place salt in a bowl or other type of vessel outside the front door. This is thought to keep witches from entering through the keyhole or cracks in the door at night. According to the legend, a witch is obligated to count every grain of salt before she can enter, and it takes her so long to count them that the Sun comes up before she is done, and she has to leave.

Exorcizing a House or Building with Salt

While walking three times around the inside and outside of the building, throw salt and recite the following:

Sale sapienza
Portaci pace, salute e providenza
Allontana fatture, malocchi e invidia
Lo chiedo e lo commando
In nome del Signore e della beata
Vergine Maria
E così sia.[10]

Salt wisdom
Bring us peace, health and providence
Keep away curses, evil eyes and envy
I ask it and command it
In the name of the Lord
and the Blessed Virgin Mary
And so mote it be.

Mazzo di Erbe (Herb Bundles)

Placing a *mazzo di erbe*, or herb bundle, on or above doors or thresholds is another way to protect entrances as well as specific rooms. These can be made with fresh or dried plants. I usually use an odd number of plants, either three, five, or nine, and I often use mugwort, sweet basil, and yarrow and tie them together with a red ribbon.

*Il Mazz de san Giuan era un mazzo di erbe raccolte la notte di san Giovanni (24 giugno). Questo mazzo era benedetto in chiesa il giorno della festa del Batttista, e usato, durante l'anno sequente, come rimedio contro le infermità dell e persone, degli animali e come scongiuro contro i temporali. Le specie variavano da zona a zona, abbiamo notizie certe dell'uso di camomilla (*Matricaria chamomilla L.*), assenzio (*Artemisia absinthium L.*), e aglio (*Allium sativum L.*); a volte si aggiungevano rami carichi di ciliege (*Prunus avium L.*) e ribes rosso (*Ribes rubrum L.*).[11]*

The Mazz de San Giuan (Giovanni) was a bunch of herbs collected on the night of Saint John (June 24). This bundle was blessed in the church on the feast day of the Baptist, and used, during the following year, as a remedy against the infirmities of people, animals and as a ward against storms. The species varied from area to area, we have reports that chamomile (*Matricaria chamomilla* L.), wormwood (*Artemisia absinthium* L.), and garlic (*Allium sativum* L.); sometimes branches loaded with cherries (*Prunus avium* L.) and red currant (*Ribes rubrum* L.) were added.

When choosing plants for herb bundles, consider using plants that live around you such as angelica, Saint John's wort, wormwood, or motherwort or some of the other commonly used apotropaic plants listed below.

EXAMPLES OF APOTROPAIC PLANTS

Alloro (Bay Laurel): Used to worship the god Apollo and celebrate victory and triumph in Greece as well as Rome, bay laurel is also known well as a culinary herb.

Artemisia (Mugwort): Known cross-culturally as a protection plant, mugwort is used for cleansing and purification and in ritual as a sacred smoke much like other artemisias and sages.

Rosmarino (Rosemary): Used to move and circulate energy in a room when burned or in the body when taken as an herbal preparation.

Achillea (Yarrow): A protection plant that has been traditionally celebrated at midsummer, yarrow is placed in plant bundles with other herbs to be hung above doorways or burned for smoke.

Ruta (Rue): Called the "herb of grace" because it is thought to provide grazia, rue can be dipped in holy water and used to sprinkle on people or the home and garden as a blessing and as a method of purification.

Aglio (Garlic): Considered by Pliny the Elder to be a cure-all, garlic is one of the plants of Saint Michael and is often added to brevi bags or simply worn around the neck as a protective amulet.

The Ethics of Protection

Below is a list of ethics to keep in mind when working with protection magic:

- There is really nothing to protect. This does not mean that others don't try to cause us harm or that we don't get hurt. It means that we are each a complete embodied expression of the eternal and a participant in the continuous play of universal forces that are unassailable and over which we always have some degree of influence. Practices that we use for protection should ultimately relax and center us in a way that brings us into full engagement with our surroundings.

- Spells, prayers, and gestures of protection, when practiced and imprinted on our psyche, signal a shift of consciousness that concentrates and centers our energy, enabling us to become more present to our fullness of being. They allow us to fill up our righteous physical and psychic space with confidence and clarity, and they resolve self-doubt, distraction, and dissociation, all of which can lead us into harmful situations.

- Protection magic is not about certainty, bending reality to our will, or controlling the behavior of others. Instead, it positions us squarely in ourselves and is more about enacting our agency and confidence in our ability to weave who we are with the layers of reality. In essence, it's about creation.

❦ Apotropaic techniques and devices allow us to attune our senses and develop our receptivity and responsiveness to external conditions so that we can discern how and when to avoid entanglements that could cause us harm as well as respond to harm by gathering our energy and our creativity.

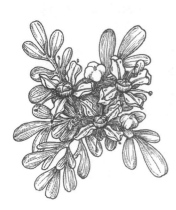

12
Portafortuna

Divinatory Arts for Good Fortune

WE'VE TALKED ABOUT DIVINATION throughout this book, but in this chapter we'll explore some specific techniques. Divination, also referred to as the mantic arts, appeared on the Italic peninsula way before even the Roman Empire. Divination is often thought of as a means of knowing and thereby controlling the future, but that's only one small sliver of the capacity of divining. It is also sometimes understood as a way to know which aspects of life are "predestined," but that assumes some type of fixedness or stagnation, as if something in this universe could be predictable. If we live in a cyclical universe that is in a continuous flow then there is nothing that is essentially predetermined. In astrology we differentiate between fate and destiny. Fate is how the chart has been laid out, and destiny is what you do with it. There is nothing that is not alive and therefore dynamic and moveable, and divination is how we learn that we are actually in that continuous flow.

Often our dominant narratives around divination lead us to believe that it is simply fortune-telling; and even sometimes the use of the word *folk* to describe nonprofessional, state-sanctioned healing practices, has taken on a diminished connotation. The idea is that "folk," or divinatory, practices are superstitious (another term with derogatory connotations) and based in fantasy instead of science. This idea of "science" is also a narrow view of what qualifies as scientific and, in fact, the mantic arts are and always have been a type of science. *Science* is defined by the Oxford dictionary as "the systematic study of the structure and behavior of the physical and natural world through observation, experimentation, and the testing of theories against the evidence obtained" and "knowledge of any kind." The mantic arts fall under both of these categories.

Etymologically, the word *divination* comes from *divinacioun*, meaning "discovering what is hidden or obscure" and from the Proto-Indo-European root *dyeu-*, which means "to shine."[1] It also comes from the Latin *divinationem*, which means "the power of foreseeing, prediction," or to be "inspired by God."

Divination was and is practiced by cultures worldwide, and the word has many connotations from fortune-telling to oracular prophecy. Daoist practitioner Liu Ming spoke about divination as a form of attunement: "Divination isn't to figure out what God wants you to do, it's to know how amazing we are, how we are spontaneously adjusting ourselves to the Feng Shui of the room."[2] In this sense, divination is a tuning fork. It is also a form of diagnosis and one could argue that all forms of diagnosis are divinatory in nature. Even our medical diagnosis requires practices that would fall under the systems of traditional diagnosis. In particular, divination is a form of pattern recognition, and all clinical diagnosis by professional medicine is based on this. Even our high diagnostic technologies require someone that can "read" the results. As Liu Ming said, "Whether it's the pulse or a lab test, it is still divination. One of them isn't more legitimate than the other."

Divination is a language or many languages that connect us to the patterns that are moving in our fields of experience. It makes us aware of the flow we're in, and a mantic practitioner, or iatromantis, is one who is in that flow of patterns of consciousness and facilitates such in the work of healing. As discussed in chapter 2, *iatromantis* is a Greek word that literally means "physician-seer,"[3] so this is a visionary doctor or what some might call a shaman. This is a person who can work with a patient or client and establish a rapport with them to determine the cyclical phase and pattern they're experiencing in the moment. Ultimately, it is a practice of "reading" time and mapping it in some way to gain clarity on what needs to be done or not. We see this in modern medicine when a diagnosis includes a disease state such as stage 1 or stage 2. This tells us the phase, cycle, or timing of a condition or circumstance.

In both ancient Greece and Rome, we see several methods of divination, including the oracular trance that was mentioned in the discussion in chapter 3 about the Sibyls and the Pythia. In the next chapter we will discuss dream incubation, which was another major divinatory art. There were many other divinatory practices and skill sets that were used for not just medical or healing purposes but also for sociopolitical quandaries. Examples include augury (reading the direction taken by a flock of birds), haruspicy (reading animal entrails), and bibliomancy (reading a random passage in a book).

Some of the most well-known examples of bibliomancy is the reading of the Sibylline Books by the priests of the Roman Kingdom (pre-Roman Empire; likely Etruscan). This practice is quite resonant with some of our modern divination practices, such as shuffling tarot cards and pulling one at random. In this case, the prophecies of the Sibyl of Cumae, who had written them on a series of either oak leaves or papyrus, were read when the future or current conditions were in question. The priests "spread out the rolls and chose a passage at random, allowing fate or the will of the gods to choose the remedy to be applied."[4]

Portafortuna (Bringing Luck)

Included under the umbrella of divination is what is known in Italian folk medicine as *portafortuna*, which literally means "to bring (*porta*) luck (*fortuna*)" and refers to specific practices that will bring good luck, and *cleromanzia*, or cleromancy, which is the practice of "following the signs." Both practices are included in divination as they are methods requiring contact with the continuity of time. These practices do not place humans as victims or subjects without agency. Although they can be perceived or applied that way, it is more effective to apply them as a form of communication and a means of self-direction whereby we can move and shift ourselves in the way we are flowing with the universe.

Along with portafortuna, we have its contrary force of *sfortuna* or "bad luck," and all that comes to us as misfortune. These are not essentially binary but instead are part of cyclical nature, or losing and receiving in relationship to reciprocal exchange. This is expressed in the common phrase "you reap what you sow," which tells us that there is some natural order of things. When we apply techniques of portafortuna we are calling in something extra in the form of abundance. In this sense, portafortuna and sfortuna are not binary, separate forces but are both expressions of relationship that can be shifted one way or the other using various techniques.

Both good luck and bad luck are extreme poles in the cycle of giving and receiving, so when someone has an intention of receiving good luck they are hoping for something more or extra beyond the balanced cycle of exchange, or cause and effect. A good-luck charm, for example, will shift the balance of exchange toward fortune. This corresponds to the concept of grazia, or grace, that provides or magnetizes something in a supernatural manner, and so is beyond the natural cycles. When we receive good luck, we are being touched by fortune outside of direct cause and effect.

Here we can circle back to the idea that lucky charms in the form of words, phrases, actions, and of course various lucky objects must be given. A gift is a form of grazia and good luck in that it is a form of abundance for which we did have to lose or give anything to receive. We see this happen in Italian folk magic in another, more controversial way, and that is in stealing. By stealing we are receiving abundance for which we did not have to give anything:

In these ideas, we again find the extra in the sense of extra-economic. If a person buys a horse-shoe, for instance, he participates in an economic transaction in which objects of value are exchanged. In stealing something or receiving it as a gift, a person gains without losing. The value so stolen or received is separate from, and additional and extra to, the transactional exchanges of ordinary economy. The incidentally found, stolen or gratuitously received object embodies the notion of the extra and is therefore believed to promote it in the form of good fortune.[5]

Good luck and bad luck are also tracked by following certain signs and omens. Every region and even every family will have their own system of signs but the lists below provide a number of common ones:

Good Luck Signs
- ❧ Bird droppings falling on a person
- ❧ A four-leaf clover being found in the grass
- ❧ A two-tailed lizard appearing on the path
- ❧ A bee buzzing around a person
- ❧ A cricket jumping on a person

Bad Luck Signs
- ❧ A broken mirror
- ❧ A missed train
- ❧ The number 17
- ❧ Spilled salt, oil, or wine
- ❧ A black hornet or a bird found inside a house

At the center of all this is the vital force, as we discussed in chapter 5. Portafortuna and sfortuna are ways in which people act to facilitate the vital force. In particular, when people such as Southern Italians have been subject to a long-term lack of finite resources and economic prosperity, these are the ways in which they empower their agency, for better or worse.

Tarocchi and Cartomanzia
(Tarot and Cartomancy)

Other common forms of divination were and continue to be part of Italian culture to this day. The following divination practices are not exclusive to Italian culture, but while they are common in many cultures, they have taken on their own form in Southern Italy and the Italian diaspora. One of the most common forms of divination is the use of the tarot. The tarot has become a controversial topic that I have to address in order to have any discussion about tarot divination. The origins of tarot divination are not completely known. The word *tarot* comes from the Italian word *tarocchi*, which means "foolishness" and refers to a card game called *Trionfi*, which was played in fifteenth-century Italy.

How it became used as a tool for divination, or cartomanzia, is not clear but the Romani claim to be the first group of people to have used it as such. There is no documented evidence that supports this, but because it's an oral tradition and because the Romani have been and continue to be oppressed, it is not something that would have made it to the ethnographic archives.

We know that marginalized groups don't generally have access to resources that document their history and, in fact, their history is often erased. I don't believe myself to have the tools or knowledge to make an informed determination on the origins of tarot divination as I was not present during the fifteenth century, and oral tradition is utterly subjective. That said, it is common knowledge that the Romani have been primary carriers of tarot divination and that fortune-telling has been one of their means of economic survival for centuries. I suggest that anyone who is considering starting a tarot practice or, in particular, a business reading tarot, do some research to make your own assessment of the information.

I am not a tarot reader, but I do use the tarot for personal divination, and it is an important divinatory tool in Italian folk magic and part of our oral tradition.

Cartomancy in Italy

Contributed by Gina Miele

While scholars dispute the origins of tarot due to a lack of written documentation, one thing is clear: cards of all sorts were popular across Europe during the Renaissance, and in Italy in particular, beautifully designed decks were produced for the powerful courts of the period ("Gli antichi tarocchi siciliani" n.d.). The cards, called *trionfi* (triumphs/trumps) were used to play games, including the Gioco dei tarocchi, or Game of Tarot. From the *Visconti-Sforza Tarot* in Milan to the *Minchiate fiorentine* of Florence and the *Tarocchino bolognese* of Bologna, tarot played a significant cultural and historical role on the land that is now known as Italy. In the nineteenth century, the association of the decks with divination and the occult in a practice called *cartomanzia*, or cartomancy (fortune-telling with playing cards) gained currency, with kings and illustrious figures consulting the cards before making political or military moves (Barbadoro). At the same time, in southern Italy, fortune-telling by way of card reading primarily utilized regional playing cards, specifically the Neapolitan (*le carte napoletane*) and Sicilian (*il tarocco siciliano*) decks.

The oldest surviving tarot cards on record are three decks produced in Milan in the mid-fifteenth century. The oldest, the *Visconti di Modrone Tarot*, was commissioned by Duke Filippo Maria Visconti, Duke of Milan. It was followed by the *Visconti Brambilla Tarot* and the *Visconti Sforza Tarot*, made for Francesco Sforza, Filippo Maria Visconti's son-in-law. Historical tarot lovers can view surviving Visconti tarot cards at the Accademia Carrara in Bergamo, the Pinacoteca di Brera in Milan, the Morgan Library and Museum in New York, and the Beinecke Rare Book and Manuscript Library at Yale University (Husband 2016). Fifteenth-century Ferrara also produced two important tarot decks under the duchy of Borso d'Este: the *Mantegna Tarot*, created by Andrea Mantegna, and the *Sola Busca Tarot*, which likely inspired some of Pamela Colman Smith's illustrations for the *Rider-Waite-Smith Tarot Deck* of 1909 ("A Renaissance Riddle" n.d.).

In the nineteenth century, an explosion of tarot decks in Italy coincided with a renewed interest in the occult and the utilization of the cards for fortune-telling. Many of these historical decks have been reproduced by artists at Milan's Il Meneghello Edizioni and Turin's Lo Scarabeo, including the *Gumppenberg Tarot* (1810), the *Soprafino Tarot* (1835), the *Sibilla Oracle* (1850), the *Minchiate Fiorentine Tarot* (1850), and the *Naibi Tarot* (1893).

While some sources indicate that the divinatory use of Neapolitan playing cards began as early as the Middle Ages by *fattucchiere* (women who practiced magic) in the poorest districts of Naples ("Tarocchi

Napoletani" n.d.), others locate the origin of the practice in Naples to the Spanish domination, beginning in the early sixteenth century. In her research on cartomanzia in Naples, Alessia D'Anna claims card reading reached its height under the Bourbon dynasty's reign from 1734 to 1861. She suggests that soldiers' wives may have been the first to scrutinize the cards for news of their husbands' fates in battle. The older women of the city closely guarded their knowledge, orally passing down the secret skill to their children and other young women who wished to practice the art of cartomancy (D'Anna).

Similarly in Sicily, *il tarocco siciliano* was (and is) used both for card games and fortune-telling. Like the Neapolitan deck, the cards are divided into four suits: *spade* (swords), *coppe* (cups), *denari* (coins) and *bastoni* (clubs). Since the mid-twentieth century, a renewed interest in the practice, both in Italy and the Italian diaspora, has fueled the creation of websites and books with instructions on how to couple intuition with prophecy through cartomancy. In his article on the *guaratrici* (healers) in Ragusa, Sicily, Salvatore Battaglia shares that his mother revealed the art of reading cards to him on the condition that he practice it only to help others. Card readers, he cautions, may accept goods in kind, but never money (Battaglia, 2021).

Works Cited

"A Renaissance Riddle: The Sola Busca Tarot Deck (1491)," The Public Domain Review (website).

Barbadoro, Giancarlo. "I Tarocchi." Libreria ASEQ (website).

Battaglia, Salvatore. "Ragusa. tra medicina e tradizione popolare: in sicilia c'era "a signura cha cuogghia i viermi' e ca leggia i Tarocchi." Libertà Sicilia (website), March 15, 2021.

D'Anna, Alessia. "Divinazione con le carte napoletane: la storia." *Figli del Vesuvio* (blog), November 1, 2019.

"Gli antichi tarocchi siciliani," Nuovo Sud (website).

Husband, Tim. "Before Fortune-Telling: The History and Structure of Tarot Cards." The Metropolitan Museum of Art (website), April 8, 2016.

"Tarocchi napoletani: esempio di facile lettura delle carte." Villaggi Campania (website).

Other forms of divination are multiple and varied. Almost any form or function of nature can be determined to be part of nature's pattern and therefore interpreted as an expression of the divine.

Favomanzia (Favomancy)

Favomanzia, or favomancy, is bean divination or "throwing the beans." This involves the use of some type of whole legume, usually fava beans or chickpeas, and throwing them so that they randomly scatter. Then the pattern is read and interpreted. This is another practice that has unclear origins but likely came from Russia and/or Mongolia. Favomancy is a form of cleromancy that involves the throwing of any small objects such as grains, bones, pebbles, and even dice. Fava beans in particular are thought to bring good luck and are often added to amulet bags or just carried in a pocket.

Fava bean (vicia fava) may be served in a frittata or in garlic sauce. When dried, roasted and blessed, it becomes the very popular "lucky bean." Legend has it that you will never be broke as long as you carry one. Some people believe that if you keep one in the pantry, there will always be food in the kitchen. The legend of the fava bean began during the famine in Sicily, where the bean was used as fodder for cattle. To survive, the farmers prepared them for the table. Hence, they considered themselves lucky to have them. The bean is also a symbol of fertility, since it grows well even in poor, rocky soil. Italians would carry a bean from a good crop to ensure a good crop the following year. The blessed dried beans are distributed at altars along with pieces of blessed bread.[6]

Caffeomanzia (Caffeomancy)

This is the reading of coffee grounds and is similar to reading tea leaves. The process involves using unfiltered coffee such as Turkish style. There are many versions of how to do this but basically you pour a cup of unfiltered coffee, drink it halfway so that much of the liquid is gone, and you can see the thick grounds on the bottom of the cup. Then turn the cup upside down, turn it three times, then lift it up and read the pattern that has been made by the grounds.

Ring and String Divination

This is one of the most popular divination tools that I've noticed in Italian-American communities. The ring and string divination tool can be used anywhere with nothing but a wedding ring (or other preferably gold ring) and a piece of string. Basically, you string a ring onto a string, thread, or piece of yarn and use it as a dowsing tool. This can be done with any pendulum type instrument, a crystal, or a charm. Again, there are many ways of interpreting the way the ring moves but the best way to determine this is by asking the ring. You hold the string, with the ring strung on it, so that the ring can swing. You bring the ring to a center and nonmoving position and then ask it which way is which. For example, this is often used to determine the sex of an unborn baby (this obviously started before sonograms and gender reveal parties). To do this, ask the ring, "Which way is for female?" and note the way that it swings. The ring will move itself. You can then ask, "Which way for male?"and note that. Then you can ask what the gender of the baby will be and see which way it swings. Any question can be asked and answered through this process.

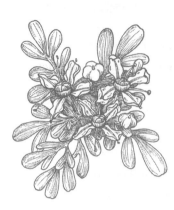

13

Dream Incubation

Healing through Communal and Individual Practices

Dream Incubation remained central to western medicine from about 600 BCE until about 500 CE when the church ended it because they wanted to have the franchise on revelation.

PETER KINGSLEY

[The doctor] ought to be able to bring about love and reconciliation between the most antithetic elements in the body. . . . Our ancestor Asclepius knew how to bring love and concord to these opposites, and he it was, as the poets say and I believe, who founded our art.

PLATO, *THE SYMPOSIUM*

THE WORD *INCUBATION* is from the Greek, ἐγκοίμησις or *enkoimesis*, which means "to sleep within" and was translated to Latin as *incubatio* or *incubare*. Dream incubation is an ancient practice that likely first emerged in the Near East (Mesopotamia, Anatolia, and the Levant) and then spread to Egypt 4,000 years ago and to Greece where various practices that induced trance and sleep states brought people into contact with the divine in order to invoke healing.

Incubation is basically the healing received in a dream, usually by a deity. It is a mantic art and in the Greek and Roman world was a form of physical and spiritual healing as well as a divinatory practice. A "dream temple" is a temple devoted to the practice of incubation and includes places for those in need of dream healing to enter into the process. It is thought that the Latin translation only came into use during the medieval period when people would go to sacred sites and shrines to sleep and receive healing from a saint as part of the cult of the saint's traditions.

There is both ritual incubation and "unintentional" incubation. Ritual incubation includes customs and specific steps or practices that intentionally cultivate a dream for a specific reason. Frequently, when one decided to take a pilgrimage to a dream temple it was because they were "called," often in a dream. In order to take on a journey such as this required a certain amount of resources so it was not possible for everyone. Yet dreaming is always available to us all and unintentional incubation happens spontaneously, during sleep, anywhere.

Incubation was often generated collectively with several people or groups of worshippers sleeping in the same place. This was a time in history when individuality was far less extreme. Dream temples were designed so that many people could incubate in the same area together. These temples were located within sanctuaries or healing centers. The sanctuary was often dedicated to different gods or goddesses, but the dream temple itself was usually dedicated to Asclepius, the god of healing. Not only were the temples dedicated to Asclepius, but they were designed to invite him in.

Incubation was practiced in the area of the temples known as an *abaton* (a word derived from *ábatos* meaning "inaccessible") or *enkoimeterion* (meaning a place to sleep), which was a secluded section of the temple where people went to dream. Often these were built into complexes where several places of worship were constructed near each other. Those that were dedicated to healing were centers where human and more-than-human wisdom could be channeled through a "therapeutic landscape" and merge with those seeking cures and knowledge as well as a greater understanding of their place in the world.

There were dream temples all over the Greco-Roman world. Here are a few of the locations:

Greece
Kos/Cos: Greek island

Epidaurus: Now the modern towns of Palaia (Ancient) Epidaurus and Nea (New) Epidaurus

Trikka: Now Trikala in northwestern Thessaly

Italy
Rome: On the Isola Tiberina (Tiber Island)

Velia: Now Ascea, Salerno

Akragas: Now Agrigento, Sicily

Pompeii: Now a preserved city near Naples

Enkoimesis

Enkoimesis, also called "dreamless sleep," is the state of consciousness desired to achieve direct realization of the eternal/divine. Many people made a pilgrimage to the dream temples to receive healing for acute and/ or specific conditions or circumstances, while others were devoted to the lifelong practice of dream incubation. Often these were people who might be called the priests or priestesses of the temple, or the iatromanteis. For the devoted dream practitioner, the ultimate goal of incubation was to acquire a state of complete awareness and consciousness beyond dualistic reality. This state is sometimes thought of as "Christ consciousness" or, in Hindu tradition, *turiya*, and is the most attuned state of sensory perception. It is a state of utter stillness that is considered to be near death or similar to death, and it was practiced by high initiates in the cult of Asclepius as a method of staying aware during the transition of death as well as a tool for enlightenment.

Oneiromancy

Dream incubation can also offer oneiromancy—from the Greek *oneiros* (dream) and *manteia* (prophecy/seeing)—or divination based on dreams, which ultimately is intended to lead to healing. Dream incubation invites a "visitation," or contact with a divine spiritual force, usually the god Asclepius. It was embedded in the cultural context and often part of a person's spiritual path, a greater plan in their healing journey, or an aspect of collective connection to God and to community healing. It is also a form of divination as we discussed in the last chapter. Divination, again, is a means of orienting ourselves in the flow or continuum of time and becoming clear on the patterns that are moving through our field of experience. Incubation, or dreamwork, is yet another ancient technique to engage with the living world in such a way.

Dreaming is one of our access points to our unconscious realms, and our dreams bring what's unconscious into consciousness in a symbolic manner. When we interpret and understand these symbols, they can help us integrate their meanings into our psyche and soma, body and soul, so that we can live in optimal embodied presence, health, and relations.

Integration of these meanings occurs as a result of the following:

1. Identifying the basic quality, type, and conditions of the dream. This includes assessing the scene, place, symbols, feelings or basic energy, and characters of the dream.
2. Determining what's happening, what your position is in the dream, what others are doing, and what the pattern of the narrative is.
3. Interpretation of all the elements in 1 and 2.

The value of dreamwork was one of the core tenets of the work of psychiatrist and psychoanalyst Carl Jung, and his framework for dream interpretation has become part of a vast source of knowledge in the Western world. While dreams to the ancient Greeks and Romans were just as real as waking life and were believed to be on a spectrum that could be integrated and woven or sewn together, our modern ideas around psychology have created a polar template whereby the unconscious and conscious are at opposite positions. Polarity is a creation pattern or a tool that pulls a single force into opposite directions so that the tension/energy created between them births something new and emergent.

Polar Creation Pattern

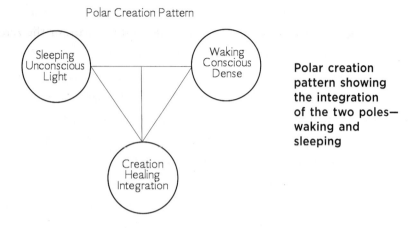

Polar creation pattern showing the integration of the two poles— waking and sleeping

In terms of Jungian psychology, the goal of dream incubation is to access one of the poles (waking or sleeping), the unconscious, or the divine, so that we can understand whether the two poles are working together in service of healing and creation or not. The unconscious side of this is usually unknown to us until we act in some way to bring it to our awareness. The desire to do this usually arises from some problem or situation that makes us uncomfortable or causes pain in such a way that we are driven to understand the underlying forces connected to it. Jung is famous for saying, "The psychological rule says that when an inner situation is not made conscious, it happens outside as fate." In other words, the unconscious realms are always present and have an impact on our lives whether we are consciously aware of them or not.

> *Waking and dreaming are in relationship to each other. One is the outer experience, one is the inner experience. They are the two wings of the butterfly. They require each other to stay aloft and you are at the center . . . that is where the substance of your character is ripened.*
>
> TOKO-PA TURNER

The dream spectrum figure was adapted from a rendering of Carl Jung's concepts as described in *Dancing in the Flames* by Marion Woodman and Elinor Dickson. This image shows the relationship of the electromagnetic spectrum and the subtle body and where soma (body) meets pneuma (spirit) at the midground of the soul (psyche), or the zero point. The zero point is where transformation occurs with the dream/ trance experience being the bridge. Dreamwork and incubation provide us with access to the unconscious forms and symbols that our experience takes. Healing occurs when we understand the meanings of those forms and can integrate them with the forms that our experience takes in our waking life. In this tradition, healing emerges when there is alignment/ coherence between the imaginal/spirit/divine/unconscious realms and the material world. Symptoms, illness, distress, and disease are all rooted in the dissonance between ourselves and the divine.

In ancient Greek this was called *soma kai psyche*, which literally means "body and soul" but implies the union of both through alignment or resonance within both psyche and soma. Whatever brings psyche and soma together is the *sympatheia*, which translates to "symptom" and is the *coniunctio natura*, or bridge point/link between the worlds. This has been compared to Jung's concept of synchronicity where outer experience or synchronicities/coincidences arise naturally from the contact zone of the realms. From this view we can see how illness, strife, and trauma can all become gateways or beacons toward healing.

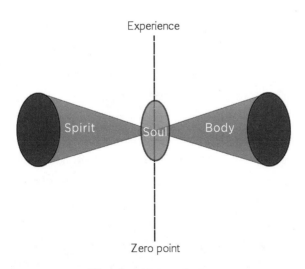

The dream spectrum

Steps of Dream Incubation

We all can dream and there are no "rules" about how to dream. Dreaming is a basic human function and, in fact, it is merely a state change. We experience different states of consciousness all day, every day. In this sense, we are always dreaming in some way. This means that we are receiving sensory and symbolic information with meanings attached to them all of the time. When we are in a dream state the symbolic propensity of our psyche is increased, and when we are awake it is lessened, but it still always present. Everything we see, hear, and do has symbolic meaning. By symbolic I am referring to the form that something takes vs. what that form is associated with in our psyche. Every letter on this page is a symbol that represents a sound and when several sounds are put together they form a word, which also makes a sound that we have attached a meaning to. Therefore, every word is a symbol.

Because our symbolic awareness is largely personal and based on our own life experience and the associations we have with symbols, dream interpretation is not well accomplished using generalized dream books. Every dream symbol will have different associations to every person, depending on their own unique experience with it. This is particularly true in our modern world whereby we have become far more individualistic than our ancestors were. As a traditional practice in Italian folk medicine there are specific dream symbols that have a collective meaning. In my own family we had common dream symbols that, if one saw them in a dream, they had a universal meaning for our family. However, these meanings might be different for different families.

Familial dream practices in Italian folk medicine usually involved the sharing of dreams that had significance for either the family or the individual. In Italian families, a significant dream had by an individual is significant for the entire family because we operate as one unit in many ways. Significant dream symbols in Italian folk medicine are predictive, often related to the warning of an upcoming death or a visitation from a loved one who has already passed and is letting someone know that they are doing okay, or if they are not okay, what they might need from the living in order to complete their transition. Dreams can also indicate the outcome of important circumstances or help discern an action needed to resolve an issue.

The seven ancient steps to dream incubation are based on the ethnographic information that's been collected from various translations and texts. These steps can be adapted to create a dream practice. One of the foundational components of dream incubation is that the quest for a dream is timely and aligned with the divine will. Sometimes we only have the energy/capacity to perform an "abridged" version of the steps. This is completely fine to do as any effort at all toward making that connection will be beneficial.

The seven traditional steps I've listed here are my own adaptations from the book *Where Dreams May Come* by Gil. H. Renberg.[1] Each of these steps is described in detail in the sections below.

1. Incubation
2. Preparatory period
3. Offerings, sacrifice, and consultation fee
4. Ritual and prayer
5. Sleep/dream
6. Dream interpretation/prescription
7. Ex-votos (votive offerings)

Step 1: Incubation

Incubation began with a question or a longing for healing and wisdom. It is often recorded that the dream querent would have to be called by Asclepius to the dream temple in order for the dream to be effective. In other words, one couldn't just decide they needed healing; the healing process and form of treatment had to be aligned with the will of the gods.

Step 2: Preparatory Period

The prepatory period began outside of the abaton and usually involved prayer and purification. Often a sacred bath would be performed as well as sacrifices and offerings to the gods and goddesses. Dream incubation could be an intense ordeal, and the idea of "preparation" assured that the individual was ready for the experience on both a spiritual and neuro-emotional level. Once the pilgrim arrived at the temple, an assessment was made as to what they needed to do in order to be prepared to enter the abaton. This often involved the following:

- ❧ Purifying baths
- ❧ Specific diet
- ❧ Prayer and meditation
- ❧ Herbal preparations
- ❧ Theater*

This was a healing process where storytellers and actors would bring people into the imaginal/mythic realms so they could give meaning to their own similar psychological experiences through the understanding of a myth. The passage of time-time as healer, or just spending time at the sanctuary, resting, and being with the spiritual community was thought to prepare the person for what was to come.

Step 3: Offerings, Sacrifice, and Consultation Fee
Offerings were part of the preparatory process and made as part of the reciprocal energy exchange. They could be one or more of the following:

- ❧ Cakes
- ❧ Prayers
- ❧ Animal sacrifice
- ❧ Fee payment

Offerings, considered a form of sacrifice, were often carried in a *kanoun*, or ritual basket, that contained cakes and fruits. These cakes were known as *popanon* and were made with a specific recipe designed to be offered at altars and to specific gods and goddesses. A small fee was sometimes offered and according to the Pergamum *lex sacra* (sacred law) it was three obols.

---

*Every sanctuary included a theater area where myths and stories were portrayed.

Step 4: Ritual and Prayer

The Pergamum lex sacra provides a description of incubation at the Oropos Amphiareion that included

> what one was to wear—presumably the wreath that is mentioned in the surviving portion, and the white robe apparently mentioned in the other lex sacra just before what appears to be a reference to an olive wreath—as well as what not to wear, since in addition to one or two other prohibitions now lost this other inscription appears to indicate that neither rings nor belts were acceptable and that one was to go barefoot.[2]

Here's an example of a prayer that was said in preparation for incubation from the Greek Magical Papyri:

> :κύριοι θεοί, | χρηματίσατέ μοι ¹ ερὶ τοῦ δεῖνα ¹ ράγματος | ταύτῃ τῇ νυκτί, ταῖς ἐ¹ ερχομέναις ρ[αις]. | ¹ άντως δέομαι, ἱκετεύω, δοῦλος ὑμέτερος | καὶ τεθρονισμένος ὑμῖν.[3]
>
> *Lord gods, reveal to me concerning such-and-such a matter this very night, in the coming hours. I completely beg, I supplicate, as your slave and the one enthroned by you.*

Step 5: Sleep/Dream

Once the first four preparatory steps were completed, the person would be welcomed into the abaton of the temple to begin their sleeping/dreaming. At this point they would lie on a *klinē* (a type of couch) that was placed next to the *agalma* (statue of the god) and then fall asleep, hoping to receive a dream or visitation from Asclepius.

Often the abaton housed both snakes and dogs as they were seen as intermediaries between the worlds as well as healing forces. The lick of a snake or dog would often become the healing remedy, or a snake or dog could appear in a dream and heal the patient.

The expectation was that either Asclepius himself or another god or goddess from Asclepius's family, including his children Hygeia and

Panacea, would come. The sleeping individual could also be attended by other gods or spirits.

Step 6: Dream Interpretation/Prescription

Sometimes the dreamer would be given a divinatory dream that provided them images and symbols, and sometimes they received instructions as to what they needed to do in order for healing to occur. It is thought that these prescriptions would then be brought to the temple healers to be carried out or interpreted.

Step 7: Ex-Votos (Votive Offerings)

When healing or a request was fulfilled, ex-votos, or votive offerings, were typically made. As mentioned in chapter 9, *ex-voto* comes from Latin *ex voto suscepto*, which means "fulfillment of a vow." Ex-votos are still made to the saints and angels as well as to the Virgin Mary. At the ancient dream temples, the gift or offering—often a replica of the body part that was healed—would be made to Asclepius or any deity or spirit that had come in the dream and healed the person.

Elements of Divination

Ancient Greek and Roman dream incubation has six elements, or *stoicheia*, as defined by Artemidorus Daldianus, a Greek diviner who lived in the second century CE and wrote the five-volume treatise Oneirocritica (The Interpretation of Dreams). These elements are not universally symbolic at all but are dependent on the way they converge with the holistic nature of the person and can be found in the scenes, situations, characters, feelings, and perspective of the person in their dream. While all six elements can appear in a dream, most dreams will have one element as a primary focus.

The six elements are as follows:

1. **Nature** (*physis*): Anything that is unconditioned, eternal, expansive or unlimited such as the fundamental nature of the dreamer, a wild or natural place, or any natural element

2. **Convention, law (*nomos*), and social structure:** Culture, written law, and anything that is constrictive or conditioned

3. **Customs and habits:** Collective or individual patterns and routines, which could include daily habits, community celebrations, vernacular phrases and greeting customs, styles of dress, and so on

4. **Occupation, skill, and art:** The person's gifts and how they use them in service to their culture, job, hobbies, creative expressions

5. **Time:** The past, present, future, season, era/age, and so on

6. **Name:** The etymology of words, for example a word is received in a dream and the dreamer discovers that the etymology of the word has a message for them, names of phenomena, and all nouns

Analyzing the stoicheia was one of the fundamental methods of dream interpretation used by the ancients, who compared these dream elements to the waking life of the dreamer to determine whether they were harmonious with it or contrary to it. This meant that the diviner or dream interpreter would need to understand the context of the dreamer's life, including their character, life and situation, mood, personal history, social or cultural identity, economic status, marital status/domestic partnerships, and any other biographical data or pertinent qualities, as well a full description of the dream. Once all this was known, the interpreter would determine whether or not the elements of the dream were *kata physis* (in accordance with) or *para physis* (in opposition to) the same element in waking life.

If the stoichiea in the dream conformed to or was in accordance with the dreamer's experience of them in waking life (kata physis) it was determined to be "good," or auspicious; if they diverged or where oppositional (para physis), it was "bad." This technique was often used to predict future events as well as give meaning to life situations and relationships. It could also help determine where the dreamer needed to establish more balance and where problematic issues needed to be made conscious.

Dream Examples of the Six Elements

The following examples will help illustrate how each element could be represented in a dream and what it might mean to the dreamer.

NATURE (PHYSIS)

If you dream you have three eyes, and obviously you don't in the waking world, that dream would be para physis, or opposed to, your natural state. This could mean that you are not seeing something clearly.

If you dream that you put your hand in a fire, and it feels cold, not hot, that would also be para physis and could tell you that something isn't what it seems in waking life, or perhaps that whatever you believe is "warming" you in life isn't really doing so. Also, often with fire we think of creativity, so it could be that you're not actualizing your creative fire.

If, on the other hand, you build a fire in a dream, and it keeps you warm, then it is kata physis, or in accordance with, your waking life and could mean that whatever you're building will work out.

CONVENTION, LAW (NOMOS), AND SOCIAL STRUCTURE

If you are breaking a law or social norm in a dream that would be para nomos, as the action would be discordant or conflict with the societal law of your waking life.

CUSTOMS AND HABITS

If you normally drink coffee every morning and in your dream you are drinking tea, that would be para and could mean that you should switch to drinking tea. If, on the other hand, you always drink tea in the morning, and you are doing so in your dream, that would be kata and could mean that drinking tea is supportive to you and that maybe you should continue doing it or drink more.

OCCUPATION, SKILL, AND ART

If you're an herbalist in waking life and in your dream you are using a specific herb to heal someone, that would be kata to your skill and could mean that you should use that herb. However, if you're a mechanic in waking life, and you're pouring herbal tea in the engine of a car, that would be para and could mean that you are either in the wrong profession or that your skill needs improvement.

TIME

If you dream of eating an apple when apples are in season that's kata. If you dream of eating an apple, and there's snow on the ground, that's para and could mean that you're not in seasonal or cyclical harmony with one of your behaviors.

NAME

If you dream of a name, particularly a story character or title, find out the etymology of it and see if the meaning matches up to a circumstance in your waking life. If you dream of the word *storm*, and you are planning an outdoor party in your waking world, that would be para. But if you dream of Bacchus, the god of wine, that would be kata.

Ancient Dream Examples

Most often in our dreams more than one or even all six of the stoicheia will appear and therefore we need to assess how they are aligned with each other.

Here are two examples from Artemidorus in *An Ancient Dream Manual* by Peter Thonemann[4]

> Water is cold by nature, so to dream of drinking cold water is always auspicious; to dream of drinking hot water is usually malign, unless it is your personal custom to drink hot water, in which case it is auspicious.

> A man dreamt that he beat his mother, and the dream turned out to be auspicious: the dream-symbol was contrary to law (element 2) but accorded with art, since the man was a potter by profession and one's mother is like the earth.

Combining the elements and interpreting them using this method requires experience, which comes from practice. It's ultimately about knowing yourself (or the dreamer) well, identifying harmonious and inharmonious life patterns.

Asclepius

Asclepius (also spelled Asklepios) is the god of healing, and the Asclepiadic cults began to emerge in 300 BCE onward. The name Asclepius, (/æsˈkliːpiəs/; Greek: Ἀσκληπιός Asklēpiós [askleːpiós]; Latin: Aesculapius) or Hepius, means "unceasingly gentle" based on the interpretation by mythologist Robert Graves.[5] Other interpretations come from the Greek verb *asko or askeo, which means "to practice, to adorn, to work in regards to making art."*[6]

> *Doctor of our ailing, Asklepios, I begin your praise,*
> *Son of Apollo, awakened through Mother Koronis*
> *Of the Dotian Plains, daughter of King Flegion,*
> *Great to humanity, soother of cruel suffering.*
> *And thus are you welcomed, Master. By this song I*
> *beseech you.*[7]
>
> HOMERIC HYMN TO ASKLEPIOS

The origins of Asclepius are not known for sure but most historians believe he emerged first from Thessaly in the form of a pre-Greek god. His name then being Aischlabios or Aislapios. In this phase of his evolution he was what would be called a chthonic god, which as we established in chapter 3 means "in, under, or beneath the earth," or subterranean. Asclepius at this time was also sometimes thought of as a genius loci, or god of place.

The chthonic gods do not live in the sky or heaven, they live here with humans, and in order to have contact with them we must make pilgrimages to their dwellings to meet with them. These dwellings are most often openings such as caves, wells, the hollow trunks of trees, and groves.

There are some accounts that Asclepius was, before anything, a mortal physician who first became a legend and only later became a god. The divine story of Asclepius goes something like the following (please keep in mind that there is a patriarchal overlay here that has shaped the myth over many centuries):

The god Apollo slept with the mortal woman Coronis who became pregnant. She, however, was not in love with Apollo or she was ashamed at her predicament and sought to marry the mortal man Ischys in an effort to legitimize her pregnancy. Apollo got wind of this, apparently from a raven, and killed Coronis. He then rescued his son [Asclepius] from her dead body by performing a cesarean section.

Another version of the story tells us that Coronis abandons Asclepius near Epidaurus on Tittion Mountain where he was cared for by a goat and a dog. It was quite common in Southern Europe for people to substitute goat's milk for mother's milk. There he was found by a shepherd who took him to Apollo.

In both versions, Asclepius was taken to Chiron, the centaur, to be raised and tutored in the healing arts. Chiron was the student of Artemis and the teacher of Asclepius.

Asclepius became so skilled in the art of healing that he began to bring people back from the dead. This upset the balance of birth, death, and rebirth, angering Hades who went to Zeus to complain. Zeus then killed Asclepius with a thunderbolt and then deified him, bringing him up to the sky with the ascended gods and making him into the constellation Ophiuchus, the serpent bearer.

For no one who is slain by a thunderbolt remains without fame. Thus he is also honored as a god.

ARTEMIDORUS

As a sky god, Asclepius was no longer bound to specific locations on Earth and performed miracles from heaven including being in attendance to those seeking his healings in dreams. Shrines and sanctuaries built for gods were intended to either provide an opening for chthonic gods to meet with those on the surface or as containers/vessels for sky gods to come to Earth.

Asclepius did eventually emerge in Christianity as both a saint and as a Christ figure, the archetype of the "divine man" and healer/savior known for his compassion and gentleness.

The Rod of Asclepius

One of the most famous images associated with Asclepius is his staff with the snake wrapped around it. The snake and the dog are totemic symbols of Asclepius and both are considered to have mantic medicine powers. It is thought that nonvenomous snakes inhabited the dream temples, crawling around freely, and lulling patients into their dreams with the repetitive sound of their hiss. Another speculation on the symbolism of the snake, at dream temples and in association with Asclepius, is that their venom was used to induce an oracular trance. The chthonic gods were considered to be oracular healers. The snake is also thought to symbolize regeneration because it sheds its skin.

The rod of Asclepius also resembles the caduceus of Hermes where we see two snakes entwined, symbolizing the resolution of duality as Hermes drove his rod between two fighting snakes to break them up. They then converged and entwined around his staff. It is believed that this snake and staff imagery is probably much older than the staff associated with Aslcepius, dating back to ancient Mesopotamia.

Dogs are also often depicted at the side of Asclepius. A dog that comes in a dream is often considered to be Asclepius himself and, if one is licked by a dog in a dream, it is believed they are healed by them. Dogs in mythology are also often portrayed as psychopomps, or guides into other worlds.

In several inscriptions it is directly conveyed that an animal cured a suffering individual. Two of the inscriptions demonstrate healing by dogs. In the first one . . . there is only a brief statement that a blind boy called Lyson was cured by a dog in the vicinity of the sanctuary.[8]

🌿 Create a Dream Incubation Ritual

To create your own dream incubation ritual, follow the seven steps below.

Step 1: Incubation

This starts with the initial desire or longing to deepen in to dream practice. Or it could be the result of a need or want to understand yourself more. Sometimes there is a specific question or concern that you many want answered or to gain insight about.

Write down your question on paper. Or sit with the questions in your heart and mind.

Step 2: Preparation

Do the following to prepare the day before you want to have a healing dream:

1. Eat a nonaggravating diet of foods that nourish you.
2. Spend time in solitude and contemplation (e.g., meditation, journaling).
3. Take a bath before going to bed with epsom salt and/or healing herbs.
4. Add your own desired preparatory activity here.

Step 3: Offering

Make an offering to a god/goddess/saint/or other spirit being that is associated with dreamers or who you may be petitioning to come to you in your dream.

1. Place some food on your altar (e.g., a sacred ancestral food such as pomegranate seeds)
2. Write a poem to the god Asclepius and read it out loud.
3. Pour a libation (offering of a drink to a deity). This can be a bit of wine or juice poured outside on the ground, in a bowl of salt or soil and placed on an altar, or just poured from one cup to another.
4. Add your own offering ideas here.

Step 4: Ritual and Prayer

Create a ritual and a prayer in preparation for incubuation.

1. Burn incense or a candle.
2. Take a flower essence.
3. Say a prayer to Asclepius or whatever magical or divine being you wish to invoke.
4. Ask a question of Asclepius or another deity.

Step 5: Sleep/Dream

Prepare for a nap or bedtime. Part of this step includes sleep hygiene and preparing the room that you'll be going to sleep in. I suggest learning about sleep hygiene and incorporating what works for you to enable you to relax and slip into the dreamtime. Your sleep location should be comfortable and removed from noise and potential interuptions as much as possible.

1. Before you go to sleep, hold the intention that the answer to your question will come to you when you wake from sleeping/dreaming.
2. Relax and go to sleep.

Step 6: Dream Interpretation

As soon as you start to wake up, search your mind for an answer to your question or a memory of a related dream.

1. Write down the answer you received or describe the related dream with as much detail as possible in your journal.
2. Analyze the answer or dream for any messages, predictions, advice, or instructions that you find helpful.

Step 7: Ex-voto (Votive Offerings)

If you received an answer to your question or had a related dream, it's time to thank your deity.

1. Make an offering of thanks using any of the above ideas for offerings.
2. Draw a symbol, image, word(s), or anything else that you received from your dream and place on your altar.

3. Light a candle.
4. Say a prayer of thanks.

Plants and Flower
Essences for Dreaming

Plants and flower essences can be used for various purposes while practicing dreamwork. Below are some suggestions followed by lists of herbs to use for some of those purposes.

- For help in conjuring/incubating a dream
- For initiating relaxation as we fall asleep
- For protection and grounding when entering the dream world
- As allies in the process of emotionally and neurobiologically integrating the information and messages we receive in dreams
- As plant spirits that show up as dream characters or visitors

Dream Incubation

Artemisia (Mugwort): Enhances dreaming and visions. Place a sprig of mugwort under your pillow or use as a tincture. Caution: Mugwort is contraindicated during pregnancy.

Erba di San Giovanni (Saint John's Wort): Provides spiritual protection from nightmares when used as a flower essence.

Non ti Scordar di Me (Forget-Me-Not): Facilitates or enhances communication between the dreamer and spirit guides/messages in the dream world. Use in the flower-essence form.

Caglio Zolfino (Our Lady's Bedstraw): Calms, enhances sleep, and stimulates dreaming when used as a flower essence.

Oleandro (Oleander): Use for divination, dreamwork, and plant journeying. Brings the dreamtime or unconscious mythic wisdom into our waking consciousness by removing or carving away the outer shell or veils of resistance just as a sculptor releases the being within the clay. Oleander is one the plants supposed to have been used by the Mediterranean Sibyls to induce a prophetic trance and as such is a sacred power plant. Caution: Oleander is known to be toxic and is safe to use as a flower essence only.

Relaxation and Sleep Promotion

Lavanda (Lavender): A calming, relaxing nervine. Take as a tea or tincture or use a small amount of essential oil in bathwater or on your pillow. Caution: Too much lavender can act as a stimulant rather than a relaxant. Use essential oils sparingly or try making an infused oil instead.

Camomilla (Chamomile): Muscle relaxant and antispasmodic. Relieves tension, calms, and cools sympathetic overdrive and hyperarousal of the vagus nerve. Also known to eliminate nightmares and night terrors. Use as a tea, tincture, or flower essence.

Papavero (Poppy): In Italy we would use *Papaver rhoeas*. Here in the United States we might instead use *Eschscholzia californica* (California poppy). A tincture of California poppy before bed can aid sleep.

Protection and Grounding

Rosa (Rose): Protects the heart center and counteracts nightmares; use as a tincture, tea, flower essence, or pretty much any other preparation desired.

Ruta (Rue): For protection while you sleep, place a sprig above the bed, at the bedside, or in an amulet.

Rosmarino (Rosemary): Use as an incense for protection in the dream world. Contraindication: Rosemary can be stimulating in a tea or tincture, so it is not recommended for internal use before bed.

Achillea/Millefoglie (Yarrow): Place a sprig of yarrow under your pillow for protection or take yarrow flower essence.

Alloro (Bay Laurel): Use as an incense for protection and grounding.

Angelica (Angelica): For protection as well as receptivity to visionary messages, use as a flower essence, oil, or amulet.

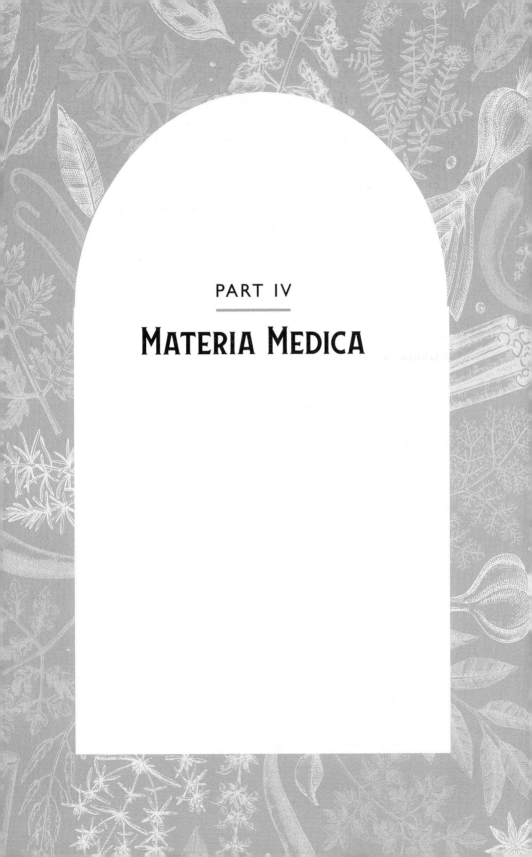

PART IV

MATERIA MEDICA

Introduction to the Materia Medica

The following materia medica includes some of the most common plants used in Italian folk medicine. I have ongoing relationships with these plants and each one is different. The information from each plant doesn't come in consistently, it's an emergent and dynamic experience; I encourage you to make your own relationships with each plant and follow the areas where called to learn more. For example, sometimes we learn about a plant by growing it or by making preparations. Sometimes it's research. They are multidimensional beings as are we, and our relationships aren't textbook. Therefore, you'll see that some of the areas discussed for each plant have more or less information than others because that's what is prominent either in my lived experience or my research. My own efforts to balance this and give a more comprehensive picture of each plant comes from wanting to express their full scope and thus each one is presented in a basic monograph that includes a description of the plant from the following perspectives:

- Taxonomy, etymology, and general description
- Folklore, mythology, and ancient uses
- Current herbal medicine uses
- Italian folk medicine uses—this is a mere sampling of each plant's uses because, of course, there are many and they vary from region to region
- Energetics and correspondences
- Emotional and psychospiritual benefits
- Magical uses
- Preparations and recipes

But these plants are dynamic, and if you are curious about areas that lack information, please listen to that call and step deeper into that area and see what's there.

You will find some herbal terms in the monographs that may not have been discussed in depth in the previous chapters but are included because they are often part of Traditional Western Herbalism descriptions. In some of the monographs you will see the term *doctrine of signatures*, which is an old way of learning the potential actions of a plant by the way it appears, and there is a great deal of information on this if you should want to explore it further.

Please note that although the Italian names are listed first as elsewhere in the book, the plants are in alphabetical order by their English names shown in parentheses to make them easier to reference should you wish to find a particular plant.

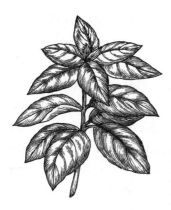

BASILICO (BASIL)
Devil Plant

Family: Lamiaceae
Genus: *Ocimum*
Species: *basilicum*
Italian vernacular names: *Arancio del ciabattino, erba reale*[1]
English vernacular names: Sweet basil, Genovese basil, Italian basil

Where basil grows, no evil goes.—OLD ADAGE

The word *basil* is from the Latin *basillicum* and Greek *basilikon* meaning royal or king. Also, basil is associated with the word *basilisk*. The basilisk is a mythical serpent from Roman legend, and the basil plant is said to be the antidote for its venom.

Basil is an ancient medicinal plant found in apothecary cupboards worldwide as well as in almost every herbal materia medica published now and throughout history. Basil is native to India and Asia, and *Ocimum sanctum*, also known as tulsi or holy basil, is a sacred plant in the Hindu tradition. Genovese basil, or sweet basil, which is the one associated with Italian cuisine, is a cultivar of *Ocimum basilicum* and is protected by the European Union with Denominazione di Origine Protetta certification and is considered a unique species of basil.[2]

Folklore, Mythology, and Ancient Uses

An old folk use of basil from the Middle Ages was to divine the chastity of a woman by placing a basil leaf beneath her bowl. If she ate her meal it meant she was chaste.

The earliest accounts of basil's attributes are associated with anger and hatred and, in some accounts, it was believed that scorpions would grow wherever a basil leaf was placed. It was considered a fiery plant and was often incorporated into myths about Satan. This may be how it came to be known as the devil plant. The Greeks and Romans believed that in order for basil to grow properly you had to curse and yell while planting its seeds.

Basil has, alternately, been associated with love, and it became the feature of folklore and story when Giovanni Boccaccio wrote about it as a balm for lost love in *The Decameron*. This story inspired the poem "Isabella, or the Pot of Basil" by John Keats where he describes how Isabella, when finding out about the murder of her lover Lorenzo, unearths him and buries his head in a pot of basil plants. Basil has often in myth and folklore been associated with love and death, and it has been referred to as the plant of "love washed with tears." The death aspect corresponds to the Mediterranean ritual of placing basil in the hands of the dead to protect them on their journey to the otherworld. It was also thought to protect one from poisonous snakes and evil spirits:

Ma per contrapposizione la stessa pianta avrebbe la facoltá di allon-tanare serpenti, scorpioni e insetti, cosí come gli spiriti malgni. Anche il solo bere un vino al basilico sarebbe utile contrastare i morsi delle vipere e degli altri animali velenosi.[3]

But by contrast, the same plant would have the ability to ward off snakes, scorpions and insects, as well as evil spirits. Even just drinking a wine with basil would be useful to counter the bites of vipers and other poisonous animals.

It has been said that witches drank the juice of basil before they took flight. This is likely because of its protective properties as well as its use on the bridge between life and death.

The legend of the empress Helena, also known as Saint Helena or Saint Helena of the True Cross, is a story of the mother of Roman emperor Constantine the Great, who reigned from 306 to 337 CE. Helena was herself known as the Warrior Queen, with her own army and entourage of priests accompanying her on a pilgrimage to Palestine to recover lost sacred Christian sites. During the process of her explora-tion, she uncovered the "true cross" of Jesus Christ. Legend varies, but it is said that she was attracted to a strong fragrance that led her to a hillside covered in sweet basil plants. Some versions tell that this was the site where a temple dedicated to the goddess Venus was demolished in order to build Constantine's church. It was beneath these ruins that she discovered pieces of three crosses. The Empress divined the true cross by bringing a sick woman to the site and having her touch each cross until she was healed by one, the true cross.

Herbal Medicine Uses

Medicinally, basil has anti-inflammatory and antibiotic properties and can improve digestion. It can be taken as a tea, tincture, or included in cooking recipes.

Italian Folk Medicine Uses

Basil is used in indigenous Italian folk medicine as a facial steam to resolve headaches. It is also used in amulets for protection.

Emotional and Psychospiritual Benefits

Basil comes into our lives when we need to move and release internal obstacles to abundance. If we have grief from love lost or heartbreak that we have resisted feeling, basil can invoke the fire or inspiration, as well as confidence we need to allow the pain of loss to flow, resolve, and integrate as a natural consequence of being alive. It may mean that it's time to take initiative to actualize our own autonomy. It can also mean that we need to address an issue with clear and direct communication. Since this plant falls under the rule of Mars, we may need to confront something whether within or without and transmute it into a force of creation rather than conflict.

Energetics and Correspondences

Energetics: Hot and dry in the first degree
Astrological influence: Mars
Element: Fire
Tarot card: The tower, the suit of wands, and the suit of swords
Deity: Mars, Lucifer

Magical Uses

Basil has long been known as an herb to invoke love and activate love spells. This aspect in modern terms is not about coercing someone into an otherwise unwanted love relationship. It more accurately eases the emotional heart of deeply held trauma and grief that may be stuck or stagnant, making movement and the processing of emotions difficult. This stagnation and lack of dynamic motion can become an obstacle to the reception and generation of attraction as well as the ability of the heart to be a vessel for the reciprocal and reflective exchange of love. Basil stimulates the motion and flow of emotions through the sacred heart so that they may be resolved, integrated, and embodied allowing the heart to regain full capacity and thereby give and receive love and become open to romantic relationships. It is from this that basil is magically known as an herb of attraction.

Basil is used in spells to attract wealth, abundance, customers in business endeavors, inspiration, and joy by alleviating our internal blocks to receiving such blessings. To invoke the power of basil, you can do one or more of the following:

- Place a sprig of fresh basil or a handful of dried basil in a bag in your wallet to attract financial abundance.
- Place a sprig or sprinkle dried on your desk or near your computer to attract business.
- Burn it as incense for protection.
- Wear a sprig as an amulet to strengthen and clear the emotional heart.
- Drink a cup of basil tea daily to release lost love and invite in new love.

Preparations and Recipes

Ocimum basilicum, basil, sweet basil, or as my father says, *basilico* (which sounded to me like basil-LEE-gol) is a commonly known cooking herb that is used in many, if not all, Italian cooking recipes. The leaves are used.

🌿 Basil Honey Vinegar

1 pint jar
1 cup of fresh basil leaves or ½ cup of dried basil
Apple cider vinegar
Honey to taste

1. Chop basil leaves and add to jar.
2. Pour apple cider vinegar over the basil and fill the jar.
3. Leave for two weeks in a cool, dark place, then strain and add honey to taste.

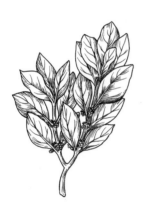

ALLORO (BAY LAUREL)
The Excellent Plant

Family: Lauraceae
Genus: *Laurus*
Species: *nobilis*
Italian vernacular names: *Lauro, melauro, òiro, orbàga*[1]
English vernacular name: *Sweet bay*

Bay laurel, or *alloro* in Italian, is an evergreen tree or shrub that can potentially reach up to sixty feet tall and grows best in warm climates such as that of the Mediterranean. In Latin, the laurel wreath is called *laurus* or *laurea*, from which comes *baccalauréat* in French, *laureato* in Italian, *baccalaureate* in English, and *bachillerato* in Spanish. The word *bay* simply means "berry," and *laurel* originates from Latin as a variation of the Greek name Daphne but with the *D* changed to *L*. This would make it *Daurus*, or from Old Latin, *Dacrus*.[2]

Folklore, Mythology, and Ancient Uses

Bay laurel was used to worship the god Apollo and celebrate victory and triumph in Greece as well as Rome. According to mythology, Apollo fell in love with a nymph named Daphne who did not love him. She tried to run from him, but he chased her. Daphne prayed to Gaia to make her disappear, so Gaia rescued Daphne and, in her place, left a laurel tree.

Pliny recommended alloro leaves made into a decoction for bowel pains, and the berries for liver conditions. Greek physician, Soranus of Ephesus, wrote that it was used as a vaginal suppository that could cause an abortion.[3]

Nicholas Culpeper wrote about bay laurel by beginning with "This is so well known that it needs no description." He went on to list its many uses that include the breaking up of kidney stones and other calcifications, as well as an aid to labor, childbirth, and menstrual issues and said that when "given to a woman in sore travail of child-birth, do cause a speedy delivery, and expel the after birth, and therefore not to be taken by such as have not gone out their time, lest they procure abortion, or cause labor too soon."[4]

Bay laurel is one of the ingredients in the medieval remedy called the *potio Sancti Pauli*, or "drink of Saint Paul" that was supposedly created by him. The formulation was given in wine to "epileptics, cataleptics, analeptics, and those suffering in the stomach." It was also given along with an ancient Babylonian formula called *Esdra magna* for malaria.

Herbal Medicine Uses

Bay laurel is not popular in modern Western herbalism but is still used by many Italians and Italian Americans for digestive issues and respiratory infections. In addition to its use as a digestion aid, it is helpful for bronchitis and makes a beneficial analgesic when infused in oil or some other fat and used externally to treat bruises and sprains. It is also known to be anti-inflammatory, antioxidant, anticonvulsive, and antiepileptic, and research has shown it to be active against fungal and bacterial infections. Bay laurel is also carminative and can reduce high blood sugar.[5]

Italian Folk Medicine Uses

The leaves of bay laurel are used as a decoction for digestive upsets and respiratory issues and are infused for herbal baths and hair rinses.

L'infuso delle foglie era bevuto nelle affezioni gastriche e nelle affezioni respiratorie, in particolare ne raffreddori; con la stessa droga si

*preparavano dei bagni aromatici contro i dolori reumatici. Una forma
più diluita d'infus delle foglie era somministrato ai bimbi per allevia-
tre le coliche gassose. Il cataplasma di foglie di alloro e foglie di nocciolo
era applicato, molto caldo, sulla pianta dei piedi nel caso di febbre e di
dolori conseguenti all'influenza.*

*Pediluvi con infuso di foglie di laruo erano molto apprezzati per togliere
la stanchezza a gli indolenzimenti. Il decotto di foglie era frizionato sul
capo per contrastare la caduta die capelli e curare l'alopecia.*[6]

The infusion of the leaves was drunk in gastric and respiratory ailments, in particular colds; with the same drug they prepared aromatic
baths against rheumatic pains. A more diluted form of infusion of the
leaves was given to children to relieve gaseous colic. The poultice of
bay leaves and hazel leaves was applied, very hot, on the soles of the
feet in case of fever and pain following the flu.

Footbaths with infusion of lauro leaves were much appreciated to
relieve tiredness and soreness. The decoction of leaves was rubbed on
the head to counteract hair loss and cure alopecia.

Emotional and Psychospiritual Benefits

Alloro aids in trancework and meditation and is said to promote prophetic visions. It's also thought to be an ally in higher thinking or intellectual pursuits as we see in the tradition of wearing a laurel wreath when
someone graduates with a Bachelor's degree or a *baccalaureate.*

Energetics and Correspondences

Energetics: Warm and dry in the second degree
Astrological influence: The Sun
Element: Fire
Tarot card: The star
Deity: The nymph Daphne

Magical Uses

Bay laurel is thought to promote invisibility, and it is burned to clear
spaces, bestow blessings, and grant wishes. One can light a bay leaf, make

a wish, then blow it out or write a wish or prayer on a bay leaf, light it, and allow it to burn fully. Prayers or intentions can also be written on a bay leaf and added to a brevi bag.

Preparations and Recipes

The leaves and fruit of bay laurel can both be used. The leaves can be collected all year but are best during the summer, and the fruit is gathered in the autumn. The following is recipe for a decoction used for respiratory infections and flu-type illnesses.

🌿 Laurel Decoction[7]

1 quart of water

3 to 5 bay leaves

A handful of olive leaves

2 to 3 slices of lemon

2 to 3 chopped figs (dried or fresh)

1. Place all the ingredients in a pan.
2. Bring to a boil and simmer for 20 minutes.
3. Strain and drink throughout the day.

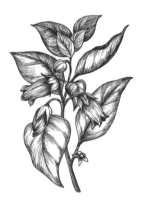

BELLADONNA (BELLADONNA)

The Witches' Plant

Family: Solanaceae
Genus: *Atropa*
Species: *belladonna*
Italian vernacular names: *Morella furiosa, ciliegia dell follia*[1]
English vernacular names: Deadly nightshade, devil's berry, wolf cherry, flower of the forest, lady of the forest, black cherry, great morel, banewort, sorcerer's cherry

Belladonna is in the Solanaceae, or nightshade, family along with tobacco, tomatoes, eggplant, potatoes, henbane, mandrake, ashwaganda, brugmansia (angel's trumpet), datura, and more. These plants all contain alkaloids called tropanes: atropine, scopolamine, hyoscyamine, and others, including solanine, which is found in all parts of potatoes except the tubers and unripe tomatoes.

The botanical name for belladonna is *Atropa belladonna*. *Atropa* comes from the Greek goddess Atropos, meaning "the unturnable," who is one of the three Fates (Moirai in Greek). Atropos is the last Fate. After the first Fate, Clothos, spins the thread of life, and the second Fate, Lachesis, measures how long the life will be, Atropos cuts it at the end.

Atropine, also from the Greek goddess Atropos, is belladonna's most active ingredient. This is the chemical that causes pupil dilation. Atropine, scopolamine, and hyoscyamine are all active ingredients in all parts of the plant—roots, leaves, flowers, ripe berries, seeds, and nectar, which can make honey contain the same alkaloids.

These alkaloids are anticholinergic, which means they block the action of the neurotransmitter acetylcholine responsible for involuntary muscle movements. Basically, anticholinergics are muscle relaxers and antispasmodics.

The overall effects of belladonna are on the central nervous system. The plant acts as a sedative, depressing cardiac function and causing drowsiness, dry mouth, hallucinations, confusion, slurred speech, tachycardia, loss of balance, amnesia, and potentially death. Atropine has a biphasic effect, either slowing or accelerating cardiac function depending on the dose. Scopolamine is generally a sedative, and hyoscyamine is a stimulant.

Belladonna is native to Southern Europe, North Africa, and Western Asia, and its name, which means "beautiful woman," is derived from the Italian language. Belladonna is a highly toxic plant, and it has been much maligned not so much for its toxicity but more for its common use as a hallucinogen and for its association with witchcraft and witches.

Belladonna, n.: In Italian a beautiful lady; in English a deadly poison. A striking example of the essential identity of the two tongues.

AMBROSE BIERCE, *THE UNABRIDGED DICTIONARY*

Hildegard von Bingen strongly purported its negative image:

> Belladonna has a coldness in it, but this coldness also holds evil and barrenness, and in the earth and at the place where it grows, a diabolic influence has some share and participation in its craft. It is dangerous for a person to eat or drink, since it will disorder his spirit, as if he were dead.[2]

Belladonna can be grown in North America and prefers a more alkaline soil, such as mine, which is rich in limestone. It's a forest plant that likes some breakthrough sunlight. Belladonna is rhizomatous, so it will spread underground via underground rootstalks, and it is perennial. It is also hermaphroditic; each plant has both male and female organs that are either wind or insect pollinated.

Folklore, Mythology, and Ancient Uses

The name *belladonna* has been associated with the Roman goddess of war, Bellona, and possibly comes from its notable use by women to dilate their pupils which was, apparently, considered to be beautiful:

> Drops prepared from the belladonna plant were used to dilate women's pupils, an effect considered to be attractive and seductive. Belladonna drops act as a muscarinic antagonist, blocking receptors in the muscles of the eye that constrict pupil size. Belladonna is currently rarely used cosmetically, as it carries the adverse effects of causing minor visual distortions, inability to focus on near objects, and increased heart rate. Prolonged usage was reputed to cause blindness.[3]

Clothos spins the thread of life and Lachesis measures how long the life will be; Atropos cuts it at the end. Atropos meaning "the unturnable."

Herbal Medicine Uses

Belladonna is considered an entheogen and psychedelic. It is also a sedative and an antispasmodic. It has a long history of medicinal and psychotropic use, and tropane derivatives continue to be used in modern medicine today. The dosage of belladonna varies, but anything over 100 mg is considered potentially lethal.

Dale Pendell, in his book *Pharmakognosis*, says he took 8 drops of seed tincture and didn't feel that much. According to Finnish herbalist Henriette Kress, the tincture is prepared from the leaves and root with a dosage of ¼ to 1 grain. A grain is 60 millligrams.*

The most common use of Belladonna in traditional herbal medicine is for pain relief either internally or externally. It has been traditionally used externally for pain related to neuralgia, gout, sciatica, and arthritis. Its antispasmodic properties have been used to treat spasmodic asthma, and the leaves were even once an ingredient in a cigarette formula made for those with asthma.

Italian Folk Medicine Uses

Belladonna is known to be one of the main ingredients in witches' flying ointments, *unguentum sabbati*, or witches' salves. These salves were imbued with hallucinogenic substances and applied to the skin to produce "flight" to the witches' Sabbath.

Non sempre le streghe, come abbiamo visto, sono state indicate come figure negative. Essendo collegate al mito della Luna, che tra le sue facce ha Persefone, o Prosperpina, dea dell'oltretomba, e Artemide, o Diana, dea vergine delle fertilità, hanna ovuto nel tempo aspetti contrapposti, inizialmente senz'altro positivi. Eloquente, in tal senso, l'espressione francese con cui spesso erano identificate: le belle femmes, esspressione a cui, probabilmente, si richiama il nome "belladonna" riferito a quest'erba; molto utilizzata ne preparati magici, nel Medioevo era anche detta più esplicitamente "erba delle streghe." Era, infatti, un

---

*These dosages are highly speculative. Please do no experiment based on them.

ingrediente irrinunciabile nella preparazione di quegli unguenti che, spalmati sul corpo, davano la sensazione di volare, per la presenza di agenti allucinogeni.[4]

Witches, as we have seen, have not always been indicated as negative figures. Being connected to the myth of the Moon, which has among its faces Persephone, or Prosperpina, goddess of the underworld, and Artemis, or Diana, virgin goddess of fertility, over time they have had opposing aspects, initially undoubtedly positive. In this sense, the French expression with which they were often identified is eloquent: le belle femmes, an expression to which, probably, the name "belladonna" to this herb refers; widely used in magical preparations, in the Middle Ages it was also more explicitly called "witch's herb." It was, in fact, an indispensable ingredient in the preparation of those ointments which, spread on the body, gave the sensation of flying, due to the presence of hallucinogenic agents.

It's not clear what is meant by "flying" in the old legends about witches. It was likely a form of trance induced by some type of hallucinogenic substance, but there are instances when the stories about witches flying seem to be literal including trial testimonies from the inquisition.

Belladonna is many things: a deadly poison, a potent medicine, a sacred plant since prehistory, a plot device in ancient and modern literature, and the ultimate witches' herb. It is so beloved of the Devil, it's said he only leaves it unattended on May Eve while he is busy being worshipped at the witches' Sabbath. Of the witches' flying ointment recipes surviving today, almost all of them contain belladonna and it is usually the main active ingredient. The tropane alkaloids in belladonna can cause heart palpitations in large doses which can make one feel like they are flying or falling and this herb can also cause very vivid lucid dreams. This combination creates an effect similar to a shamanic otherworld journey, but the witch's flight is astral, not physical. Belladonna is a dream herb par excellence.[5]

Emotional and Psychospiritual Benefits

The belladonna flower essence helps with cord cutting and release. It also brings clarity of vision and focus of mind.

Energetics and Correspondences

Energetics: Cold and dry in the fourth degree
Astrological influences: Saturn and Mars
Element: Earth
Tarot card: The magician
Deities: Hecate, Persephone

Magical Uses

Magical uses include "flying," divination, and "seeing" or prophecy.

Preparations and Recipes

It is best not to use this plant except as a flower essence because it is very poisonous.

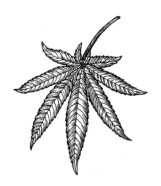

CANAPA (CANNABIS)

The Little Star

Family: Cannabacea (same family as hops)
Genus: *Cannabis*
Species: *indica* or *sativa*
Italian vernacular names: *Erba, Maria, 'o piccirillo*[1]
English vernacular names: Marijuana, pot, weed

Indica and *sativa* are the most common varieties of *Cannabis. Ruderalis* is also well known, and it is lower in THC (tetrahydrocannabinol) and higher in CBD (cannabidiol) than *indica* or *sativa,* although there is some debate among botanists whether or not *ruderalis* is a separate species or not. The etymology of cannabis comes from the Greek word *kannabis*, which means "hemp." Another line of etymology comes from the Hebrew *kaneh bosem* with *kaneh* meaning a "reed "or "stalk" and *bosem* meaning "fragrant."[2]

In Southern Italy, hemp has been one of the main agricultural crops throughout history. Italian farming of hemp, largely for textiles and fiber, made Italy the second largest producer of hemp just before Russia until the 1930s when hemp illegalization laws started to go into effect around the world.

> In the best period in our country, over 120 thousand hectares were grown on hemp with an annual yield of about 800 thousand quintals. In 1914 the province of Ferrara produced 363 thousand quintals of hemp, compared to 157 thousand in the province of Caserta, 145 thousand in the province of Bologna and 89 thousand in the Neapolitan. In many Italian regions it is still easy to come across small and characteristic artificial ponds, the so-called stingy or rotted, where hemp drums were once soaked for the first phase of processing.[3]

Folklore, Mythology, and Ancient Uses

It is believed that cannabis originated in central Asia, and its first documented use as a medicinal plant dates back to 2800 BCE in the pharmacopeia of the emperor Shen Nung[4] and based on our most recent genetic data it is believed to have emerged about twenty-eight thousand years ago on the Tibetan plateau.[5]

We find evidence of cannabis cultivation in Italy dating back 2000 years ago, and there is evidence of it having grown wild there long before then, even back into the late glacial period through the Holocene. How it managed to be transported there from the East is still in question.[6] There is a theory that the use and cultivation of cannabis in the Greco-Roman world started with their contact with the Scythians, nomads from central Asia who migrated west.

> The Scythians, as I said, take some of this hemp-seed [presumably, flowers], and, creeping under the felt coverings, throw it upon the

red-hot stones; immediately it smokes, and gives out such a vapour as no Grecian vapour-bath can exceed; the Scyths, delighted, shout for joy.[7]

Asterion, which means "little star" is one of the ancient names for cannabis according to Dioscorides. In ancient Greece it was used as an offering to the goddess Hera as well as an entheogen that induced a trance. The portrayal of cannabis in this context "suggests that it was thought to bring users in contact with the astral realms."[8]

Cannabis is thought to be one of the entheogenic substances used by the Pythia and Sibyls to induce a prophetic trance according to American archaeologist Leicester B. Holland. The theory is that the oracle stood over an omphalos, or opening, where smoke would rise from an underground cavern or basement.

> Down there, by the spring waters, the priestess would light a fire and throw on the psychoactive ingredients. The hemp plant, Cannabis sativa, and its seeds, Holland wrote, might have produced the desired effect. He noted that the Scythians, an ancient nomadic people who lived north of the Greeks, had used hemp in various rites. Hemp, too, had a pungent, sweet odor, perhaps not unlike the intermittent fragrance that Plutarch had reported.[9]

Cannabis was used by the ancient Greeks in incense formulas for the rites of the cults of Asclepius and called Scythian fire.[10] Claudius Galen wrote that it was customary in Italy to serve small cakes containing marijuana for dessert.[11]

The people of the cannabis or the ancient shamans that allied with cannabis were known as the Kapnobatai and were associated with the Mysians of Thrace who once inhabited Southeast Europe. *Kapnobatai*, or *capnobatae* in Latin, means "smoke walkers"[12] or "those that walk in/on smoke/clouds." The Kapnobatai are also associated with the god Dionysus, the god of wine and intoxication. The wines used in the rites associated with their worship were often infused with psychotropic substances such as opium poppy and cannabis. The famous wine of the Greeks known as *nepenthe* is believed by scholars to have been infused with cannabis.[13]

Herbal Medicine Uses

The use of cannabis as a medicinal plant is becoming more and more recognized as laws and prohibitions around its use are starting to be removed. Cannabis is being used as an herbal preparation to address multiple health concerns from anxiety to muscle-skeletal pain and even as a cancer treatment. Its main active ingredients are called cannabinoids, and the two most well-known of these chemicals are THC and CBD. THC is the psychoactive component of the cannabis plant. Both chemicals bind receptors in the human body called endocannabinoids by mimicking our own endogenous endocannabinoid chemicals and activating our internal endocannabinoid system, which is "our own internal cannabis system."[14]

Italian Folk Medicine Uses

The folk medicine uses of cannabis in Southern Italy for external sprains or strains often refer to the "tow," or "la stoppa," which is the fiber extracted from the plant. Below is a formula for using cannabis fiber as a poultice.

La Signora Adele Cambiaghi di Induno Olona ricorda un metodo terpeutico contro le storte, messo in atto da sua mamma. Si sbatteva lungamente del bianco d'uovo, con questa preperazione si imbeveva abbondantemente della stoppa di canapa. La stoppa, cosi medicata, era applicata sulla parte dolente, si fasciava e si lasciava la medicazione in sito per alcuni giorni.[15]

Mrs. Adele Cambiaghi of Induno Olona recalls a therapeutic method against sprains implemented by her mother. Egg white was beaten for a long time, then abundantly soaked in hemp tow. The tow, thus medicated, was applied to the painful part, bandaged and the dressing was left in place for a few days.

The use of cannabis as an entheogen is also well documented but often with condemnation and references to witchcraft as the church became more powerful.

Nell'Europa del Basso Medioevo, l'uso della canapa, in campo erboristico, era esclusivo della stregoneria, tanto che nel 1484, papa Innocenzo VIII condannò quest'erba come sostanza satanica, perché le presunte streghe se ne serviavano per i loro riti. Era infatti uno degli ingredienti che componevano i vari miscugli per favorire le trasformazioni e i "voli" magici, in quella che qualcuno ha definito una religione "psichedelica."[16]

In the Europe of the Late Middle Ages, the use of hemp, in the herbal field, was exclusive to witchcraft, so much so that in 1484, Pope Innocent VIII condemned this herb as a satanic substance, because the alleged witches used it for their rites. It was in fact one of the ingredients that made up the various mixtures to favor magical transformations and "flights," in what someone has defined as a "psychedelic" religion.

Emotional and Psychospiritual Benefits

Cannabis flower essence changes how we relate to linear time, making our experience of time passing more cyclical and circular and enabling us to drop in to the moment without urgency. It makes us aware that there is no need to rush and that everything will unfold in perfect timing when we allow ourselves to stay in the fullness of the present instead of being in the past and future.

Energetics and Correspondences

Energetics: Cold and dry in the third degree.*
Astrological influence: Saturn
Element: Earth
Tarot card: The fool
Deities: Hera, Dionysus

Magical Uses

The magic of cannabis is based in its ability to invoke shifts of consciousness, connection with the sacred, and its association with "flight" or transformation.

Preparations and Recipes

The flowers of cannabis are typically used, but the stalks can be also be used as fiber, and the resin (hashish) and the leaves can be used medici-

---

*This will change slightly depending on the part of the plant and where it is grown as well as if it is dried or not. While this is true for all plants, the range of preparations of Cannabis makes it especially relevant here.

nally. The seeds and seed oil are a food source. Cannabis buds or the "shake" leaves can be used too as well as all above-ground parts of male plants. The leaves will be less potent.

Unguento alla Canapa (Cannabis Ointment)

    4 ounces of Cannabis-infused oil

    .75 ounces of beeswax

1. Heat the oil gently.
2. Melt the beeswax and add it to the oil.
3. Pour it into glass or tin jars.
4. Use for sprains, strains, and muscle or joint pain.

To make cannabis infused oil:

The cannabis must be decarboxylized. There are many methods of doing this that can be found on the internet. Basically, it must be heated first.

1. Place decarboxylized cannabis in a clean glass canning jar, a measuring cup, or double boiler.
2. Place the jar in a hot water bath or over the bottom of the double boiler on the stove for several hours.
3. Strain through a cheesecloth and store in a glass jar.

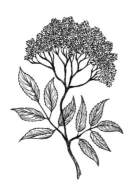

SAMBUCO (ELDER)

God's Stinking Tree

Family: Adoxaceae
Genus: *Sambucus*
Species: *nigra* or *canadensis*
Italian vernacular names: *Fiori di Maggio, sambucaro, sambugo marino, sambüch, mascé, papcüca, savucha*[1]
English vernacular names: Black/European elder, boretree, Scot tree, pipe tree, devil's wood, American/common/ sweet elder

The word *sambucus* is derived from the Greek *sambuce*, which is an ancient musical instrument made from elder wood as the pith is easily removed to create a hollow wind instrument. This instrument was said to be the flute played by Pan, the mythic god of shepherds, fertility, and nature. Other ancient names for elder include *amatilla, atrapasse* (Latin), *aeld* (Anglo-Saxon).

The doctrine of signatures for elder says that because it grows in low moist places, it is moistening and will treat moist, wet, drippy conditions such as a runny nose and edema/dropsy. The pith of elder, when pressed with the fingers, makes an indent similar to what happens when you press on the skin of someone with edema, "doth pit and receive the impress thereon, as the legs and feet of dropsical persons do."[2] The lenticels on the stem indicate that it can be used to sew up skin lesions.

Folklore, Mythology, and Ancient Uses

Archeological excavations have found that elder wood has been used in the making of tools, and the berries/seeds have been used as medicine since the Neolithic period. Charlemagne decreed that in his empire every household must grow an elder tree because of its medicinal value.

> *Nell'area del Mediteranneo il legno di sambuco era considerato sacre e con esso, nel Medioevo, si costruirono molte Madonne nere, statue lignee dallo sguardo fisso, spesso custodite nelle cripte di chiese che avevano sostituito antichi luoghi di culto della Madre Terra.[3]*

In the Mediterranean area, elder wood was considered sacred and with it, in the Middle Ages, many black Madonnas were built, wooden statues with a fixed gaze, often kept in the crypts of churches that had replaced ancient places of worship of Mother Earth.

Elder is one of the sacred trees of ogham (pronounced oh-um or oh-wum), the Celtic tree alphabet that corresponds to the months of the year. The month of December belongs to elder, or the letter *r* for *ruis*. Its association with the god Pan also aligns with the Roman celebration of Saturnalia that happens in honor of the god Saturn and begins on December 17.

The name Saturn comes from the Latin word *serere*, which means "to sow," again referencing the time of year for planting. It also comes from the Latin *satyros*, from which we get the word *satyr*. A satyr is a half human, half goat divine being; that is, the god Pan.

Herbal Medicine Uses

Elder flowers are especially helpful for all types of respiratory allergies like hay fever and asthma. They're also used to treat ear infections and eczema. Elder is known to reduce excessive heat and inflammation by opening the eliminatory channels of the body: the skin, lungs, colon, kidneys, and blood vessels. This improves and balances the overall flow and circulation of fluids in the body, thus bringing in freshly oxygenated blood that can move and disperse phlegm. Elder also stimulates, meaning that it moves and disperses stagnation, and with open eliminatory channels, energy can be released.

Elder is also mucostatic, so it affects the secretion of mucus. This is thought to be because it contains the flavonoids rutin and quercetin, which are known for their anti-inflammatory and antiallergic actions. Elder is trophic to the respiratory tract, which means that it feeds and nourishes it and supports a condition that is in a balanced state of fluidity: not too dry and not too mucousy. It is known to cool fevers with its dispersing and opening action. It moves heat out toward the periphery, making it diaphoretic, or sweat promoting.

Elderberry in particular has been studied for its immune and antiviral properties. Most of the antiviral studies have been done with influenza viruses, and they show that elderberry cuts off one of the spike proteins that the flu uses to get into our cells. Elderberry has been more recently study for its effects on SARS-CoV-2, and it has been found that "*S. nigra* cell cultures constitute a promising biotechnological system to produce anti-inflammatory agents with inhibitory activity against SARS-CoV-2 and ACE2 binding for complementary treatments."[4]

Italian Folk Medicine Uses

Italian folk medicine, too, uses elder flowers to prevent mucous buildup and certain types of headaches. Cures often include prayers and gestures.

Si mettevano, in un recipiente, fiori di sambuco, miele e aceto, il tutto era infuso con acqua bollente, la preparazione era bevuta contro il catarro.[5]

Elder flowers, honey and vinegar were placed in a container, the whole was infused with boiling water, the preparation was drunk against the phlegm.

Elder is also involved in both the cause and the cure for a specific type of headache called *cigli alla testa* where the pain is at the top center of the skull. In this treatment, the practitioner runs

her thumb down the center of the skull, from the center of the forehead to the posterior base, and returns to make the sign of the cross on the area of acute pain. After several repetitions, small strands of the hair at the base of the head are lightly tugged (beginning at the center, then pulling hairs on the left and then the right). Next a prayer is spoken:

Buon giorno cumpa'Savuchə
Ciglia aggə e ciglia t'adduchə,
Ti giuro e ti prometto,
Che 'ndufuchs nu ti mettə.

Good morning cumpa' Savuchə,
I have the headache and I give it to you,
I tell you the truth and I promise you,
In the fire I'll not place you.

In the procedure, the illness is presented either to *cumpa'* (close family member, padrino or godfather) or San (Saint) Savuchə/Sambuco. The latter is not a Catholic saint, but this does not alter his power in the minds of helpers and patients. Savucha is a local name for *Sambucus nigra* L. (Adoxaceae), the elderberry tree; inhalation of smoke from a burning elderberry tree is said to cause such headaches. . . . The prayer acknowledges the tree's ability to inflict pain, and in order to placate the entity the sufferer vows never to burn the tree for firewood. Some helpers reported that the healing ceremony for cigli alla testa may be conducted under an elderberry tree, which serves as an altar for accessing the mythic entity of San Savucha. Normally only one treatment is necessary, but the patient can return for treatment if the symptoms persist.[6]

Emotional and Psychospiritual Benefits

As clinical herbalist and flower essence practitioner Kate Gilday says, the flower essence of elder, "Holds the joy and exuberance, the magic and mystery of the plant spirits. Offers protection on the etheric and spiritual planes."*

Energetics and Correspondences

Energetics: Cool and moist, stimulating, sedating
Astrological influence: Venus, sometimes Saturn
Element: Water
Tarot card: The devil
Deity: Pan, San Savucha

Magical Uses

Elder is often used for protection and hung on the doorways of houses. It is believed that if you fall asleep under an elder you may end up in the faery world, but stand under one in a storm, and you won't be struck by lightning. If you want to bless someone, scatter elder leaves and berries in the direction of the wind while saying the name of person you want to bless.

Preparations and Recipes

All parts of the elder can be used, but because the leaves, roots, and bark are emetic (cause vomiting), the most common parts used are the flowers and berries.

🌿 Elderflower Tea

1. Add 1 cup of boiling water to 2 teaspoons of fresh or dried elder flowers.
2. Drink 2 to 3 times per day for hayfever

---

*Her Woodland Essence website is a wonderful resource for flower essences.

🌿Elderflower Tincture

1. Fill a glass jar with elder blossoms. Tamp down.
2. Pour 100 proof vodka over the blossoms.
3. Cover and leave in a cool, dark place for 4 to 6 weeks.
4. Strain and rebottle. Store in a cool, dark place.
5. Take 15 to 20 drops 3 times per day for hayfever and seasonal allergies.

🌿Elderberry Tincture

Elderberries have many of the same properties as the flowers, but they are sweet and more tonic/nutritive. Elderberry is considered helpful for treating anemia and the flu.

1. Follow the same method as for the elderflower tincture above. I usually grind the berries in a blender or they can be mashed with a potato masher type tool instead.
2. Take ¼ to ½ teaspoon 3 times per week to prevent the flu or ¼ to ½ teaspoon 3 to 4 times per day if you have the flu.

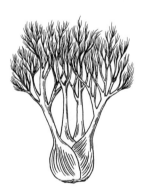

FINOCCHIO (FENNEL)
The Towering Plant

Family: Apiaceae
Genus: *Foeniculum*
Species: *vulgare*
Italian vernacular names: *Finocchietto*
English vernacular names: Sweet fennel, sweet anise

Fennel is native to Southern Europe and the Mediterranean. It's a member of Apiaceae family (same family as parsley) and so is a relative of carrot, parsnip, coriander, angelica, Queen Anne's lace (wild carrot), and poison hemlock. Because it is in this family, it's good to be careful if you should be harvesting it wild.

Fennel is called the towering plant because of its height, which can be up to six feet or more depending on the variety. It is a perennial or biennial and thrives in Mediterranean-type climates but can be planted as an annual in northern locations.

Fennel, *finocchio*, is generally referring to Florence fennel, or *Foeniculum vulgare* var. *azoricum*. This is a cultivar with a large bulb that is sweeter than wild fennel. The botanical name for fennel comes from the Latin *feniculum*, or *foeniculum*, which means "hay." It's thought that the Romans gave the plant this name, which became *fenol* or *finol* in Old English and eventually became *fennel*. Other names for fennel are sweet cumin and anise (when mislabeled). Fennel is likely called anise at times because of its famous taste and smell that is reminiscent of both anise and licorice.

There are, generally speaking, two types of fennel: the wild and the garden varieties. The wild type is more bitter. The garden varieties are numerous, but here are a few: *vulgare* is the standard type for fresh and dry leaf production, *purpureum* has bronze leaves and *Rubrum* has deep bronze to red leaves and both are used as ornamentals.[1]

The giant fennel, or *Ferula communis*, also known by its common name narthex, is part of the fennel family and grows from seven to ten feet tall in wooded areas and in shrublands in the Mediterranean and East Africa. Although it is generally considered poisonous, the young, blanched shoots were eaten by ancient Romans and are still eaten by some folks today. Don't eat the leaves.

Both fennel and giant fennel can be easily grown. Even here in a cold climate I grow fennel each year from seed. And below are instructions for growing giant fennel.

[The] plant prefers full sun and fast draining soils. Sow in spring by laying seed flat on potting soil, cover with 1/4 inch of compost, tamp securely and keep evenly moist until germination, which can take several weeks. Individuate seedlings and work up in pots until sufficiently sized to transplant out to the landscape.[2]

Folklore, Mythology, and Ancient Uses

Fennel is well known for its association with both Italian cooking and culture:

> It has followed civilization, especially where Italians have colonized, and may be found growing wild in many parts of the world upon dry soils near the sea-coast and upon river-banks. It flourishes particularly on limestone soils and is now naturalized in some parts of this country, being found from North Wales southward and eastward to Kent, being most frequent in Devon and Cornwall and on chalk cliffs near the sea. It is often found in chalky districts inland in a semi-wild state.[3]

The uses of fennel can be found throughout folklore and mythology. Giant fennel was used by the gods to make a scepter called a thyrsus made from a fennel stalk, topped with a pine cone, and entwined with ivy. It is most often associated with the staff of Dionysus. Thyrsi were carried by people as wands during religious festivals and ceremonies. It's thought that they represent prosperity, fertility, and hedonism. It's believed that the maenads, followers of Bacchus, or Dionysus, carried them as well, and it's been written that honey dripped from them.

Dionysus is often portrayed holding both a staff and a vessel, or kantharos (bowl) of wine. The staff represented the masculine, and the wine cup represented the feminine as Dionysus is known as a nonbinary god. The thyrsus became a weapon with a concealed iron point at the tip in some instances, particularly in Bacchus's incarnation, as it's been called "'a spear enveloped in vine-leaves,' and its point was thought to incite to madness."[4]

> Enter Dionysus. He is of soft, even effeminate, appearance. His face is beardless; he is dressed in a fawn-skin and carries a thyrsus (i.e., a stalk of fennel tipped with ivy leaves). On his head he wears a wreath of ivy, and his long blond curls ripple down over his shoulders. Throughout the play he wears a smiling mask.[5]

According to Pliny the Elder, fennel was thought to improve eyesight:

Fennel has been made famous . . . by serpents, which taste it to cast off their old skin and with its juice improve their eyesight. Consequently, it has been inferred that by Fennel juice especially can dimness of human vision also be removed. This juice is collected when the stem is swelling to bud, dried in the Sun and applied in honey as an ointment. The most esteemed is gathered in Spain from the tear-drops of plants.[6]

> *Above the lower plants it towers,*
> *The Fennel with its yellow flowers;*
> *And in an earlier age than ours*
> *Was gifted with the wondrous powers*
> *Lost vision to restore.*
> HENRY WADSWORTH LONGFELLOW

Herbal Medicine Uses

Fennel bulbs, fronds, and seeds/fruits are all used medicinally and in cooking. Fennel is used in herbal medicine as a stimulant, diaphoretic, aromatic, stomachic, galactagogue, emmenagogue, and aphrodisiac. It's also a carminative that dispels gas and improves digestion and because it is antispasmodic in the digestive tract, it has been used for colic. Fennel thins secretions and mucus so is sometimes added to cough teas or syrups, and it is known to increase breast milk and was traditionally boiled with barley. It is also used as an eyewash for conjunctivitis and migraines.

Because of its carminative properties, fennel is often used to make a variety of digestive liquors and other drinks such as amari (bitters), a staple in Italian kitchens. These drinks are specifically beneficial to aiding digestion and supporting the healing of digestive ailments, and they fall into two categories: *aperitivo* (pl. *aperitivi*) or *digestivo* (pl. *digestivi*). We find similar practices in most, if not all, traditional cultures whereby the people use herbs, spices, and digestive herbal preparations such as finnochietto as a natural ingredient to preparing meals.

Digestivi and apertivi are standard courses in any Italian meal. *Aperitivo* means "opener," and these are drinks that are sipped premeal or with appetizers. One of the most well known aperitivos in Italian culture is the aperol spritz. The medicinal intention here is to get the digestive juices moving so that we can optimally digest our meal.

Digestivo simply means "digestive," and these are more commonly served after a meal or in between courses. Digestivi include *amaro, limoncello, nocello,* and *finocchietto,* which is also called *fennelcello.* You can find the recipe for fennelcello in the "Preparations and Recipes" section below. Postmeal digestive herbal drinks keep the digestive enzymes going to complete the process of fully integrating our food on both a physiological and energetic level. Digestive herbs such as fennel stimulate all digestive secretions to aid in the breakdown of food to increase absorption and nutrition.

Italian Folk Medicine Uses

Most of the recorded folk uses of fennel are how it's added to cuisine and as an ingredient in recipes. Otherwise, it is often used as a tea made from the seeds or added to a decoction to sweeten it and for its medicinal properties.

> *Nella tradizione popolare era consigliato per aiutare la vista e per aumentare il flusso del latte nelle donne che avevano appena partorito.*
>
> In folk tradition it was recommended to help eyesight and to increase the flow of milk in women who had just given birth.
>
> PAOLINO UCCELLO, *PIANTE E PAROLE CHE GUARISCONO*

Emotional and Psychospiritual Benefits

The fennel flower essence aids our ability to see habits that are no longer serving us. It supports us in our learning journey so that we can make mistakes and learn as we go.

Energetics and Correspondences

Energetics: Hot and dry in the second degree
Astrological influence: Mercury
Element: Fire
Tarot card: Temperance
Deities: Dionysus, Bacchus

Magical Uses

Fennel was often thought to ward off witches and other evil beings:

> In mediaeval times, Fennel was employed, together with St. John's Wort and other herbs, as a preventative of witchcraft and other evil influences, being hung over doors on Midsummer's Eve to ward off evil spirits.[7]

And according to Italian historian Carlo Ginzburg, the *benandanti*, members of an agrarian cult in Northern Italy, carried fennel stalks into their night battles: "Armed with bunches of Fennel stalks, they periodically fought for the fertility of the fields, against male and female witches armed with canes of sorghum."[8]

Preparations and Recipes

Fennel is primarily a food plant and its bulb is often used in recipes such as soups, stews, and stir fries. It is also often made into a liquor called Fennelcello, which is a digestive drink taken with meals. All parts of the plant can be used as medicine or in cooking including seeds, fronds, and the bulb/root.

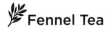 **Fennel Tea**

Fennel tea aids digestion, is a mild expectorant, and can increase breast milk.

1/2 teaspoon of fennel seeds
1 cup of water

1. Bring water to a boil in a kettle or pan.
2. Pour boiling water over the fennel seeds.
3. Steep for 10 minutes and drink.

🌿Fennelcello

Fennel, or *finocchio,* is both sweet and bitter, reminiscent of the taste of licorice, and as mentioned earlier, it is used in herbal medicine as a carminative that dispels gas and improves digestion. Fennelcello is a popular *digestivo* made with fennel and taken after meals to aid in the breakdown of food.

> 2 to 3 whole fresh fennel bulbs with or without fronds*
> A glass canning jar
> 1 quart of 100 proof vodka.†
> ¼ cup of fennel seeds
> Simple syrup
> Optional: fresh fennel flowers

1. Chop fennel bulbs and fronds and add to the jar until it's about 2 inches from the top. (Fennel flowers can also be included.)
2. Add fennel seeds.
3. Fill jar with vodka and cover it with the lid.
4. Let sit for 2 to 4 weeks then strain out plant material.
5. Add 8 to 12 ounces of simple syrup (see recipe below). Adjust amount to the desired sweetness.

🌿Simple Syrup

This basic recipe is equal parts sugar and water, but you can adjust the amount of sugar to your taste.

> 8 ounces of water
> 1 cup of sugar

---

*Fennel bulbs can be purchased at the grocery store. They may or may not include the fronds. If there aren't fronds, you might want to grab an extra bulb to make sure the jar is filled up.

†I use 195 proof pure grain alcohol, diluted 50:50 with distilled water, that I have for my tinctures, but it's not worth buying if you aren't going to use a lot of it. Vodka is fine.

1. In a medium saucepan combine water and sugar.
2. Heat the mixture, stirring, until sugar has dissolved.
3. Allow to cool, then add to strained fennelcello.
4. Label and enjoy!

AGLIO (GARLIC)

The Great Protector

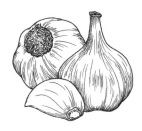

Family: Amaryllidaceae
Genus: *Allium*
Species: *sativum*
Italian vernacular names: *Aj, aj matt*[1]
English vernacular names: Camphor of the poor, poor man's treacle

Garlic, *Allium sativum*, is thought to be native to Central Asia because that is where it still grows wild. It's likely that its range was much wider at one time and probably stretched into Eastern Europe. There are multiple allium species that grow wild around the world, but they are not "true" garlic.

Garlic became a primary staple in Italian cooking and culture but is used far more in Italian-American cuisine than Southern Italian. In Southern Italy it is likely that garlic was a cheap, easy-to-grow source of sustenance and medicine for poor peasants, which is why it became so popularly cultivated. There are a several Italian "ecotypes" or *Allium sativum* cultivars that originated in Southern Italy, often known as Italian red garlic.

The etymology of the word *garlic* comes from the Old English *gārlēac*, with the prefix *gār*, which means "spear," presumably referring to the shape of the clove, but I'd suggest it is also a reference to its correspondence to Saint Michael and his sword. The second half of the word, *lēac*, means "leek." The origin of *Allium* isn't clear, but it might be from the Greek word *aleo*, which means "to avoid," possibly referring to its smell. Or it could be from the Greek *hallesthai*, which means "to jump out," referring to how quickly its shoots grow. *Sativum* simply means to "cultivate" or "sow."

Folklore, Mythology, and Ancient Uses

The Egyptians fed their slaves with garlic to make them strong and capable of doing more work. The Old Greek historian Herodotus wrote, "Inscriptions on the plates of the Egyptian pyramids tell us how much their builders used the garlic for this vegetable, 1600 talents of silver were spent (approximately 30 million dollars),"[2] and evidence that garlic existed in Egypt as far back as 3700 BCE was found on Egytian crypts:

> The Egyptian crypts are the oldest visible inscriptions for the existence of garlic. Archaeologists have discovered clayey sculptures of garlic bulbs dating from 3700 BC, while illustrations with garlic have been found in another crypt from 3200 BC. In Ebers papyrus (around 1500 BC) various medicinal plants have been mentioned, and among others the much appreciated garlic, efficient in healing 32 illnesses. The youngest pharaoh Tutankhamun (1320 BC) was sent on his trip to life beyond the grave escorted by garlic, as a patron of his soul and protector of his wealth.[3]

Pliny the Elder considered garlic to be a cure-all and said that

> it was much eaten by the Roman soldiers and sailors, and by the field labourers. It is in reference to this vegetable, "more noxious than hemlock," that Horace exclaims—
>
> "O dura messorum ilia!" (oh those hard workers)
>
> It was thought to have the property of neutralizing the venom of serpents; and though persons who had just eaten of it were not allowed to enter the Temple of the Mother of the Gods, it was prescribed to those who wished to be purified and absolved from crimes. It is still held in considerable esteem in the south of Europe, where, by the lower classes, great medicinal virtues are ascribed to it.[4]

Pliny also writes that garlic won't smell as bad if it is planted when the "moon is below the horizon" and harvested when it's conjunct.

The use of garlic in Greece has been recorded as far back as the eighth century BCE when Homer wrote about how Hermes gave Odysseus a type of garlic to protect him from Circe. This is speculative, however, as Odysseus calls it "moly," which some scholars have said is *Allium* moly, or golden garlic. Yet it is described as having a black root: "At the root it was black, but its flower was like milk."[5] Other scholars will insist that this moly was actually mullein.

The existence of garlic in Jewish history is also well documented:

Ancient Jews characterized the plant as an aphrodisiac, a nutritive and restorative food. Its telltale after-effects were also a way for other peoples, such as the ancient Romans, to recognize Hebrews by the scent they exuded after eating the plant. Hundreds of years later, garlic continued to be a mark of Jewishness: at the time of the Spanish Inquisition, those who had converted to Catholicism in order to elude death or imprisonment were identified by authorities by the smell of garlic on their breaths.[6]

Legend says that Mohammad wrote about how garlic sprang up in the garden of Eden wherever Satan stepped with his left foot: "When Satan stepped out from the Garden of Eden after the fall of man, Garlick sprang up from the spot where he placed his left foot, and Onion from that where his right foot touched."[7]

Herbal Medicine Uses

Garlic is one of the most popular herbal medicines we have, and in fact, in my opinion and experience, it is overused as is any herb that becomes commercialized. Yet this is also one of the best things about garlic, for although there are many supplements on the market, the bulb itself is inexpensive and available at any grocery store.

More than 220 studies have correlated ingestion of garlic with lower rates of stomach, intestinal, and other cancers. Here are some of the other common medicinal benefits of garlic:

- Lowers cholesterol and blood pressure
- Stimulates immune system
- Acts as an antibacterial and antiviral
- Treats ulcers, bacterial diarrhea, sinus infections, and ear infections
- Works effectively on antibiotic-resistant pneumonia

The first plant I used at the beginning of my herbal studies was garlic. My daughter had chronic ear infections, and her doctor said she needed tubes in her ears. We didn't have insurance so the surgery was cost prohibitive. I had heard of using garlic oil for ear infections, so we tried it and it worked! She never had another ear infection.

Italian Folk Medicine Uses

The use of garlic in both Italian and Italian-American cuisine and medicine is a bit controversial. Italian Americans tend to use several cloves of garlic in their cooking and take large doses when sick. However, my direct conversations and observation with Italians—both the Italian immigrants in my family and the Italians who were born in Italy—have taught me that garlic is used sparingly. Many Italians will only put one clove in a soup or sauce and some will even take it out before serving. I made a social media post about this once and received comments from Italian Americans saying that they had a different experience and that their family used many cloves in cooking. Therefore, I will leave this up to the reader.

One of the consistent inconsistencies in Italian folk medicine and cooking is that variations are regional and familial. But I will bring attention to the fact that garlic is a very powerful plant and is so strong that the body perceives it as a poison and mounts an immune response in order to eliminate it. This is why it is so good at killing bacteria and viruses. It is much more potent in its raw form than its cooked, so the extended use of raw garlic can be very depleting for some people.

Garlic is also associated with the Archangel Michael or San Michele (Saint Michael) and often during blessing or "charging," garlic prayers to San Michele will be spoken. San Michele is a protective/apotropaic deity, and garlic is believed to be an aspect of him containing his protective powers.

L'aglio benedetto il giorno di san Giovanni serviva alla preparazione dell'insalata mangiata durante il pasto di quel giorno, era considerato uno scongiuro contro la corruzione dell'organismo.[8]

The garlic blessed on Saint John's Day was used in the preparation of the salad eaten during that day's meal, it was considered an exorcism against the corruption of the organism.

Garlic is also thought to be beneficial for a toothache:

Contro il mal di denti si applica un empiastro di aglio sul polso dello stesso lato del dente sofferente.[9]

Against toothache a garlic poultice is applied to the wrist on the same side of the suffering tooth.

Emotional and Psychospiritual Benefits

Garlic flower essence is helpful for protection on all levels.

Energetics and Correspondences

Energetics: Hot and dry in the fourth degree, pungent, salty, stimulating, oily
Astrological influence: Mars
Element: Fire
Tarot card: Strength
Deities: Goddess Hecate, Archangel Michael

Magical Uses

Because garlic is so powerful, it is often used for protection and to ward off malocchio. Garlic amulets are also often worn to prevent illness.

Preparations and Recipes

Garlic preparations are one of the most popular kitchen medicines we have. Garlic bulbs are accessible because they can be purchased inexpensively in any grocery store. It is also easy to grow in many geographical regions. The flower essence is specifically used to ward off ticks and other insects.

Garlic Oil

20 cloves of chopped fresh, organic garlic
Enough olive oil to cover the garlic

1. Place the chopped garlic in a pan on top of a heat diffuser or in a double boiler.
2. Cover garlic with olive oil.
3. Turn heat on low and heat for 30 to 60 minutes. Do not simmer or cook; just heat it up on very low heat.

Alternate method 1: Place garlic and oil in a crockpot and heat for 6 to 8 hours.

Alternate method 2: Place garlic and oil in an ovenproof dish with a cover and leave in a gas oven that has a pilot light for 2 to 3 days. Note: Most modern gas ovens no longer have pilots. I bought an oven with an old-fashioned pilot on purpose, and you may also want to do so when it's time to replace your oven.

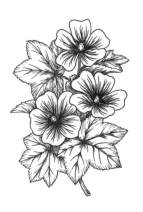

ALTEA OR MALVA (MALLOW)

The Soft Cure

Family: Malvaeacea
Genus: *Althaea*
Species: *officinalis*
Italian vernacular names: *Màlva, màlba, ariondela, narbutza*[1]
English vernacular names: Common mallow, low mallow, hollyhock

There are several species that are interchangeably called mallow or marsh-mallow, and they all belong to the Malvaeacea family. In Italian folk medicine you will find reference to both Altea (Italian spelling referring to the Althaea genus) and Malva. These refer to different plants and subspecies of the Malvaeacea familiy such as *Malva sylvestris, Malva neglecta,* and *Althaea rosea.* In Greek, *malva* means "soft," and *althaea,* from the Greek verb *althainô,* means "to heal."

In ancient Greek the word for malva is *alkeja/alkéa/alcea* which we see here:

> There is a grove in the innermost room of the enclosure,
> Where lush green wood ascends with shadowy tips,
> Laurel trees and cornelian cherry and slender platanos aloft. There
> are also many herbs in this place, arching over the deep roots;
> Klymenos, complete with the noble asfoldelos, and adiantos
> Aristereon, most tender of plants, and kypeiros with thyron,
> Kyklaminos, like the violet, and erysimon, complete with hormi-on,
> Stoichas, then paionia, surrounded by thickets of polyknemon.
> Then polion, mandragoras also, and pale diktamnon,
> Krokoa with sweet scent, and kardamom, next to kemos,
> Smilax, dark poppy, and low chamaemelon,
> Panakes and alkeja, with karpason and akoniton . . .
> And many others more poisonous rose up from the ground
> ORPHIC SONGS OF THE ARGONAUTS

Folklore, Mythology, and Ancient Uses

Pliny the Elder writes about both species of mallow in his book *Natural History*:

Both kinds of mallows, on the other hand, the cultivated and the wild, are held in very general esteem. These kinds are subdivided, each of them, into two varieties, according to the size of the leaf. The cultivated mallow with large leaves is known to the Greeks by the name of "malope," the other being called "malache,"—from the circumstance, it is generally thought, that it relaxes the bowels. The wild mallow, again, with large leaves and white roots, is called "althæa," and by some persons, on account of its salutary properties, "plistolochia." Every soil in which mallows are sown, is rendered all the richer thereby.[2]

Pliny also notes that "these herbs were highly praised, that the fresh plant is the most effective form, and that less than 50 mL of the fresh juice daily would render a person free of all diseases," and the "benefits of marshmallow . . . extend even to the place where they grow, since they fatten any ground on which they are sown."[3]

Most ancient accounts of using mallow describe it as being boiled in wine or milk: "The root boiled in milk and taken as a broth relieved a cough in 5 days."[4]

Herbal Medicine Uses

Medicinally mallow is used for almost any condition where soothing, nourishment, and softening is needed, specifically along the mucus membranes and lungs. Mallow is a superb remedy for inflammation and irritation of the digestive tract, the throat, and the skin: "The leaves, the root, and the flower of the herb provide the drug, which is applied all around the world as mucous glaze for catarrhal diseases of the trachea and the digestive organs."[5] Mallow herbal preparations are a source of mucilage used to address any inflammatory condition but especially those of the digestive and respiratory tracts such as the following:

- Sore throat
- Dry cough
- COPD
- Gastritis
- Colitis
- Ulcers
- Hyperacidity

At Pompeii today, the root and leaves of common mallow are washed, boiled together, and used for toothache, and for stomach problems; this liquid is also highly regarded as a cough medicine. The leaves alone boiled in water are used for toothache, the roots alone boiled in water for stomach problems, or for children with stomach problems, boiled with apple.[6]

Italian Folk Medicine Uses

Mallow is one of the most extensively used plants in Southern Italian folk traditions and has a reputation as a cure-all. This is likely, in part, because it has incredible cooling and moistening properties that are so needed in Southern Italy's hot, dry climate.

> *Whosoever shall take a spoonful of the Mallows shall that day be free from all diseases that may come to him.*
>
> PLINY THE ELDER

Mallow has often been used in Italian folk medicine for *mal di gola* (sore throat):

Sore throat has a natural cause; it is believed to stem from exposure to cold, wet weather. Treatment can involve prayers, a decoction of mallow leaves (*Malva sylvestris L.* [Malvaceae]), or both. When healed ceremonially, light massage of the neck is combined with prayers and crosses made with the thumb over the painful area. At the end of the procedure, the illness is presented to San Biagio (San Vlase, in south Italian dialect), protector of the throat:

San Vlasǝ glorioso,
'Ndu voschǝ stai 'nghiusǝ,
'Ndu voschǝ de castagnǝ.
Fammǝ passa' 'stu mal dǝ gola.[7]

Glorious Saint Vlase,
Inside the forest you are trapped
Inside the forest of chestnut trees.
Make this sore throat pass [go away].

Other conditions that folk medicine uses mallow to treat include muscle stiffness, eye ailments, and fever:

Le foglie cotte nell'acqua e condite con olio erano usate contro la stitche-
zza abituale. Il liquido risultante dall decozione delle foglie, o di tutta
la pianta, si usava per gargarismi, lavande, bagni e colliri emollienti; si
beveva contro la febbre.[8]

The leaves cooked in water and seasoned with oil were used against
chronic stiffness. The liquid resulting from the decoction of the
leaves, or of the whole plant, was used for gargles, douches, baths and
emollient eye drops; it was drunk against fever.

Emotional and Psychospiritual Benefits

Mallow essence has proven helpful for those people who are rigid or
overly contracted and "set in their ways." It eases "stoicness" and the lack
of connection to the emotions or the lack of the ability to express them.
It also softens intolerance and soothes the heart chakra so that it may be
more capable of responding to input from the lower chakras.

Energetics and Correspondences

Energetics: Cool and moist in the first degree, mucilaginous, salty, sweet
Astrological influence: Moon or Venus
Element: Water
Tarot card: Queen of cups
Deity: Hecate

Magical Uses

Mallow is one of the flowers of Beltane, along with hawthorne, apple,
lilacs, honeysuckle, primrose, dandelion, and others. The plant is associated with Hecate and with thresholds in some way and is often an ingredient in flying ointments, not as an active entheogen but as a guide, buffer,
and synergist. It can be carried in an amulet to attract love and is thought
to promote sexual desire:

> Mallow seed is attached to the arms of patients suffering from sper-
> matorrhoea; and, so naturally adapted is this plant for the promotion
> of lustfulness, that the seed of the kind with a single stem, sprinkled

upon the genitals, will increase the sexual desire in males to an infinite degree, according to Xenocrates; who says, too, that if three roots are attached to the person, in the vicinity of those parts, they will be productive of a similar result.[9]

Preparations and Recipes

The roots, leaves, and flowers of mallow can all be used in preparations and recipes. However, oftentimes the root is the most available on the commercial market.

The two most common mallow preparations in modern herbalism are the glycerite and the cold infusion, a recipe for which is given below.

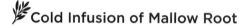

Cold Infusion of Mallow Root

Taken right before a meal, this infusion is particularly helpful for people with inflammed digestive mucosa as it creates a mucilaginous barrier along the stomach lining.

¼ cup of marshmallow root
1 pint of cold or room-temperature water

1. Place the marshmallow root in a 1 pint canning jar.
2. Pour water over it and let steep for 20 minutes, shaking occasionally.
3. Strain and drink.

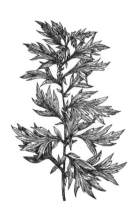

ARTEMISIA (MUGWORT)

Mater Herbarum, Mother of Herbs

Family: Asteraceae (formerly Compositae)
Genus: *Artemisia*
Species: *vulgaris*
Italian vernacular names: *Assenzio selvatico, amarella, canapaccio, brantaròn, incèns, èrba regina*[1]
English vernacular names: Common wormwood, green ginger, felon herb, Saint John's plant, moxa, sailor's tobacco

There are several hundred artemisia species around the world. They include *tridentata* (big sagebrush), *annua* (sweet annie), *absinthium* (wormwood), *dracunculus* (tarragon), and *abrotanum* (southernwood). Mugwort is a perennial that grows in marshy soils and hedgelands. It grows from two to four feet tall.

Vulgaris is Latin for "common," indicating that this is a common plant. The name *mugwort* is from the Old English *mugcwyrt*, with *mugc* meaning "midge" and *wyrt* or *wort* simply meaning "herb." Midges are a type of fly so *mugwort* could be interpreted as an herb to repel flies or pests.

Aemilius Macer, a tenth-century didactic Roman poet, called mugwort, motherwort. The use of the word *mother* here translates as "uterus" or "womb."[2] This follows because the Latin *matrix* meant "breeding female" and is derived from the Indo-European root *māter* from which came the words *matter* and *mother*.[3] *Matrix* was originally used as the word for the uterus or womb as well as "a supporting or enclosing structure."

Folklore, Mythology, and Ancient Uses

The word *artemisia* is derived from the Greek goddess Artemis (Diana in Roman mythology), to whom the plant is dedicated. Artemis has been popularly known as the goddess of the hunt, but she is also a Moon goddess. Moon goddesses generally correspond to the female reproductive system as well as to the energetic nature of human femininity regardless of the gender of the person. Feminine energy is receptive and intuitive, so this indicates that mugwort will increase receptive/intuitive capacity.

Artemis has often been associated, and some believe merged with, the Greek goddess Ilithyia, or Eileithyia (the bringer). Eileithyia's Roman counterpart is Lucina (light bringer) or Natio (birth). So Eileithyia is the goddess of labor and birth, and she brings aid and light to the process of birth in all its forms. As she and Artemis became one over time, Artemis became a protector of the birth process but not by bringing light and aid as much as by averting danger. She is said to have midwifed her brother Apollo into the world.

When racked with labour pangs, and sore distressed
the sex invoke thee, as the soul's sure rest;
for thou Eileithyia alone canst give relief to pain,
which art attempts to ease, but tries in vain.
Artemis Eileithyia, venerable power,
who bringest relief in labour's dreadful hour.

ORPHIC HYMN 2, TO PROTHYRAEIA,
AS TRANSLATED BY THOMAS TAYLOR, 1792

There are some who think that the surname [for the plant]
is derived from Artemis Ilithyia, because the plant is specific
for the troubles of women.

PLINY THE ELDER, *NATURAL HISTORY*, 25.

Once the Christian religions came into power, mugwort was no longer associated with Artemis and was instead attached to Saint John the Baptist. According to Judika Illes in *The Element Encyclopedia of 5,000 Spells*, "Allegedly John the Baptist wore a girdle (belt) woven from mugwort while in the wilderness. A similar magic belt allegedly provides you with good health."[4]

Herbal Medicine Uses

Mugwort is an emmenagogue, nervine, anthelmintic, stomachic, and oneirogen. The average dose is 1 to 2 teaspoons of dried or fresh herb to 1 cup of boiling water 2 to 3 times per day or 20 to 30 drops of tincture 2 to 3 times per day.

Mugwort is a top herb for the hormonal system with a specific affinity for the uterus. It brings heat and circulation to the pelvic region helping to relieve stagnation and distribute oxygenated blood to the tissues. This is specifically helpful for congestive dysmenorrhea (menstrual cramping). Congestive cramping is related to blood stagnation in the pelvis due to poor circulation, bloating, inflammation, lack of blood flow, or excessive blood flow. The improvement in pelvic circulation leads to healthier uterine tone and, in turn, to increased fertility.

The infused oil of mugwort is also used as a massage oil for areas of the body, including the pelvic region, where there is pain associated with stagnation and coldness.

Contraindication: Because mugwort is considered an emmenagogue and is a uterine stimulant, it is contraindicated in pregnancy.

Italian Folk Medicine Uses

Mugwort is often used to relieve pain externally as an oil, salve, or a "poultice prepared with *Allium sativum* L., *Ruta* sp., *Mentha* spp., *Artemisia* spp."[5]

> *Una leggenda cristiana la pianta germoglio ne paradiso terrestre, lungo il sentiero che doveva percorrere il serpente, allo scopo di impedirne il cammino e preservare l'uomo dal peccato. Da questo racconto l'artemisia diventa l'erba del pellegrino, di colui che percorre le strada e puó empre incorrere in brutti incontri.[6]*

A Christian legend says the plant sprouts paradise, along the path that the snake has traveled, in order to prevent humans from the paths of sin. From this story mugwort becomes the herb of the pilgrim, of the one who travels the streets and runs into dangerous encounters.

> *Artemide era anche protettrice dell strade e dei crocicchi, e quindi dei vian-danti, a cui rishciarava il cammino di notte, con luce della luna.[7]*

Artemis was also the protector of the roads and crossroads, and therefore of the wayfarers by lighting their way at night with the Moon.

Emotional and Psychospiritual Benefits

Mugwort essence empowers and awakens our intuitive ability. It is traditionally known as a dream enhancer as a well a protection plant. Mugwort guides us into the world of both our sleeping dreams and the dreams we long to actualize in our waking life. It connects us to the creative and fertile richness that comes from being grounded in our feminine center.

It is also used to "balance the transition from night to day consciousness, and to help those who have a tendency to an overactive psychic life, cutting them off from the physical world of 'reality,' remain connected to the practical, earthy aspects of life," and for those "prone to disturbed nights because of an overactive dreamlife."[8]

Energetics and Correspondences

Energetics: Hot and dry in the second degree
Astrological influence: Venus, the Moon
Element: Fire
Tarot card: The moon
Deity: Venus, Artemis, Chiron*

> *What is Venus but the Artemisia that grows in your garden?*
> PARACELSUS

Magical Uses

Mugwort is often used in magical applications for protection in the following ways:

- Applied in fumigation to protect from poisonous snakes and spiders
- Worn as an amulet around the neck
- Hung over entrances
- Carried in a satchel for protection while traveling

In the *Garden of Health*, Johann Wonnecke von Kaub writes, "Dioscorides, once again, in his chapter on Artemisia informs that the individual using Mugwort cannot be harmed by poisons or sorcery, nor can be injured by the bite of a sick animal."[9]

---

*Associated with Chiron because the goddess Diana (who tutored him on the healing arts) gave him three types of Artemisia species to use as medicines.

Preparations and Recipes

Mugwort baths are used for energetic cleansing as well as a method of imbibing the medicinal compounds of the plant through and on our skin, so both locally and systemically.

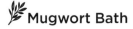

Mugwort Bath

> 1 quart of water
>
> 1 cup of fresh or dried mugwort leaves and flowers

1. Heat water in a pan and bring to a boil.
2. Remove the pan from the heat and add the mugwort to the water.
3. Cover and steep for 30 minutes.
4. Strain the water and add it to bath water.

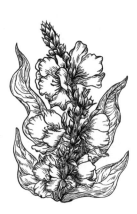

VERBASCO OR TASSO BARBASSO (MULLEIN)

The Noble Herb

Family: Scrophulariaceae
Genus: *Verbascum*
Species: *thapsus*
Italian vernacular names: *Candela da rè, fiòri da sharbàt*[1]

English vernacular names: Adam's flannel, common mullein, flannel plant, goldenrod, hare's beard, hag's taper

The Italian word for mullein is *tasso barbasso* or simply *verbasco*. Tasso barbasso is roughly translated as "bearded" or "hairy" barbasso, barbasso being derived from *barbasco* and *verbasco*.

Here'a general description in Italian with an English translation following:

> *Tasso barbasso, Verbasco a grandi fiori, Guaragnasco maggiore, Candela regia, Pan delle ser-pi, Pianta Domine. Il nome del genere è quello usato*

da Plinio (per es. in xxv, 108: Est similis verbasco herba) e forse deriva dal latino barbascum che significa barbato, con riferimento alla diffusa pelosità di queste piante.²

Tasso barbasso, large-flowered Mullein, majestic great Mullein, wavy leaf Mullein, plant of the snakes, Pianta Domine. Its genus was named by Pliny (for example in book XXV, 108 describes Mullein herb) and perhaps derives from the Latin barbascum which means bearded, with reference to the widespread hairiness of these plants.

The word *mullein* comes from the Latin word *mollis* meaning "soft." Mullein's botanical name is *Verbascum thapsus*, which is believed to refer to the prehistoric Greek city of Thapsus in Sicily. The direct translation of *thapsus* from Greek is "burial," and the Greek city of Thapsus, one of the most important cities of that time, is known for having a large necropolis of cave tombs. *Verbascum* likely means "plant," so mullein is the plant of Sicily or the plant of Thapsus.

Mythical names for mullein include Aaron's rod, named for the brother of Moses whose staff of mullein is said to have protected people from the plagues of Egypt. Mullein is also known as Jacob's or Jupiter's staff.

Mullein is native to the Mediterranean, Asia, and Northern Africa. It is a member of the Figwort, or Scrophulariaceae, family, which contains up to five thousand species, although some of those species have recently been transferred to other families. There are about 350 species of the *Verbascum* genus. *Scrophulariaceae* comes from the word *scrofula*, which refers to a plant's ability to treat scrofula, or mycobacterial cervical lymphadenitis, which is an inflammation of the lymph nodes due to a bacterial infection related to tuberculosis or any infection that causes lymph swelling.

Mullein is mostly pollinated by bees and butterflies but is also autogamous, which is a fancy word for "self-pollinating," as are most of the flowers in the Scrophulariaceae family. Mullein is a biennial/two-year plant and has a life cycle that consists of three main phases. It spends its first year as a ground-dwelling plant with leaves that circle in a basal rosette pattern. In the second year it begins to lift, and it's leaves enlarge and push upward and outward. The final, or third, phase happens during the summer of the second year as its flower stalk surges up like a torch, and its gentle yellow flowers spin themselves around it.

Folklore, Mythology, and Ancient Uses

There was a Roman agricultural practice of tying mullein around a tree as an amulet to keep pests away.[3] And it is widely believed that the herb given to Ulysses was mullein, although several other herbs may have been the "moly" given to him by Hermes, and it's likely that it was a combination of herbs. That said, many sources agree that a mullein spike was what protected Ulysses from the spells of Circe.

> *She'll mix a potion for you; she'll add drugs*
> *into that drink; but even with their force,*
> *she can't bewitch you; for the noble herb*
> *I'll give you now will baffle all her plots.*
>
> HERMES, GIVING MULLEIN TO ULYSSES
> TO PROTECT HIM FROM CIRCE

Herbal Medicine Uses

There is barely an herb that is attributed more to the lungs than mullein. This plant goes into almost every lung formula or tea that I make, and it is appropriate for any and all lung conditions. I use it alone as well. Mullein acts upon the structural capacity of the tissues to hold or release water and create dynamic equilibrium or ionic balance. It is moistening to the lungs with a secondary drying effect that is the result of expectoration. It draws water into dried-out tissues, causing a release of stagnant secretions and in doing so opens the lungs, reduces coughing and tightness, lubricates the mucosa, and relaxes the larynx. Its doctrine of signatures indicates the cilia of the lungs and upper respiratory tract as expressed in its soft, furry, lobe-shaped leaves and certainly the spine with its tall, straight, central stalk.

Mullein is known to lubricate mucosa both along the respiratory tract and within the joints, especially the vertebrae and other nerve-rich areas such as fingers and toes, enabling the full range of breath through the lungs and movement of the body.

Italian Folk Medicine Uses

In Italian folk medicine, the flower of mullein is used externally as a poultice for inflammation and gangrenous infections. The infused oil of the leaves is used for skin diseases and wound healing.[4] Mullein can also be used for respiratory and hair conditions:

> *Il decotto dei fiori era bevuto nel trattamento dell affezioni respiratorie.*
> *Il decotto delle foglie era usato per sciacquare i capelli grassi e contro la forfora.*[5]

The decoction of the flowers was drunk in the treatment of respiratory ailments.

The decoction of the leaves was used to rinse oily hair and against dandruff.

Emotional and Psychospiritual Benefits

The mullein flower essence can help you identify your current life path and an understanding of how to move forward towards it. Use mullein to align your heart chakra as any plant that tones and supports the lungs corresponds to the heart and that general area of the body. When our hearts are broken or we feel grief it can often become stuck in our lungs due to the tightening and/or holding of breath that occurs as a response to stress and fear.

Energetics and Correspondences

Energetics: Cool and damp in the first degree but has a drying element as well

Astrological influence: Saturn

Element: Water

Tarot card: Five of cups

Deity: Saturn

Magical Uses

When Mullein comes into our lives it is time to strengthen our container so that we can embrace and receive abundance and love as well as release it. It helps us to notice when our cup runeth o'er and we must either let go, share, or rearrange our excesses so that we can be clear, breathe deep, and focus. Mullein aids us in standing tall and centered as we maintain our roots while lifting straight to the sun. This can be a strong commitment to a goal, practice, or a dream. Invoke the magic of mullein by burning the stalk or by placing pieces of any part of the plant in an amulet or brevi bag.

Preparations and Recipes

The leaves, roots, and flowers can all be used in preparations and recipes. While the leaves are more attuned to the lungs, and the roots are more attuned to the joints and nerves, a mullein tincture can be made from both the roots and the leaves. The primary way I have used the flower is in infused oil for ear infections similar to how garlic oil is used.

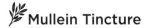 **Mullein Tincture**

Tincture is made with the leaves and sometimes the roots. Mullein root tincture is used for pain, specifically nerve pain. The leaf tincture is generally used for dry coughs and is made with the leaves of the first year plant, or the second year plant in the spring before the stalk forms.

1. Chop or cut the fresh leaves.
2. Place in a glass jar, tamp down, and add more until the jar is full.
3. Pour 100 proof alcohol to cover.
4. Leave for 4 to 6 weeks in a cold dark place, shake regularly.
5. Strain and pour into a glass jar for use.

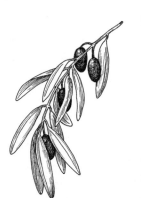

OLIVA (OLIVE)

The Tree of Peace

Family: Oleaceae
Genus: *Olea*
Species: *europaea*
Italian vernacular names: *Ulia, orbàga, uliv, olia, euli auliva*[1]
English vernacular names: Sweet oil plant

There has hardly been an herb that is as famed as olive or *Olea europaea*. Olive in all of its expressions, whether it's as an oil, a food, or a symbol, is one of the Mediterranean's greatest elixirs. In Italian-American culture, olive oil, simply called *olio*, is an ingredient in almost every recipe, and it is taken by the spoonful medicinally for almost any ailment. A spoonful can even just be good nourishment and used as a way to keep up your immune system or just for energy. It is customary in my family and community to use olive oil instead of butter on bread. We either dip the bread in the olive oil or drizzle the oil right on the bread.

The etymology of *olive* comes from the Greek word *elaia* and the Etruscan *eleifa*, both simply referring to the olive tree as well as the fruit.[2] In the Salento area of Italy, it is called *ulía*. This word also means "I'd like to." The olive is a primary sacred plant all over Southern Italy, but as I write this, the olive trees in this region are being decimated by a bacterial disease called Xylella. The people of the region have been making a great effort to save the trees and call themselves *Il Popolo degli Ulivi* meaning "the people of the olives," with their mission being to provide information and resources to stop the disease as well as create new ways of being in relationship with place:

> May the centuries-old and millennia-old olive trees of Apulia be the occasion to re-think new forms of economy and horizontal organizational models, and to rediscover, in a modern way, what our Messapic, Greek, and Roman ancestors already knew: we are the olive trees.[3]

Olive trees grow in a Mediterranean climate and don't particularly like growing in pots according to both my experience and the experience of others. The best zones for growing olive are zones 8 through 10. Olive leaves can be harvested all year long, the bark is harvested in the spring and the fall, and the fruits are picked in the fall.

Folklore, Mythology, and Ancient Uses

The olive is native to the Mediterranean, and recent DNA research has traced its probable origins to the Levant. It became domesticated between 8,000 to 6,000 years ago in the Eastern Mediterranean.[4]

The mythology of the olive appears in many of the region's cultural traditions and, of course, is the famous tree branch brought to Noah by a dove in the biblical legend of Noah's Ark. A Greek legend says that the olive first grew because of a contest between Athena and Poseidon. Both deities struck a rock; Poseidon with his trident and Athena with her spear. When Poseidon did so, water ran out of the rock, and when Athena did so, an olive tree grew out of it and hence became her gift to the people of Athens. The olive is still considered the city's primary *moria* (sacred tree), or tree protected for its spiritual significance.[5]

Olive oil attracts dirt. It was used as a cleanser as well as a healing agent, and in ancient Rome and Greece, it was used in sacred bathing rituals and external cleansing. The Roman baths, called *thermae*, were heated by a hypocaust (a system of underground pipes) and were part of daily life as well as ritual and celebration. The Romans had a bathing regimen that began with body oiling. The entire body was oiled with olive oil or olive oil infused with healing and aromatic herbs. Next, they would take a plunge in cold water, followed by warm water, and finally a soak in hot water. After the bath they would scrape their body with a strigil, which is a curved metal skin scraper.

According to Pliny the Elder, "there are two liquids that are especially agreeable to the human body, wine inside and oil outside, both of them the most excellent of all the products of the tree class, but oil an absolute necessity."[6]

Olive oil was referred to by Homer in the *Odyssey* as "liquid gold," and Hippocrates noted that it had sixty medicinal uses.[7]

Herbal Medicine Uses

Herbal preparations of olive are usually of the tincture, tea, or decoction varieties. The leaves are antiseptic and astringent, and a decoction of the leaves is used for fevers and respiratory infections. Olive leaf tincture is used for immune support and as a preventative and treatment for infections.

While olive oil is an herbal remedy on its own, often used as a demulcent and a laxative, it is also used as a carrier oil for infused herbs.

It is highly nutritive and is made up of 75 percent monounsaturated fats, which are known to lower LDL cholesterol. It is also considered to be antioxidant and anti-inflammatory.[8]

According to Victor Preedy and Ronald Watson, editors of *The Mediterranean Diet*,

> olive oil (OO) is the defining component of the Mediterranean diet (MD), which is associated with the primary prevention of several chronic diseases including cardiovascular disease, cancer, and diabetes. OO contains several bionutraceuticals including monousaturated fatty acids and polyphenols. Components such as hydroxytryrosol, tyrosol, oleocanthal, and oleuropein are responsible for several anti-atherogenic, anticancer, and antidiabetes benefits, primarily due to antioxidation and antiinflammation mechanisms.[9]

Oleuropein is thought to be the active ingredient in olive oil, and studies have shown that it decreases insulin resistance:

> Oleuropein has already demonstrated interesting blood glucose lowering properties. The results of experimental studies suggest that the hypoglycemic effects of oleuropein could be mediated by modulation of multiple intracellular signaling mechanisms that are directly involved in the regulation of blood glucose concentration.[10]

Italian Folk Medicine Uses

Italian folk medicine uses of olive oil include sty removal and menstrual pain relief:

> *Nel caso di orzaiolo, si consigliava di guardare, ogni mattina, nella bottiglia dell'olio di oliva, avvicinando il piu poosibile il collo dell bottiglia all'occhio, anzi, se possibile, toccandolo. Questa curiosa terapia era molto in voga lungo tutta la penisola.*[11]

In the case of sty, it was recommended to look at the bottle of olive oil every morning, bringing the neck of the bottle as close to the eye as possible, indeed, if possible, touching it. This curious therapy was very popular throughout the peninsula.

Per lenire i dolori mestruali si mescolavano due cucciai d'olio d'oliva con cinque cucchiai di vino e un cucchiaio di zucchero o di miele, si sbatteva velocemente e si beveva la miscela, anchi piu volte al di.[12]

To relieve menstrual pains, two tablespoons of olive oil were mixed with five tablespoons of wine and a tablespoon of sugar or honey; the mixture was whipped quickly and the mixture was drunk, several times a day.

Emotional and Psychospiritual Benefits

Olive flower essence is used for extreme fatigue whether spiritual or physical or both.

Energetics and Correspondences

Energetics: Cold and dry in the first degree; however, according to Galen of Pergamum, olive oil is "temperate and exceeds no one in quality," meaning that it has no dominant energetic quality.[13]

Astrological influence: Saturn and sometimes the Sun

Element: Earth

Tarot card: Queen of swords

Deity: Athena

Magical Uses

For protection, olive branches are often placed over thresholds, and olive wreaths are hung on doors. Olives are also used as offerings to deities, saints, and gods and to divine if a person has the evil eye.

Preparations and Recipes

The leaves, fruit, and bark of the olive plant can all be used in preparations and recipes. I mainly use straight olive oil as a preparation or as a menstruum for infused oils. The leaves can also be made into tea or tincture.

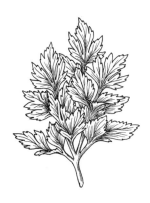

PREZZEMOLO (PARSLEY)
Herb of Death

Family: Apiaceae
Genus: *Petroselinum*
Species: *crispum*
Italian vernacular names: *Apio ortense, per-nasevel, petrosillo, petroselino*[1]
English vernacular names: Garden parsley, rock parsley

The word *parsley* comes from the Greek *petroselinon* meaning "rock parsley," with *petros* meaning "rock, stone." The botanical name of parsley is *Petroselinum crispum* and it's in the Apiaceae or Umbelliferae family along with many other plants we know of, such as celery, giving parsley one of its common names, celery of the rocks. Other Apiaceae family plants include carrot, fennel, parsnip, coriander, angelica, and poison hemlock.

> Petroselinum, the specific name of the Parsley, from which our English name is derived, is of classic origin, and is said to have been assigned to it by Dioscorides. The Ancients distinguished between two plants Selinon, one being the Celery (Apium graveolens) and called heleioselinon—i.e. "Marsh selinon," and the other—our parsley—Oreoselinon, "Mountain selinon"; or petroselinum, signifying "Rock selinon." This last name in the Middle Ages became corrupted into Petrocilium—this was anglicized into Petersylinge, Persele, Persely, and finally Parsley.[2]

There are thirty+ varieties of parsley, but the two most common are flat-leaf and curly. Flat-leaf parsley is what we often call Italian parsley, or *Petroselinum crispum* var. *neapolitanum*. Curly parsley is *Petroselinum crispum* var. *crispum*.

Parsley is a source of vitamin C, B vitamins, iron, beta-carotene, and chlorophyll. Its taste is slightly bitter, crispy, and salty. These flavors indicate the presence of minerals and sodium. Parsley is also known as a carminative and diuretic. Carminative means that it relieves gas and bloating thereby helping to improve digestion.

Folklore, Mythology, and Ancient Uses

Parsley has been called the herb of death because it was commonly used in funeral rites in ancient Greece. It is native to the Mediterranean and has been known in modern times as primarily a culinary herb, but it has a long history as a medicinal plant as well.

The original story from Greek mythology that associated the parsley plant with death is the story of Archemorus. Archemorus was first named Opheltes until, as an infant, he was left unattended and killed by a serpent. It was then that the first parsley plants on Earth grew from his spilled blood. After that he was named Archemorus, which means "beginning of death." After his death, the first Nemean Games were held in his honor, and all the participants wore crowns of parsley.

Parsley has also been called the devil's herb because of its low germination rate. According to legend, this is so because the seed goes to the devil nine times before sprouting, and the ones that don't are the ones that the devil keeps. Another form of this legend says that the seeds have to be sown nine times before they'll come up and, to preserve the soul of the gardener, should only be planted on Good Friday. The parsley that does grow is thought to be immune to evil spirits and therefore protective.

In ancient Rome and Greece, parsley was planted over graves or made into wreaths to decorate them while the saying *De'eis thaiselinon* or "To need only parsley" was often added. This meant that the person had come to their final ritual of death where the parsley plant was incorporated.[3]

Parsley is a biennial, meaning it's life cycle is two years, and according to superstition it is bad luck to transplant it. Wherever you plant it in the garden is where it must stay for its two-year life cycle. It is traditionally planted next to rue and at the border of the garden indicating its energetic signature as a threshold plant or a plant that guides us through thresholds such as death or any initiatory or transformative process. It also signifies that it appears at the beginning or incubatory stages of something. As the old saying goes, "We are only at the parsley and rue," meaning "We are just getting started."

> I never didn't transplant parsley. That's the worst thing you can go for to do. You sow some on a bed and lets it grow there, and that's all right, but if you digs it up and goes for to transplant it someone in the family's sure to die.[4]

It was also thought that giving parsley away would bring bad luck:

> Having grown a crop of parsley it was always considered unlucky to give it away because to do so was to transfer any of your good luck along with it. Therefore, to solve this problem anyone who you wanted to give parsley to must steal it from your garden, openly or covertly. In 1841, William Blackwood writes the following: "In the hieroglyphic language of flowers, the gift of parsley implies a wish of the person's death to whom it is presented; for parsley has ever been the herb with which the Greeks decorate their graves and tombs; and hence to want parsley was an expression applied to a person in his last extremity.[5]

The story of "Petrosinella" (meaning "little parsley"), written by Giambattista Basile in 1634 in Naples, is the earliest known telling of "Rapunzel" on record. In this version a pregnant woman steals parsley from the garden of an ogress.

In ancient medicinal writings, parsley and celery are often mixed up. They, along with fennel, asparagus, and butcher's broom, are the five "opening roots" of Galenic (Greek-Arab) medicine. *Opening* means that they remove obstructions to elimination.

Parsley was often made into a suppository to cause an abortion or to relieve constipation. According to hedge witch legends, a woman who wanted to end a pregnancy should eat parsley 3 times a day for 3 weeks. And while Pliny the Elder wrote that parsley caused sterility, that was more likely a reference to its contraceptive properties.

According to Dioscorides, parsley was used as "an emmenagogue, [and] also for pain in the side, and for stomach, kidney, and bladder problems,"[6] and according to Pliny the Elder,

> Parsley is held in universal esteem; for we find sprigs of it swimming in the draughts of milk given us to drink in country-places; and we know that as a seasoning for sauces, it is looked upon with peculiar favour. Applied to the eyes with honey, which must also be fomented from time to time with a warm decoction of it, it has a most marvellous efficacy in cases of defluxion of those organs or of other parts of the body; as also when beaten up and applied by itself, or in combination with bread or with polenta.[7]

Herbal Medicine Uses

Parsley is known as a carminative which means that it relieves flatulence and reduces bloating. It is also slightly bitter and therefore aids overall digestion. According to what I've learned in courses with Matthew Wood it is successful at treating bladder infections if taken as a tea, made from fresh leaves, daily. Also on advice from Matt Wood, I have been making parsley honey wine for opening the chest due to tightness caused by Covid-19 infection. This is an old recipe originally from Hildegard Von Bingen.

Contraindications: Always be careful with the parsley family. It has poisonous look-alikes in young stages of growth, so only harvest cultivated stands of parsley.

Italian Folk Medicine Uses

Parsley has many uses in Italian folk medicine now and in the past. It's uses are applied much in the same way as discussed above under the "Herbal Medicine Uses."

> *Per arrestare la montata lattea si faceva mangiare alla donna del prezzemolo, a dosi crescenti, mescolato alle pietanze.*

> To stop the flow of breastmilk, the woman would eat parsley, in increasing doses, mixed with food/dishes.

*Le foglie pestate erano applicat localmente suule contusioni e sulle pun-
ture d'insetti.*[8]

The crushed leaves were applied locally on bruises and insect bites.

Energetics and Correspondences

Energetics: Hot and dry in the second degree
Astrological influence: Mercury
Element: Fire
Tarot card: Death
Deity: Persephone

Magical Uses

Parsley is often used in rituals for communication with the dead and is
thought to protect food from contamination. Ancient magical/super-
stitious uses included feeding horses parsley before going into battle to
make them more agile and fast and eating parsley seed to make yourself
invisible.

Preparations and Recipes

All parts of the parsley plant can be used, including the seeds and roots,
but the leaves are the most popular. Although culinary use of parsley is
safe in pregnancy, therapeutic doses are cautioned against.

Parsley Wine

This is a recipe from Hildegard von Bingen, medieval Christian
mystic, also known as the "Sibyl of the Rhine," who said that this
recipe would improve cardiovascular function among other things. I
was using it during the pandemic with people who had a tight chest
from Covid-19.

    10 parsley leaves and stems
    2 tablespoons wine vinegar
    1 quart of red wine
    1 cup of honey

1. Place wine, vinegar, and parsley in a pot and bring to a boil.
2. Then turn down heat and simmer for 5 to 8 minutes.
3. Let cool until warm but no longer hot and strain.
4. Add honey.
5. Take the amount of one shot glass up to 3 times per day.

> *Whoever suffers from pain in the heart, spleen or side, drink this wine often (daily) and it will heal him.*
>
> HILDEGARD VON BINGEN

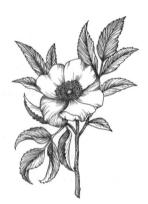

ROSA (ROSE)
Flower of Love

Family: Rosaceae
Genus: *Rosa*
Species: *canina*
Italian vernacular names: *Rosa del còcò, rösa sarvàga, rosa màta, scarnègia, rosa delle siepi, rosa spina, rosa di macchia*[1]
English vernacular names: none

There are wild roses native to every temperate region on Earth. The rose is ubiquitous but most native roses are prevalent in Asia. There are, however, thousands of rose cultivars and most of our ornamental garden roses are cultivars from China. *Rosa* spp. are probably the most cultivated flowers there are.

The birthplace of the cultivated Rose was probably Northern Persia, on the Caspian, or Faristan on the Gulf of Persia. Thence it spread across Mesopotamia to Palestine and across Asia Minor to Greece. And thus it was that Greek colonists brought it to Southern Italy.[2]

The etymology of the word *rose* comes from the Latin *rosa* and the Greek *rhodon*, both of which mean "rose," and before that probably the

Old Persian *wrda*, which means "flower" or "blossom." Searching the etymology of rose doesn't turn up any meaning other than other variations of the word for this particular flower or simply just the word for flower.

Rose in Italy is *Rosa canina*, or the dog rose. Other species include *Rosa nitidula* and *Rosa di San Giovanni*. There are also many multi-petaled cultivars.

Roses represent love, life, and humanity. I think if there were any flower that represented the archetype of a human being it would be the rose; such beauty, such thorns, so gentle, so sharp.

Folklore, Mythology, and Ancient Uses

The rose has long been a symbol of love, beauty, and the sacred heart, and throughout history it has been a ritual flower in many crosscultural celebrations and ceremonies. The celebration of roses in ancient Rome was the festival of Rosalia, also called Rosaria, or Rosatio, which means "day of rose adornment." This festival takes place anytime from May through July when the roses were blooming. On this day, garlands and wreaths of roses were made to be worn as well as offered to the gods and goddesses of love such as Venus and Dionysus.

We can see the rose associated with deities of many cultures. In Norse mythology the rose is offered to the goddess Frigga in the form of hedgerows. Even the Christians adopted the rose as primary symbol of faith: "According to Gallwitz, 'The early Christians detested the rose cult of the Romans . . . until they brought the rose's thorns into connection with Christ's crown of thorns.'"[3] The five petals of the rose were associated with the five wounds of Christ and red roses, in particular, came to represent his blood.

Roses also represent life, birth, and death. A garland of roses and the rosary are made into a circle, like birth and death and time. Birth and death are on the same place on the circle, and life contains them both. Linear time is how we string each rose or bead, one by one on the thread of the universe. It is how we navigate nonlinear Kairos.

Roses were famous funeral flowers in both ancient Greece and Rome and still are today. They were used to adorn funerary rites and were planted in burial grounds. They were also offered as bloodless sacrifices—the color red and the thorns representing blood. Blood sacrifice is a widely misunderstood component of almost every indigenous culture on Earth. When humans lived more closely with birth and death, their own and all of nature's, they understood the imperative of reciprocity and what could be thought of as a "gift economy."

Rose was the main ingredient in a compound formula from medieval times called benedicta. All of the ingredients in benedicta were blessed and given to treat multiple "infirmities." It was used for conditions of the kidneys and bladder, arthritis, gout, and all cold conditions. The ingredients from "The Trotula," a medieval compendium from the Salerno Medical School are as follows:

10 drams each of vegetable "turpeth," spurge, and sugar; five drams each of scammony, wild garlic, and roses; one dram each of cloves, spikenard, ginger, saffron, saxifrage, long pepper, poppy, watercress, parsley, gromwell, rock salt, galangal, mace, caraway, fennel, dove's-foot cranesbill, butcher's broom, and gromwell; and honey as needed. This is given in the evening in the amount of a chestnut with warm wine.[4]

Another medieval remedy is *oleum rosaceum* or rose oil that was made as follows:

One and a half pounds of slightly crushed fresh roses should be placed in two pounds of common (and in our opinion, cleaned) oil; these should be placed in a full pot suspended in a cauldron full of water. And let these boil for a while until they are reduced to a third of their original quantity. Only then should this be put into a white linen cloth and squeezed through a press.[5]

This oil was applied externally to reduce fever, headache pain, burns, digestive inflammation (applied externally on the stomach), and put on pulse points of the wrist and the bottoms of the feet to cool systemic inflammation.

The Virgin Mary is also called Our Lady of Roses, and the rose is a flower that symbolizes her and many other holy women:

> The rose was a privileged symbol for Mary, Queen of heaven and earth. One of her titles in Catholic Marian devotion is Rosa Mystica or Mystic Rose. During the Middle Ages, the rose became an attribute of many other holy women, including Elizabeth of Hungary, Elizabeth of Portugal and Casilda of Toledo, and of martyrs in general. The rose is even a symbol for Christ himself.[6]

Our Lady of Guadalupe (another name for the Virgin Mary) spoke to Juan Diego, a Chichimec peasant, and gave him a message to share with the local bishop, who did not believe him. Juan Diego met with Our Lady several more times. Each time she directs him to share the same message with the bishop, and each time he is not believed. Finally, she asks him to pick a bunch of Castilian roses (a.k.a. Damask roses, named after the city of Damascus) and carry them in his cloak to the bishop. When he opens his coat to share them there is the image of the Virgin Mary printed on the inside of it. He is then believed.

Herbal Medicine Uses

Pretty much any species of rose can be used, but I usually use my local wild rose, *Rosa multiflora*. I also absolutely love *Rosa rugosa*, and those species are the two I have the most experience with. I love using rose to treat acute anxiety or panic attacks that happen in the moment but I also use it for depression related to grief, PMS, and emotional trauma. Rose is considered a reproductive tonic and is used to promote fertility.

Italian Folk Medicine Uses

The main use of rosa in Italian folk medicine is as a food. The hips/fruit are simply eaten or made into jam as a source rich in vitamin C. The leaves are astringent and so are made into a decoction for diarrhea. The flowers/petals are added to teas alone or mixed with other plants for a variety of ailments including stomach upsets and as a laxative:

L'infuso dei fiori era assunto contro i burciori di stomaco e come blando lassativo.[7]

The infusion of the flowers was taken against heartburn and as a mild laxative.

Emotional and Psychospiritual Benefits

Rose essence builds a bridge of trust and love centered in the heart that allows us to become conscious of the ways we dilute or completely put out the fire of our passions and move or shift into the inspiration and joy that will feed them.

Energetics and Correspondences

Energetics: Cool and dry in the first degree
Astrological influence: Jupiter (red roses); Venus and the Moon (white roses)
Element: Earth
Tarot card: The lovers
Deity: The Virgin Mary

Magical Uses

In the tale *The Golden Ass*, an ancient Roman novel, the main character Lucius was turned into an ass by a witch. He goes through several ordeals until the goddess Isis appears to him in a dream and tells him that to transform himself back into a human he must eat a crown of roses that will be presented by one of her priests at the Navigium Isidis, the Roman festival for the goddess Isis, the following day. He does this and becomes human again.

Roses represent not only our capacity to become human but also our capacity for embodied transformation. In many old cultures it is understood that we are born with a human body but to truly become human we must grow, mature, and transform into our fullest potential for love, compassion, and presence.

Preparations and Recipes

Rose petals make a sweet, aromatic tea alone or added to other herbs to calm down and relax, but my favorite way to use them is as an elixir.

🌿 Rose Elixir

The amounts of each of the liquid ingredients below are to your taste. Brandy will preserve the preparation longer. It can also be completely omitted.

> Rose petals (enough to fill a jar)
> Brandy (the amount depends on how much you like the taste of brandy)
> Vegetable glycerin or honey

1. Fill a glass jar with rose petals. Tamp down, and fill again.
2. Cover the petals with brandy and vegetable glycerin or honey.
3. Leave in a dark place for 4 to 6 weeks.
4. Strain and bottle.
5. Take a dropperful up to 3 times per day or in the moment during stressful situations.

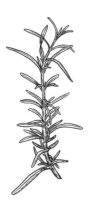

ROSMARINO (ROSEMARY)

The Memory Plant

Family: Lamiaceae
Genus: *Rosmarinus*
Species: *officinalis*
Italian vernacular names: Üsmaréen, *rusmarìn, osmarin, erba della memoria*[1]
English vernacular names: Dew of the sea, rose of the sea

The word *rosemary* comes from the Latin *rosmarinus*, with *ros* meaning "dew" and *marinus* meaning "of the sea, maritime," and perhaps it was so called because it grew near the coast. Another ancient name for this plant was *anthos*, which is the Greek word for "flower."

Rosemary is an evergreen shrub native to the Mediterranean, Northwest Africa, and Southern Asia. It has a rosette or spruce-like structure of branches with opposite leaves that can grow up to 1 1/2 inches long and ½ to 2 inches wide and small axial flowers atop a thick green stem and brown trunk. The leaves are green on top and white underneath, and the flowers are typically blue but can be white, pink, or purple if they are a subspecies or cultivar. Rosemary flowers in the spring and summer in cooler climates, but in warmer climates, it can flower constantly. The flowers are two-lobed, or labiate, like all mint-family flowers.

Rosemary is a very chemically complex plant, and one that is loaded with antioxidants (polyphenol rosmarinic acid). Most antioxidants support a healthy inflammatory response, and this seems to be the case with rosemary. Rosmarinic acid, carnosic acid, and labiatic acid, all constituents of the rosemary plant, are commonly used as a natural preservatives in the food industry in place of BHT and BHA.

According to the doctrine of signatures for this plant, its pungent aromatic smell indicates that it disinfects, deodorizes, and stimulates; its wooly roughness indicates that it has an effect on the skin; its blue flowers indicate that it's an antispasmodic (reduces stomach cramps); its needle-like leaves indicate that it's high in essential oils, and the fact that it likes to grow in warm, sunny places indicates an ability to warm, dry, and cheer.

Rosemary is a Mediterranean plant, and its optimal medicinal qualities will be present in similar climates, and although it does grow in temperate, wetter climates, this changes its potency.

Based on anthroposophy (also called spiritual science), the warming quality of any plant, such as rosemary, relates to the "I" or "self" and aids the integration of such with the other aspects of the body and psyche. From this view, rosemary integrates psyche and soma.

Folklore, Mythology, and Ancient Uses

The name rosmarinus or "dew of the sea" is thought to have originally corresponded to the goddess Aphrodite/Venus. The rosy "dew" was the blood & semen of castrated Neptune or Poseidon which impregnated the waves, causing Aphrodite to step forth from the ocean onto the Isle of Cypros. She was greeted by naiads who draped her naked body in myrtle, but not surprisingly, in ancient portraits of Aphrodite, rosemary as well as myrtle is worked into the imagery. This is undoubtedly why Rosemary is to this day regarded as an aphrodisiac. Rosemary in relative modern times was traditionally entwined into a bride's head-wreath to encourage couples to remember their wedding vows, but this really does sound like a lingering belief in rosemary as enhancing virility & fertility.[2]

Rosemary was sacred all over the Mediterranean world, including Egypt where it was used as an embalming agent. Famous Roman and Greek physicians such as Dioscorides and Pliny the Elder included rosemary in their materia medicas as one of the most valuable medicinal plants available, and Roman priests burned it for purification during ritual ceremonies. Rosemary's most well-known use is to improve memory, and it was even mentioned by Shakespeare in *Hamlet*: "There's rosemary, that's for remembrance; pray, love, remember."[3]

Rosemary was used as a part of funeral ceremonies in England and Northern Europe where there was a ritual practice of throwing a sprig into the grave or coffin of the departed so that their memory would live on:

> *Thy narrow pride, thy fancied green*
> *(For vanity's in little seen)*
> *All must be left when Death appears,*
> *In spite of wishes, groans, and tears;*
> *Nor one of all thy plants that grow,*
> *But Rosemary will with thee go.*
> GEORGE SEWELL, "THE DYING MAN
> IN HIS GARDEN"

Rosemary's virtue of improving memory was well known by Greek scholars who wore rosemary crowns on their heads to help them concentrate on their studies. English physician Nicholas Culpeper noted that rosemary "helps a weak memory, and quickens the senses. It is very comfortable to the stomach in all the cold griefs thereof."[4] Rosemary was also worn by brides as a crown or bridal wreath to symbolize fidelity and fertility, and its branches were often added as wedding decorations.

The Virgin Mary is said to have worn rosemary bound to her clothes to protect her when she fled to Egypt and, legend says, that rosemary flowers were once white but became blue when Mary draped her cloak over them.

Herbal Medicine Uses

You could call Rosemary the Queen of Antioxidants, as she boasts at being one of the strongest herbal antioxidants. In other research, scientists have pinpointed that Rosemary contains the constituent carnosic acid, which can prevent free radical damage in the brain. Carnosic acid has been shown to protect the brain from stroke, Alzheimer's disease, and other effects of aging on the brain. Furthermore, as a circulatory stimulant it can dilate blood vessels and increase blood flow to the brain.[5]

Rosemary is considered a nervine as it warms and relaxes internally and can help release tension. It helps with mental fogginess and also increases our memory and concentration, so it can be good for when we have to stay focused, but it won't overstimulate like coffee. Because it stimulates the vagus nerve, it can build energy by moving and circulating it around the body. It also "increases muscle activity via the parasympathetic, thus strengthening the arteries, stomach, intestines, gall passages, and heart, while relaxing the sympathetic and voluntary muscles."[6]

Rosemary also helps with the metabolism of sugars, warms the stomach, and stimulates digestion. It reduces bloating and water retention and cardiac edema and is helpful for headaches and sinus congestion. Externally, rosemary makes a great hair wash for thinning hair and the infused oil is beneficial for fungal infections and sore joints.

Contraindications: Avoid the therapeutic use of rosemary during pregnancy (it's fine in cooking). It can also aggravate conditions of heat such as hot flashes and certain types of nervousness. Avoid if you have high blood pressure. Because it's drying, it can also tend to dry up breast milk.

Italian Folk Medicine Uses

In mainstream herbalism the leaves/needles of rosemary are the most common part used, but Italian folk medicine does use the twigs as well. The twigs are like small, woody branches.

> *Con i rametti, per favorire la digestione, stimolare la diuresi e calmare la tosse si perpara un infuso con 1 g di prodotto per 100 ml d'acqua. Se ne beve una tazzina o una tazza dopo i pasti.[7]*

Use the twigs, to promote digestion, stimulate diuresis and calm a cough, an infusion is prepared with 1 g of product per 100 ml of water. A shot or a cup is drunk after meals.

> *La pianta era impiegata come espettorante, in infusi insieme a issopo e timo; per le bronchiti e le febbri più devastanti si usava metttere sotto il letto del malato una bacinella d'acqua con rami di rosmarino perchè si credeva che la pianta e l'acqua fossero in grado di assorbire la febbre.[8]*

The plant was used as an expectorant, in infusions together with hyssop and thyme; for bronchitis and the most devastating fevers it was customary to place a basin of water with rosemary branches under the sick person's bed because it was believed that the plant and the water were able to absorb the fever.

Emotional and Psychospiritual Benefits

The rosemary flower essence brings a sense of clarity and integration. It also grounds us in our creativity by making us aware of both sensory and extrasensory information in a way that provides insight and even epiphany.

Rosemary can also be used to treat depression and a lack of motivation or inspiration, and according to FES (Flower Essence Services), rosemary can also help with patterns of imbalance such as "forgetfulness or poor learning ability, [being] loosely incarnated in body, lacking physical/etheric warmth, especially in bodily extremities, [and] traumatic out-of-body spiritual experiences."[9]

Energetics and Correspondences

Energetics: Hot and dry to the second degree, stimulating, astringent
Astrological influence: The Sun
Element: Fire
Tarot card: Queen of wands
Deity: The Virgin Mary

Magical Uses

Rosemary has long been used as a protection plant. It can be burned as incense or worn as an amulet or talisman. It can also be woven into a wreath and hung on a doorway.

Burn rosemary before saying prayers and/or casting spells, especially those to enhance memory, and use rosemary essential oil to cleanse sacred spaces and ritual tools.*

Rosemary is influenced by Aries, the sign of the ram, which in medical astrology represents the head; hence rosemary has an effect on that area of the body and is used to treat headaches and neurosynaptic dysregulations such as depression.

Preparations and Recipes

Rosemary can be harvested any time of year if it grows in your region. It does not grow all year long in the Northeast where I live, so while it does quite well in the summer garden, it must be brought in for the winter. Even then, not too many folks have success keeping it alive throughout the cold season. Both the leaves and the flowers stripped from the branches can be used for preparations and recipes, including the following:

---

*Use all essential oils sparingly as they require large quantities of plant material to make.

- Tinctures made from fresh leaves and flowers (take 15 to 20 drops 3 times a day)
- Tea from dried or fresh leaves and flowers (1 teaspoon of rosemary to 1 cup of boiling water)
- Infused oil
- Burn bundles
- Hair rinse
- Queen of Hungary's water

Rosemary Hair Rinse

1 quart of water

2 or 3 6-inch sprigs of fresh rosemary or 1/4 cup of dried
rosemary leaves

1. In a pot, bring water to a boil.
2. Turn off heat, add rosemary, and cover with a lid. Allow to sit for at least 20 minutes.
3. Let cool and then strain.
4. Pour the liquid into an old shampoo bottle and use as a final rinse after washing your hair.

Queen of Hungary's Water

The fourteenth-century queen of Hungary, Isabella, was given this recipe by someone who is believed to have been either an angel or a hermit or both. It was given to her to wash her face and limbs with as she aged so she could retain her youthfulness and beauty. We know now that rosemary does in fact slow the aging process due, at least in part, to its high antioxidant compounds. The following recipe is adapted from Rosemary Gladstar's original recipe found in her book, *Herbal Healing for Women*.[10]

6 parts lemon balm

4 parts chamomile

1 part rosemary

3 parts calendula

4 parts roses

1 part lemon peel

1 part sage

3 parts comfrey

Witch hazel and/or apple cider vinegar to cover (Use one
or both at any proportion you prefer.)

1. Place all the herbs in a wide-mouthed jar and cover with witch hazel extract (and/or vinegar). Be sure there is about 1 to 2 inches of witch hazel/vinegar above the herb mixture.
2. Cover tightly and let sit in a warm spot for 2 to 3 weeks.
3. Strain and add ½ cup of rosewater to each cup of herbal liquid.
4. Rebottle and use as a facial toner and astringent, foot bath, aftershave, and so on.

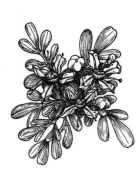

RUTA (RUE)

Herb of Grace

Family: Rutaceae
Genus: *Ruta*
Species: *graveolens*
Italian vernacular names: *Rùga, àrba rüga, ruta commune*[1]
English vernacular names: Common rue, herb of grace

The etymology of the botanical name isn't clear, and in the New Testament, rue is mentioned by its Greek name, *peganon*. The species name, *graveolens*, is from Latin *gravis* ("heavy") and *olēns* ("smelling"). *Ruta* is probably from the Greek word *rhyte*, a word that's meaning is not known for sure, but some sources say it means "bitter" or "to set free." Interestingly, its family, Rutaceae, is the citrus family.

When the Romans introduced the rue herb plant to England, they called it by its Latin name (now the generic name), Ruta. When

Anglicized and shortened to "rue," the name sounded just like the word meaning "sorrow," but that word comes from an Old English word, hreow. (Some believe that the word Ruta comes from a Greek word meaning "to set free.") The specific name, graveolens, is Latin for "having a strong or offensive smell" (dill is Anethum graveolens). Whether rue's odor is either strong or offensive is open to debate; usually, it's described as "musty." Ruta is the genus belonging to the family Rutaceae, members of which include aromatic citrus trees as well as gas plant (Dictamnus albus), a lovely white- or pink-flowered perennial.[2]

Rue was called the herb of grace because it was dipped in holy water and used to sprinkle on people as a blessing and as a method of purification. It was an herb apparently desired by God in the Bible as an offering/tithe:

Woe to you Pharisees, because you give God a tenth of your mint, rue and all other kinds of garden herbs, but you neglect justice and the love of God. You should have practiced the latter without leaving the former undone. (Luke 11:42)

Rue is native to Southern Italy and all of Southeast Europe.

Folklore, Mythology, and Ancient Uses

King Mithridates of Pontus (120–63 BCE) is said to have made rue the main ingredient in his famous panacea, which included "20 Rue leaves, 2 dried walnuts, 2 figs, and a pinch of salt."[3]

In the Middle Ages, rue was considered a cure for the plague, and in the seventeenth century, it was thought to be good for eyesight:

Pliny, John Evelyn tells us, reported Rue to be of such effect for the preservation of sight that the painters of his time used to devour a great quantity of it, and the herb is still eaten by the Italians in their salads. It was supposed to make the sight both sharp and clear, especially when the vision had become dim through over-exertion of the eyes. It was with "Euphrasy and Rue" that Adam's sight was purged by Milton's Angel.[4]

Herbal Medicine Uses

Rue is an antispasmodic, so it can be used for menstrual cramping as well as afterbirth pains. It's also an analgesic and when infused in oil can be used topically for strains, sprains, and bruises. It is thought to relieve stagnation in the cardiovascular system and in acute as well as chronic conditions such as rheumatism.

Contraindication: Rue is an emmenagogue and an emetic, so it should be taken with care at low doses. A tincture dose is around 1 to 5 drops. Rue is also known to be irritating to skin when used directly. I've seen this contraindication downplayed, but I can personally attest that rue can cause contact dermatitis in sensitive people, as I am one of them. I get a severe, itchy rash from contact with rue.

Italian Folk Medicine Uses

Rue is most known in Italian folk medicine for its protective and magical properties as well as its roles as a medicinal plant and cooking herb. It's been hailed as a cure for the malocchio and is central to one of the most famous charms of Southern Italy: the *cimaruta*, or charm of rue.

> *Come altre piante dall'odore intenso, per la presenza di oli essenziale, la ruta era ritenuta di allontanare streghe e spiriti maligni, tanto che, nel Rinascimento, venne definita "herba de fuga demonis" perché, come l'aglio, aveva un'importante funzi-one scacciadiavoli. Persino nei processi contro le streghe spesso gli stessi proces-santi usavano pro-teggersi dai malefici della presunta strega con erbe benedette, tra cui proprio la ruta.[5]*

Like other plants with an intense smell, due to the presence of essential oils, the rue was believed to ward off witches and evil spirits, so much so that, in the Renaissance, it was defined as "herba de escape demonis" because, like garlic, it had the important function of banishing devils. Even in trials against witches often the inquisitors protected themselves from the evil of the alleged witch with blessed herbs, including rue.

In the Italian folk medicine literature rue is often prepared as one of the following:

- An oleolite, in which the plant is infused in olive oil and used in topical applications for pain
- A macerate (tincture) in a grape distillate (grappa)[6]

Rue is used to treat a condition called *mal d'arco*, which is a type of hepatitis that is believed to be contracted by urinating outside either in the direction of a rainbow or at a crossroads where a treatment for a urinary condition occurred. The treatment is for the afflicted person to wake each day and add a handful of white ashes to a *pignatta* (terracotta pot). Then they must urinate into the pot. Next, they make a decoction of rue while saying specific prayers. After the decoction is made, the rue leaves are removed and laid out to make the sign of the cross. After the three days of treatment the pignatta is taken to a crossroads late at night and broken.[7]

Emotional and Psychospiritual Benefits

Rue flower essence can help protect us when we are learning to identify and work with our psychic powers. It strengthens our will and our identity so that we are less susceptible to external forces.

Energetics and Correspondences

Energetics: Hot and dry in the third degree
Astrological influence: The Sun
Element: Fire
Tarot card: The high priestess
Deity: Diana

Magical Uses

Rue is typically used for protection. Here are a few suggestions for doing so:

- ❧ Tie a sprig of rue above doorways, entrances, and thresholds for general protection.
- ❧ Place rue on an altar to protect and sanctify the altar and surrounding prayer space.
- ❧ Dip a sprig in holy water and use to sprinkle objects and spaces. I use this process to bless and protect my gardens.
- ❧ Use as a lucky charm and place it in an amulet bag to carry with you.

Preparations and Recipes

In addition to medicinal preparations, rue leaves are sometimes used in cooking as well. They impart a bitter flavor and can be added to salads, tomato sauces, and other dishes in small amounts. This ultimately works as a preventative medicine.

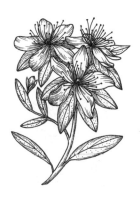

IPERICO (SAINT JOHN'S WORT)

Herb of the Sun

Family: Hypericaceae
Genus: *Hypericum*
Species: *perforatum*
Italian vernacular names: *Erba di San Giovanni, scacciadiavoli, fugademonio, bàlsamin, pilatro, pelico*[1]
English vernacular names: Goatweed, klamath weed

Saint John's wort is known as the herb of the Sun. Its botanical name is *Hypericum perforatum*. Hypericum is derived from the name of the Greek god Hyperion, meaning "the high one," and perforatum describes the small perforations seen in the leaves.

Saint John's wort has a bright, golden yellow flower with stamens that look like rays. The plant flowers in midsummer in sunny locations. It generally grows in clusters and I have found it difficult to cultivate. It seems to have a mind of its own and will grow abundantly in one area for two or three years and then slowly disappear. Its popularity on the commercial herb market has unfortunately lead to its overharvesting in some places.

Folklore, Mythology, and Ancient Uses

Saint John's wort is the plant at the center of one of the most celebrated feasts in Italy: La festa di San Giovanni Battista. Held on June 24 in Southern Italy, it is celebrated with processions and community gatherings. Bonfires are often lit at crossroads, particularly in front of or near churches where the celebrations are focused.

According to Charles Killinger in his book *Culture and Customs of Italy,*

In the fourth century AD, when the Christian religion was legalized, the Catholic Church began the process of superimposing Christian symbols on pagan feast days, an important step in establishing the church's influence on the peninsula. The festivals maintained some of their original character but now were celebrated in the names of saints and, in many cases, the Virgin Mary. San Giorgio (St. George) replaced Perseus, the more ancient serpent slayer; St. John the Baptist, bearer of the traditional ritual immersion, now assumed a saintly presence at Rome's summer water festival.[2]

And as author Carol Field describes in her book *Celebrating Italy,*

Christianity simply grafted the pagan fires to the celebration of the Feast of San Giovanni. The prophet was born precisely at midsummer, just as Jesus was born six months later at the turning point of winter, two moments in the calendar that mark passage across a critical threshold. Bearded and dressed in animal skins, subsisting on honey and locusts, San Giovanni also resembles an ancient god of the fields, or the mythical King of the Wood who married the Great Goddess in dark mid-winter. Six months later, the King of the Wood was put to death beneath a great sacred oak by his successor. So this sacrificial death, with its intimations of rebirth and renewal, was meant to encourage the fertility of the fields.[3]

Saint John's wort, along with many other medicinal plants, was found carbonized by the eruption of Mount Vesuvius giving us invaluable information about the flora that surrounded the ancient Romans.[4]

Herbal Medicine Uses

In modern herbal medicine Saint John's wort is used for pain relief, especially when it involves injuries or inflammation of the nerves and nerve-rich areas of the body. It's also often used as a remedy for sciatica and can be helpful in weaning people off of NSAIDS.

Although it was been much acclaimed for its use as an antidepressant, much of the attention its gotten for this is due to commercial marketing. While it can be helpful for certain types of depression, it is generally not used alone and is instead mixed in a formulation with other herbs. Its effectiveness seems to be specifically for "melancholic" or "black cloud" types of depression and SAD.

There have been hundreds of randomized controlled studies on St. John's Wort extract. The majority do favor a positive effect on mood, particularly when whole plant extracts are used. The flavonoids hypericin and hyperforin have been the most lauded chemicals contained in St. John's Wort that may be responsible for its pharmacological activity; yet with all the research, it is still unclear which chemicals, if any, are responsible for its activity. The flowers contain many antioxidants such as Rutin, Quercetin, and Lutein. One of the best reviews published in Phytomedicine in 2002 compiled results from 34 controlled, double blinded studies on over 3000 patients and found positive results when using between 300 and 1000 mg of extract per day. More research is needed to determine the exact mechanism of therapeutic action in this plant.[5]

Saint John's wort can also be helpful for digestive upset due to neuroemotional dysregulation via the vagus nerve and is known to aid in assimilation. It has also been shown to affect serotonin levels as well as MAO (mono-amine oxidase) and chatechol methyl-transferase, the two enzymes that break down serotonin in the brain.

Contraindications: Do not use Saint John's wort if you are on SSRIs or any other psychiatric medication. Saint John's wort increases liver function and therefore the metabolization of any medication, which reduces their effectiveness.

Italian Folk Medicine Uses

There is a tradition around Europe of hanging Saint John's wort plants, gathered on midsummer's eve, above pictures or doorways and making crowns of them to wear. They are also worn on the body and made into charms and flower waters, and garlands of Saint John's wort are still made and thrown into the bonfire at midnight.

La pianta di iperico, gettat nel focolare duranti i temporali prteggeva la casa, legata alle culle evitava scambi di neo-nati, inserita in amuleti o sotterrata all'in-gresso delle stalle preservava da fatture. In tempi piú recenti sembra che le donne lo abbiano usato per proteggersi dalle violenze carnali, durante le guerre, e che i soldati fossero soliti spalmare la linfa rossastra sui fucili, per avere una mira infalibile.[6]

The hypericum plant, thrown into the hearth during thunderstorms, protected the house, tied to the cradles, avoided exchanges of newborns, inserted in amulets or buried at the entrance to the stables, preserved from curses. In more recent times it seems that women have used it to protect themselves from sexual violence and that soldiers during war used to spread the reddish sap on their rifles to have an unwavering aim.

Emotional and Psychospiritual Benefits

Saint John's wort flower essence is known to repel negativity before it can even touch you, and at the same time it embodies matter with spirit using threads or rays of light. It has a stabilizing and focusing potential yet is also illuminating.

Energetics and Correspondences

Energetics: Hot and dry in the first degree
Astrological influence: The Sun
Element: Fire
Tarot card: The sun
Deities: San Giovanni, the Green Man, Hyperion

Magical Uses

Saint John's wort, celebrated at the summer solstice, has been used magically in many European cultures as apotropaic plant. It represents the illumination that occurs when the Sun reaches its highest point during the year. This constellation of the sky and seasons crosses both Earth and heaven, converging the energies of matter and spirit.

One of Saint John's wort's ancient names is *Fuga daemonum*, which means "scare devil" or "demon's flight" because it has always been used to vanquish unwanted spirits and as a tool of exorcism. It is often hung over doors and thresholds to ward off evil.

Preparations and Recipes

The flowers, leaves, and stems of Saint John's wort can all be used in preparations and recipes like the one below for holy water.

L'Acqua di San Giovanni (Saint John's Wort Holy Water)

This holy water is gathered the morning of June 24 and is considered magically potent for protection. The dew is placed in a sacred bowl and several aromatic leaves and flowers are added to it. It is left outside overnight in the moonlight.

1. On June 24, gather nine flowers and/or leaves of any variety including St. John's wort. You can use plants that grow in your bioregion but I usually add (along with St. John's wort): yarrow,

roses, mugwort, lemon balm, rosemary, sage, primrose, and/or comfrey. It's suggested to choose aromatic plants. Ideally you want to gather them in the morning while the dew is still on the ground.

2. Add the flowers and leaves to a quart of water in a sacred bowl.
3. Leave outside under the moonlight overnight.
4. Strain and place in a jar to be used for blessings, in spray bottles, or as holy water on an altar.

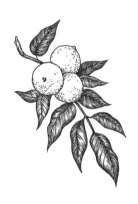

NOCE (WALNUT)
The Witches' Tree

Family: Juglandaceae
Genus: *Juglans*
Species: *regia*
Italian vernacular names: *Nùs, nós, nòs sangiovànn, núsa*[1]
English vernacular names: Common walnut, Jupiter's acorn, Jupiter's nut

The walnut tree, or *Juglans regia*, is a deciduous tree that can grow up to 100 feet tall. It is native to Southeast Europe and China and is a major cultivated food crop today. (Note: In the United States we often use the black walnut, which is *Juglans nigra* and native to North America.)

The Old English word for walnut is *walhnutu*, which means *"foreign tree."*[2] The etymology of *Juglans* is from the Latin *Ju*, which stands for Jupiter, and *glans*, which means "nut," making it "Jupiter's nut." And *regia* means royal so the walnut is Jupiter's royal or noble nut.

The association of this nut and tree with Jupiter has to do with abundance and good fortune. Jupiter is the god of light and daytime, which is interesting as this was the tree most famous for being at the center of witches' Sabbaths held in the middle of the night.

The doctrine of signatures of the walnut fruit leaves no doubt that it must have some effect on the brain. The wrinkles and folds on the nut look much like the neocortex and they are divided in two halves, just like our human brain. Research has shown that walnut does indeed improve cognitive function and memory:

> Our recent study in CE-tg (Alzeimer's disease) mice has shown that a walnut-enriched diet significantly improves antioxidant defense and decreases free radicals' levels, lipid peroxidation, and protein oxidation when compared to a control diet without walnuts. These findings suggest that a diet with walnuts can reduce oxidative stress by decreasing the generation of free radicals and by boosting antioxidant defense, thus resulting in decreased oxidative damage to lipids and proteins.*[3]

Folklore, Mythology, and Ancient Uses

The association of the walnut to royalty can be found in the writings of Herodotus, who says that it "was sent to us from Persia by the Kings, the best kind of walnut being called in Greek the 'Persian' and the 'Royal.'"[4]

Pliny also said that walnuts are not the best food because they are "oppressive to the head"[5] but instead they were used medicinally. There is some record of it being considered beneficial only in small doses such as this saying from the Salerno Medical School: "una noce fa bene, due fanno male, tre portano all morte" or "one walnut is good, two is bad, and three brings death."

As described in chapter 7, the walnut of Benevento is one of the most famous witchcraft legends of Europe. It has been the focus of many legends and the book *De nuce maga Beneventana* written in 1639 by chief physician of Benevento Pietro Piperno. This particular walnut tree is believed to have grown along the Sabato River just outside the city of Benevento, and it was were witches from all over Italy and even other places in Europe "flew" to join in the rites of some form of pagan religion, perhaps brought to Benevento by the Lombards (a Germanic people

---

*Please note that while these are interesting findings, I do not support inhumane research on animals, and it should also be noted that the biochemistry of a human is not the same as the biochemistry of a mouse.

who conquered much of what is now Italy and established a kingdom in from 568 to 774 CE) or a ritual continued from the ancient time of the cult of Diana and the Samnites who were the original tribes of the area. This tree is symbolic of the tree of life in many ways, including the folklore about it continuing to grow back even after being cut down, dug up, and utterly destroyed. The original walnut tree was said to have been uprooted by Beneventan priest Saint Barbatus. The exact location of the original walnut is not known.

The association between witches and the walnut isn't clear except that walnuts were considered to be somewhat toxic, not the greatest food source, and the leaves, bark, and wood do contain a toxin known as juglone that affects other plants. The etymology of the word *noce* comes from the Latin *nocere*, which means "harmful, to harm, or to hurt." It could be that the walnut tree was assigned as the witches' tree for this reason.

The nineteenth-century Neapolitan poem titled "La Storia della famosa noce di Benevento" describes the walnut of the witches as follows:

> *Vicino alla città di Benevento*
> *Vi sono due fiumi molto rinomati*
> *Uno Sabato, l'altro Calor del vento;*
> *Si dicono locali indemoniati,*
> *Un gran noce di grandezza immensa*
> *Germogliava d'estate e pur d'inverno;*
> *Sotto di questa si tenea gran mensa*
> *Da Streghe, Stregoni e diavoli d'inferno.*[6]

> *Close to the city of Benevento*
> *There are two very renowned rivers*
> *One Sabato the other Calor of the wind;*
> *They say the locals are demon-possessed,*
> *A large walnut of immense grandeur*
> *It sprouted in the summer and even in winter;*
> *Under this was held a large table*
> *From witches, sorcerers and devils of hell.*

Herbal Medicine Uses

Most of the herbal uses of walnut, at least in the United States, will be referring to black walnut, or *Juglans nigra*. The common walnut, *Juglans regia*, is more associated with being a food, although black walnuts are edible and tasty. The two are generally considered to be interchangeable.

Walnut is highly antifungal and antibacterial, both externally and internally. It is astringent, nourishing, and anti-inflammatory. It is also known to be an intestinal stimulant and a laxative and is antiparasitic.[7] The ripe hull of a walnut can be made into both a tincture and an infused oil that can be applied to the skin to treat ringworm and other fungal skin infections as well as candida.

There are some noticeable differences between black walnut and common walnut. One is that black walnuts' hulls will stain your hands with a black-iodine-looking color, and they are, in fact, high in iodine. Also, their flavor is stronger and more pungent. The hulls of both species contain a chemical compound called juglone, which, as mentioned earlier, is a toxic compound, but common walnut produces less compared to black walnut.[8] It is because of this toxicity that walnut preparations, and particularly black walnut, are only recommended for short term use internally.

Contraindication: Walnut preparations are contraindicated in pregnancy and nursing.

Italian Folk Medicine Uses

The most universal method of walnut preparation in Italian folk medicine is *nocillo*, a liquor made with nuts harvested on the eve of Saint John's Day, June 23–24. It is also known as the *elisir delle streghe*, the "elixir of the witches" as it was made on the night of their famous annual Sabbath. Nocillo was even made and distributed by pharmacies at one time as a known remedy for a variety of illnesses including fever, as a sedative, digestion, and toothache. There are many recipes and most were considered "secret" at one time, and many still are.[9]

Il giorno di San Giovanni si raccoglievano tre noci fresche, si pestavano e si lasciavano a macerare nell'olio, al sole, per quaranta giorni; questo oleito si appplicava su ecchimosi e contusioni.[10]

On Saint John's day three fresh walnuts were gathered, crushed and left to macerate in oil, in the Sun, for forty days; this oleito was applied to bruises and contusions.

The walnut tree is mentioned in a Lucanian prayer for "wind illness" and points to its significance as a tree of luck or blessing:

> *Mal vinde*
> *Sotto acqua e sotto vinde*
> *'Stu mal vinde*
> *Portalo sotto lo noce del buon vinde.*[11]

> *Bad wind*
> *Under water and under wind*
> *This bad wind*
> *Bring it under the walnut tree of the good wind.*

The walnut also had many uses pertaining to digestive upsets:

L'infuso della corteccia dei rami giovani era impiegato come lassative. Le foglie, in infuso, erano usate come astringente intestinale per fermare le dissenterie e, a dosi minori, come depurativo generale. . . . L'acquavite da santi Giuvannn si preparava mescolando acquvite con i gherigli sminuzzati di noci colte il giorno di san Giovanni, il preparato si beveva, a piccole dosi, contro i dolori addominali.[12]

The infusion of the bark of the young branches was used as a laxative. The leaves, in infusion, were used as an intestinal astringent to stop dysentery and, in smaller doses, as a general purifier. . . . The brandy of Saint John, was prepared by mixing brandy with the chopped kernels of walnuts picked on Saint John's day, the preparation was drunk, in small doses, against abdominal pains.

An old Mithridatic remedy that includes walnut goes like this:

Take two dry walnuts, and as many good figs, and twenty leaves of rue, bruised and beaten together with two or three corns of salt and twenty juniper berries, which taken every morning fasting, preserves from danger of poison, and infection that day it is taken.[13]

Emotional and Psychospiritual Benefits

Walnut flower essence can provide protection and support during times of major life transitions and help to cultivate innovation and adaptation during times of upheaval.

Energetics and Correspondences

Energetics: Warm in the second degree, dry in the third
Astrological influence: Jupiter and the Sun
Element: Fire
Tarot card: The hierophant
Deities: Jupiter, Diana, San Giovanni (Saint John)

Magical Uses

The magic of walnut is first and foremost its place at the center of the witch's sabbath, which is an example of its ability to magnetize and strengthen any spell, curse, or even our desires and intentions. Walnut shells have been used in divination and carried as talismans. Adding any part of the walnut tree, leaves, shells, nuts, or bark to a working altar will increase the potency of and sanctify the altar space. Walnut shells can be used as part of cleansing or purification rituals. Walnut shell powder can be used in amulet bags and sprinkled around the edges of sacred areas such as a garden, a home, or any other location.

Preparations and Recipes

The leaves, hull, ripe or unripe fruit, and sometimes the bark of the walnut are used in preparations and recipes like the one below for nocillo.

❦ Basic Nocillo

    30 unripe green walnuts, the whole fruit with the hull. Black
        walnuts can also be used.

    Vodka or brandy

    ½ teaspoon cinnamon

    5 to 10 cloves

    2 tablespoons orange peel

    A dozen coffee beans, vanilla beans, or another spice that
        sounds good to you

1. Chop walnuts into quarters, place in a clean glass jar with spices, and
   cover with alcohol.
2. Let set for 2 to 4 weeks (some people say 40 days) then strain.
3. Make a simple syrup (see recipe under fennel on page 324, combine
   it with the mixture, and bottle.

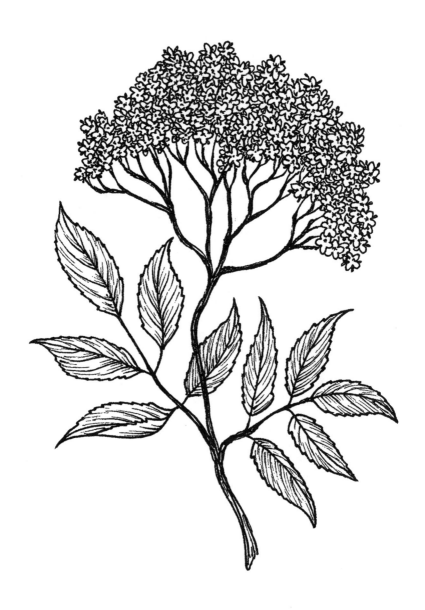

Resources and Further Reading

Below are suggestions for further reading and research. I have placed them under headings for basic herbal information, botanical information, and cultural resources. I have also included individual practitioners, teachers, and organizations that are sources of traditional knowledge. I have tried to largely include sources in English or those that have been translated, but a vast amount of information is only printed in Italian, and I have placed a few of my favorites in here as well.

Italian Folk Medicine in English and Italian

Italian Folk Medicine by Mary-Grace Fahrun
Magic: A Theory of the South by Ernesto De Martino
Power and Magic in Italy by Thomas Hauschild
Healing Journeys with the Black Madonna by Alessandra Belloni
The Things We Do: Ways of the Holy Benedetta by Agostino Taumaturgo
Italian American Folklore by Frances M. Malpezzi and William M. Clements
Italian Folk: Vernacular Culture in Italian-American Lives edited by Joseph Sciorra
Folk Medicine: La struttura psicomagica nelle medicine popolari by Micaela Balice
Il sacro al femminile by Barbara Crescimanno
Stregoneria popolare italiana by Andrea Romanazzi

Herbals and Plants in English and Italian

A Pompeian Herbal: Ancient and Modern Medicinal Plants by Wilhelmina
Feemster Jashemski
Persephone's Path: A Guide to Sicily's Roadside Plants by Charles
Sacamano
Le erbe delle nonne by Mariangela Bisanti
Le erbe delle streghe nel medioevo by Rosella Omicciolo Valentini

Italian-American Cultural Organizations

The descriptions below mainly come from the organizations' websites
where more information can be found.

Calandra Italian American Institute
calandrainstitute.org
The purpose of the John D. Calandra Italian American Institute is basic
to the central mission of the City University of New York (CUNY).
Italian Americans represent the largest European ancestral group in New
York State, New York City, and at CUNY. Thus, the primary purpose
of the Institute is to foster higher education among and about Italian
Americans. In so doing, the Institute serves as an intellectual and cultural center by (a) stimulating the study of Italian Americans through
its research, scholarship, public programming, media outlets, counseling
services, study abroad, and, ultimately by (b) bringing together a community of scholars who can focus on and enhance the Italian-American
experience both within and beyond the Italian-American community.

I AM Books
iambooksboston.com
I AM Books is an independent bookstore located at 124 Salem Street, in
the heart of Boston's historic North End neighborhood that serves as a
cultural hub for everyone interested in diving into the rich world of Italian
and Italian-American literature, history, research, art, and more. Labeled
as an "Italian-American cultural hub," I AM Books was originally located

at 189 North Street, Boston, MA, from 2015 to 2020. In late 2020, due to the Covid-19 pandemic, I AM Books switched its operations to online only. It reopened in its current space in December 2021. I AM Books sells primarily fiction and nonfiction by Italian and Italian-American authors, books in Italian, cookbooks and books on travel, history, sports, Italian-American studies, and titles by local authors. The store also features a children's section, with books, learning material, games, and toys. In 2018 and 2019, I AM Books organized the two-day literary festival called IDEA Boston, which was directed by I AM Books cofounder Nicola Orichuia.

The National Organization of Italian American Women (NOIAW)
www.noiaw.org
The mission of the NOIAW is to create a thriving, inclusive community that embraces Italian culture and supports the personal fulfillment and professional advancement of its members. The vision of NOIAW is to unite, celebrate, and empower each other.

The Coccia Institute
www.montclair.edu/coccia-institute/
The Joseph and Elda Coccia Institute is a component of Montclair State University's College of Humanities and Social Sciences. It is named in honor of Cav. Joseph Coccia, Jr. and his wife Elda. In founding the Coccia Institute, Mr. and Mrs. Coccia and Montclair State University share the vision for an entity with the flexibility to respond to new opportunities as well as network and collaborate with existing organizations in areas of shared interest. The Institute's director, Mark Rotella, along with the Coccias and the University, welcomes promising new concepts that support the Institute's mission.

Italian Folk Medicine Practitioners and Teachers

The descriptions below mainly come from the practitioners' websites where more information can be found.

Marybeth Bonfiglio
www.marybethbonfiglio.com
Marybeth Bonfiglio is an Italian-American writer, teacher, and ancestralist. She guides ancestral pilgrimages to Sicily with her organization Radici Siciliane.

Kara Wood
www.cimarutaremedies.com
Kara Wood is a folk herbalist who works with those who wish to deepen and activate the ancestral connections inside their bodies. Her ancestors were Calabrian on her mother's side, and English, German, Scottish, and Irish on her father's side. She believes the elements, plants, trees, and mushrooms are our ancestors. She believes it all is energy exchange. Epigenetics, mythology, and living folk culture direct and inform her work. She holds classes and workshops in person and online, works one-on-one with folks, and makes herbal products with plants she grows. She lives with her family on the California Central Coast.

Summer Minerva
www.summerminerva.com
Sacred Gender Project founder and creative director, Summer Minerva, is an independent researcher, multidisciplinary artist, public speaker, and educator working on the reclamation of the dignity of gender fluidity within the folk traditions of Napoli and other indigenous traditions. Summer facilitates ancestral remembrance workshops for the queer Italian American community, which includes teaching about the devotional practices of the third gender group of Napoli, the femminielli. Participants connect with esoteric aspects of their ancestral culture that have been erased due to assimilation. Summer also produces and leads annual pilgrimages for queer Italian Americans to Napoli in order to connect with ancient queer traditions and is the coeditor of an anthology of Italian transpeople's narratives titled *Italian Trans Geographies*.

Sabina Magliocco

Sabina Magliocco, Ph.D. grew up in Italy and the United States. She received an A.B. from Brown University in 1980 and a Ph.D. from Indiana University, Bloomington in 1988. She has taught at the California State University, where she served two terms as department chair, as well as the University of California, Berkeley, the University of California, Santa Barbara, UCLA, and the University of Wisconsin, Madison. A recipient of the Guggenheim, National Endowment for the Humanities, Fulbright, and Hewlett fellowships and an honorary fellow of the American Folklore Society, she has published on religion, folklore, foodways, festivals, and witchcraft in Europe and the United States and is a leading authority on the modern pagan movement. Her current research is on nature and animals in the spiritual imagination. Professor Magliocco has appeared as an occasional guest on a number of popular television series about modern legends and beliefs. You can learn more about Professor Magliocco's writing, research, and courses on her page on the University of British Columbia website.

Dr. Angela Puca

drangelapuca.com

Angela Puca holds a bachelor's and a master's in philosophy. In 2021, the University of Leeds awarded her a Ph.D. in the anthropology of religion. Her research focuses on magic, witchcraft, paganism, esotericism, shamanism, and related currents. Author of several peer-reviewed publications and coeditor of the forthcoming *Pagan Religions in Five Minutes*, she hopes to bridge the gap between academia and the communities of magic practitioners by delivering related scholarly content on her YouTube channel and TikTok Angela's Symposium.

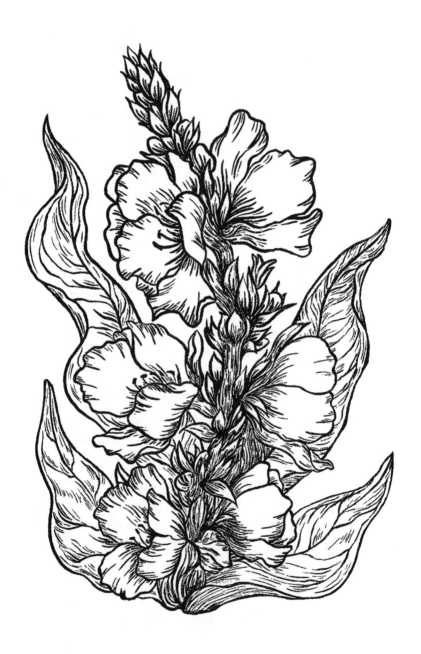

Acknowledgments

My gratitude goes out to the multitudes of people, places, spirits, and all manner of beings that have touched me in my life in such a way as to lead to the writing of this book. This section of the book has been the hardest as I want to include everyone that I have been so blessed to know and be supported by. My prayer is that I have not overlooked anyone here, but if I have, please know I love you and am eternally grateful.

To mia famiglia:

To Scott Ferguson for your ongoing and constant support during the writing of this book as well as your faith in me even when I didn't have faith in myself.

To my beloved children and grandchildren: Druseph, Hannah, Caitlin, Aidan, Ravi, and Kiran.

To my father, Nick Fazio, for insisting on turning our tiny city backyard into a vegetable garden full of ancestral plants even though I wanted a swimming pool.

To my mother, Theresa Fazio, for reading me that poem by Emily Dickinson that inspired her work as a nurse, as it also inspired my own as an herbalist. This taught me that it's not ambitions to greatness that matter, but simple kindness toward others. Mom, I believe with this poem/ prayer you have started a legacy:

> *If I can stop one heart from breaking,*
> *I shall not live in vain;*
> *If I can ease one life the aching,*
> *Or cool one pain,*

Or help one fainting robin
Unto his nest again,
I shall not live in vain.

EMILY DICKINSON

To my cugini (cousins) who have been a part of my ancestral journey or had caffé with me somewhere along the way:

Larry Fazio, Rudolfo Donato, Patrizia Donato, Gabrielle Donato, Eugenio Donato, Luciano Rocca, Lino Rocca, Cecilia Nardo Hamel, Vic Nardo, Marco Caselli.

To my teachers:

To Barbara Crescimanno of Sicily, my teacher of Sicilian music, dance, drumming, mysteries, and the ninfe of the sacred waters.

To Alessandra Belloni, my teacher of traditional Italian drumming and the Black Madonnas.

To Roberto Pellino "Zio Bacco" of Benevento for teaching me the names of the plants in the Appennini (Apennine Mountains).

To Pasquale Orso of Benevento for being part of our "team" and teaching me all the things about Guardia Sanframondi that you'll never read in any book.

To Luciana Smaron of Trentino for spending years teaching me Italian and for help with some of the more difficult translations in this book.

To my herb teacher, mentor, and friend Kate Gilday who let me follow her around for twenty years, but especially for that one day when I thought all was lost, and she told me "I believe in you."

To Pam Montgomery for letting me know that the strange familiarity I felt with the little Veronica plant in her yard was due to it being an ancestral plant.

To my paesani:

To Marybeth Bonfiglio for writing the forward to this book, but more importantly, for being the way she lives and embodies the fullness of Italian American. For inspiring me to more fully embody it myself.

To Gina Miele for her contribution on tarot and for her consult on various aspects in this book as well as for all of the books and resources she shared with me during this process.

To Kara Wood for her contribution on death practice/lutto and for bringing me into ancestral relationship with cannabis.

To Jade Alicandro for trusting me to drive in Southern Italy on dirt paths and up the sides of sheer cliffs and for being the best travel companion ever.

My deepest appreciation to my Italian-American friendships past and present and especially the following: Mary Delorenzo Wood, Jen Violi, Nico Rossi, Lupo Passero, and Jon Meehan.

My thanks to the following:

To Teri Dunn Chase whose help with the proposal for this book is why it ever even happened.

To Christine Shahin who kept telling me, "You got this" every single time I texted and said, "I quit".

To Lena Moon for being my companion in ancestral journey work with plants.

To the influences:

The Virgin Mary, Jesus, Dionysus, the Archangel Michael, Rumi, Asclepius, Tom Porter (Sakokwenionkwas—"The One Who Wins"), the Mohawk (Kanien'kehá:ka) Nation, Carl Jung, Michael Meade, Marion Woodman, Baba Muktananda, Antonio Gramsci, Marija Gimbutas, Patrick Johnson (Utica, NY), San Antonio, Santi Cosma e Damiano, the Rosary, La Madonna di Dopidi, La Madonna di Montevergine, the Peacemaker, Saint Kateri, Alexis Pauline Gumbs, Tyson Yunkaporta, Donna Haraway.

To the other-than-human influences:

The Kuyahoora Valley, the West Canada Creek, the Mohawk River, Bald Mountain, Dolgeville, NY, the cave of the Sibyl of Cumae, the cave of Leonessa in the province of Benevento, the Sabato River, Feroleto Antico, the Ionian Sea, the Tyrrhenian Sea, Il cinghiale (wild boar) of Benevento, Il lupo (wolf) of Avellino, and the white-tailed deer, coyotes, and black bear that live in the Adirondack mountains.

Notes

Introduction. Wild-Foraged and Garden-Grown Remembrances

1. Ursula Le Guin, "The Carrier Bag Theory of Fiction," in *Dancing at the Edge of the World* (New York: Grove Press, 1989), 165–70.
2. Le Guin, "The Carrier Bag Theory of Fiction."
3. Michael Meade, Facebook/Instagram post, "Michael Meade Mosiac Voices" page, posted February 18, 2023.
4. Peter Kingsley, *In the Dark Places of Wisdom* (Point Reyes, CA: The Golden Sufi Center, 1999), 191–92.

1. La Medicina Contadina

1. Rhitu Chatterjee, "Where Did Agriculture Begin? Oh Boy, It's Complicated," NPR website, July 15, 2016.
2. Wendy Holloway, *Interrogative Themes—Critical Social Psychology* (4/30), OpenLearn from the Open University, YouTube video, accessed November 16, 2022.
3. Great Secret: Peter Kingsley interviewed by Emmanuel Vaughan-Lee (Excerpt), YouTube video, accessed November 16, 2022.
4. David Graeber and David Wengrow, *The Dawn of Everything* (New York: Farrar, Straus and Giroux, 2021), 122.
5. Graeber and Wengrow, *The Dawn of Everything*, 123.
6. Graeber and Wengrow, *The Dawn of Everything*, 22.
7. "Ecosystem Profile: Mediterranean Basin Biodiversity Hotspot," Critical Ecosystem Partnership Fund (website), July 2017.
8. Serena Aneli et al., "Through 40,000 Years of Human Presence in Southern Europe: The Italian Case Study," *Human Genetics*, 140 (2021), 1417–31.
9. Aneli et al., "Through 40,000 Years of Human Presence in Southern Europe," 1417–31.

10. World History Encyclopedia, s.v. "Phoenician Colonization," accessed February 22, 2023.

11. Ryan Schleeter, "First Rulers of the Mediterranean," National Geographic (website), accessed February 22, 2023.

12. Gerhard W. Weber et al., "The Microstructure and the Origin of the Venus from Willendorf," *Scientific Reports* 12, no. 2926 (2022).

13. Katerina Douka et al., "On the Chronology of the Uluzzian," *Journal of Human Evolution* 68 (2014): 1–13.

14. Douka et al., "On the Chronology of the Uluzzian," 1–13.

15. Giuseppe Vercellotti et al., "The Late Upper Paleolithic Skeleton Villabruna 1 (Italy): A Source of Data on Biology and Behavior of a 14,000 Year-Old Hunter," *Journal of Anthropological Sciences* 86 (2008): 143–63.

16. "European Kingdoms: Ancient Italian Peninsula," The History Files (website), accessed November 16, 2022.

17. World History Encyclopedia, s.v. "Etruscan Language," accessed November 16, 2022.

18. "Where Did the Ancient Etruscans Come From?" *Smithsonian Magazine* (website), accessed November 16, 2022.

19. "Unemployment Rate in Italy from the 2nd Quarter to the 4th Quarter of 2020, by Region," Statista (website), accessed November 16, 2022.

20. "When Did They Come?" PBS (website), accessed November 16, 2022.

21. Edward Shills, *Tradition* (Chicago: University of Chicago Press, 2006), 12.

22. "Text of the Convention for the Safeguarding of the Intangible Cultural Heritage," Unesco (website), accessed February 1, 2024.

23. Edward Shills, *Tradition*, 12.

24. Donna Haraway on Staying with the Trouble, interview by Ayana Young, August 7, 2019, podcast audio, For the Wild (website).

25. Per Binde, *Bodies of Vital Matter* (Göteborg, Sweden: Acta Universitatis Gothoburgensis, 1999), 6.

26. Tyson Yunkaporta, *Sand Talk (First Harper One*, 2020).

2. A Fusion of Knowledge

1. Matthew Wood, "Traditional Elements Unique to Western Herbalism," American Herbalists Guild (website), accessed December 3, 2022.

2. Marc Williams, "African American Herbalism: A Blog Series," Chestnut School of Herbal Medicine (website), accessed December 3, 2022.

3. "Traditional Complementary and Integrative Medicine," World Health Organization (website), accessed March 6, 2024.

4. Phyllis D. Light, *Southern Folk Medicine* (Berkeley: North Atlantic Books, 2018), 9.

5. Adrienne Maree Brown, *Emergent Strategy* (Chico, CA: AK Press, 2017), 13.

6. Per Binde, *Bodies of Vital Matter* (Göteborg, Sweden: Acta Universitatis Gothoburgensis, 1999), 4.

7. Francesco Scaroina, "Tra terra e cielo: quando il popolo si faceva dottore," *Giornale Della Accademia di Medicina di Torino* 2014, 100.

8. Nicola Luigi Bragazzi et al., "Asclepius and Epidaurus: "The Sapiential Medicine as Divinatory Art between Therapeutic Landscapes and Healing Dreams," *Cosmos and History: The Journal of Natural and Social Philosophy* 15, no. 1 (2019).

9. "Ancient Greek Medicine," National Library of Medicine (website), accessed December 3, 2022.

10. Jeremy M. Norman, "Traditions & Culture of Collecting," History of Science (website), accessed February 22, 2023.

11. Peter Kingsley, *In The Dark Places of Wisdom* (Point Reyes, CA: The Golden Sufi Center, 1999), 142–43.

12. Wolf-Dieter Storl, *The Herbal Lore of Wise Women and Wortcunners* (Berkeley: North Atlantic Books, 2012), 15.

13. Claudia Müller-Ebling, Christian Rätsch, and Wolf-Dieter Storl, *Witchcraft Medicine* (Rochester, VT: Inner Traditions, 1998), 80.

14. David Hoffmann, *A Call to Herbs: From Rhizotomoi to Radicle with David Hoffman, Part 2*, YouTube video, October 18, 2012.

15. Leanne McNamara, "'Conjurers, Purifiers, Vagabonds and Quacks?' The Clinical Roles of the Folk and Hippocratic Healers of Classical Greece," *Journal of the Classical Association of Victoria*, n.s., 16–17 (2003–4): 2–25.

16. Marguerite Rigoglioso, *The Cult of Divine Birth* (New York: Palgrave Macmillan, March 2011), 93.

17. McNamara, "Conjurers, Purifiers, Vagabonds and Quacks?'": 2–25.

18. Wolf-Dieter Storl, *The Herbal Lore of Wise Women and Wortcunners*, 17.

19. Alice Sparkly Kat, *Postcolonial Astrology* (Berkeley: North Atlantic Books, 2021), 209.

20. Roger Beck, *A Brief History of Ancient Astrology* (Malden, MA: Blackwell Publishing, 2007), 17.

21. "Unani Tibb Traditional Medicine," American Botanical Council (website), accessed February 22, 2023.
22. Stanford Encyclopedia of Philosophy, s.v. "Ibn Sina [Avicenna]," accessed February 22, 2023.
23. Bashar Saad and Omar Said, *Greco-Arab and Islamic Herbal Medicine* (Hoboken, NJ: John Wiley and Sons Inc., 2011), 84.
24. "Trotula," Brooklyn Museum (website), accessed November 16, 2022.
25. "Matteuccia da Todi: The Witch Hunt Began with Her," Hotel Fonte Cesia (website), accessed November 16, 2023.
26. Mike Dash, "Aqua Tofana: Slow-Poisoning and Husband-Killing in 17th Century Italy," Mike Dash History (website), July 20, 2011.
27. Genevieve Carlton, "Meet the Woman Who Poisoned Makeup to Help Over 600 Women Murder Their Husbands," Medium (website), March 2, 2018.
28. Dash, "Aqua Tofana."
29. Dash, "Aqua Tofana."

3. Animism, Totemism, Oracles, and Chthonic Gods

1. Nicola Luigi Bragazzi et al., "Asclepius and Epidaurus: The Sapiential Medicine as Divinatory Art Between Therapeutic Landscapes and Healing Dreams," *Cosmos and History: The Journal of Natural and Social Philosophy* 15, no. 1 (2019).
2. Etymonline, s.v. "sacred," accessed December 5, 2022.
3. Alkistis Dimech, "Dynamics of the Occulted Body," Alkistis Dimech (website), accessed December 5, 2022.
4. Katherine Swancutt, "Animism," *The Open Encyclopedia of Anthropology*, edited by Felix Stein. Facsimile of the first edition in *The Cambridge Encyclopedia of Anthropology* (2019), 2023.
5. Morten A. Pedersen, "Totemism, Animism and North Asian Indigenous Ontologies," *Journal of the Royal Anthropological Institute* 7, no. 3 (2001): 411–27.
6. Troy Markus Linebaugh, "Shamanism and the Ancient Greek Mysteries: The Western Imaginings of the 'Primitive Other'" (master's thesis, Kent State University, 2017), 72–73.
7. Herbert Jennings Rose, "Nvmen inest: 'Animism' in Greek and Roman Religion," *The Harvard Theological Review* 28, no. 4 (October, 1935): 237–57.
8. Cyril Bailey, *Phases in the Religion of Ancient Rome* (Berkeley: University of California Press, 1932), 7.

9. Herbert Jennings Rose, "Nvmen inest," 237–57.

10. Troy Markus Linebaugh, "Shamanism and the Ancient Greek Mysteries," 72–73.

11. Sabina Magliocco, *Witchcraft, Healing, and Vernacular Magic in Italy* (Manchester, UK: Manchester University Press, 2018), 161.

12. Mario Alinei, "Evidence for Totemism in European Dialects," *International Journal of American Linguistics* 51, no. 4 (October, 1985): 331–34.

13. "Pausanias, Description of Greece," book 10, Perseus Digital Library (website), accessed February 20, 2023.

14. Eloise McKinney Johnson, "Delphos of Delphi: An Ethiopian Journal," accessed December 5, 2022.

15. Mama Zogbe, *The Sibyls: The First Prophetess' of Mami (Wata)* (Martinez, Georgia: Mami Wata Healers Society of North America, 2020), book description.

16. "Pythia," Hellenic Period (website), accessed December 5, 2022.

17. John Barry, ed. "Sibylline Oracles" in *Lexham Bible Dictionary* (Bellingham, WA: Lexham Press, 2016), 3.

18. Haralampos V. Harissis, "A Bittersweet Story: The True Nature of the Laurel of the Oracle of Delphi," *Perspectives in Biology and Medicine* 57, no. 3 (Summer 2014): 351–60.

19. William J. Broad, *The Oracle: Ancient Delphi and the Science Behind its Lost Secrets* (New York: Penguin Books, 2007), 101.

20. Jelle Zeilinga de Boer and John R. Hale, "The Oracle of Delphi—Was She Really Stoned?" Bible Archaeology Society (website), accessed January 4, 2023.

21. John R. Hale et al., "Questioning the Delphic Oracle: Overview/An Intoxicating Tale," *Scientific American*, August 1, 2003.

22. James Hastings, ed., *Encyclopaedia of Religion and Ethics: Sacrifice-Sudra* (New York: Charles Scribner's Sons, 1921), 404.

4. Mothers of Grain

1. Wordnik, s.v. "peasant," accessed January 8, 2023.

2. Martin Prechtel, *The Unlikely Peace at Cuchumaquic: The Parallel Lives of People as Plants: Keeping the Seeds Alive* (Berkeley: North Atlantic Books, 2012), 375.

3. Pliny the Elder, in Benoît Vermander, *Wheat and Religions* (Paris: Lavoisier, 2016), 1461.

4. University of Pennsylvania, Department of Classical Studies, (website; under "Tools" and "Dictionary"), s.v. "Avral Brothers," accessed January 5, 2023.

5. Benoît Vermander, *Wheat and Religions* (Paris: Lavoisier, 2016), 1440.

6. Marija Gimbutas, "The Earth Fertility Goddess of Old Europe," *Dialogues d'histoire ancienne, 13* (1987), 11–69.

7. Gimbutas, "The Earth Fertility Goddess of Old Europe," 11–69.

8. Marguerite Rigoglioso, *The Cult of Divine Birth* (New York: Palgrave Macmillan, 2011), 159.

9. Gimbutas, "The Earth Fertility Goddess of Old Europe," 11–69.

10. John M. Allegro, *The Sacred Mushroom and the Cross* (Gnostic Media Research & Publishing: 2009), 22.

11. Naoe Kukita Yoshikawa, "Symbolic Grain and Symbolic Bread: Relationships Between the Ancient Grain Goddess and the Virgin Mary in the Late Middle Ages," *Atchison* 3, no. 1 (Summer 1997), 108.

12. Naoe Kukita Yoshikawa, "From the Ancient Grain Goddess to the Virgin Mary: Iconography of the Bake Oven in the Late Middle Ages," *The Profane Arts of the Middle Ages/Les Arts Profanes du Moyen Âge: Les stalles de Picardie* 6, no. 1, 85–95.

13. "The Festival of Madonna of the Mountain of Polsi," Turismo Reggio Calabria (website), accessed January 8, 2023.

14. Giovanni Orlando, "The Pilgrimage of our Lady of Polsi," accessed through Internet Archive Wayback Machine on January 8, 2023.

15. Barbara Crescimanno, *Il sacro al femminile* (Palermo, Sicily: Istituto Poligrafico Europeo, 2021), 141.

16. Lorenzo Ferrarini, "Sounds and Images of Nostalgia: The Revival of Lucanian Wheat Festivals," *Sonic Ethnography*, December 15, 2020.

5. Birth-Life-Death

1. Per Binde, *Bodies of Vital Matter: Notions of Life Force and Transcendence in Traditional Southern Italy* (Göteborg, Sweden: Acta Universitatis Gothoburgensis, 1999), 19.

2. Giovanni Battista Bronzini, *Vita tradizionale in Basilicata* (Galatina, Italy: Congedo Editore, 1987), 52.

3. Margaret E. Kenna, "Houses, Fields, and Graves: Property and Ritual Obligation on a Greek Island," *Ethnology* 15, no. 1 (1976): 21–34.

4. Caroline Oates, "Review of *Bodies of Vital Matter: Notions of Life Force and Transcendence in Traditional Southern Italy*," *Folklore* 115, no. 2 (August, 2004), 233.

5. Binde, *Bodies of Vital Matter*, 204.

6. Binde, *Bodies of Vital Matter*, 221.

7. "Recipe: The Cuccìa di Castelmezzano," e-borghi (website), accessed January 10, 2023.

8. Oats, "Review of Bodies of Vital Matter," 233.

9. Charlotte Gower Chapman, *Milocca: A Sicilian Village* (Rochester, VT: Schenkman Publishing Company, 1971), 195.

10. Binde, *Bodies of Vital Matter*, 67.

11. Binde, *Bodies of Vital Matter*, 57.

6. Renaissance Medicine

1. Frederick Newsome, "Black Contributions to the Early History of Western Medicine: Lack of Recognition as a Cause of Black Under-Representation in US Medical Schools," *Journal of the National Medical Association* 71, no. 2 (February 1979): 189–93.

2. H. N. Sallam, "Aristotle, Godfather of Evidence-Based Medicine," Facts Views, and Vision in *Obgyn* 2, no.1 (2010): 9–11.

3. Matthew Blair, "Points and Spheres: Cosmological Innovation in Dante's Divine Comedy" (thesis, Baylor University May 2015).

4. "Dante Alighieri," Revolutionary People from the Renaissance (website), accessed January 12, 2021.

5. Wolf-Dieter Storl, *The Herbal Lore of Wise Women and Wortcunners*, (Berkeley: North Atlantic Books, 2012), 103.

6. David Alexander, "Dante and the Form of the Land," *Annals of the Association of American Geographers* 76, no. 1 (March 1986), 38–49.

7. Fritjof Capra, *The Tao of Physics* (Boulder: Shambhala Publications, 2010), 365.

8. Jostein Gaarder, *Sophie's World* (New York: Farrar, Straus and Giroux, March 2007).

9. Matthew Wood, *The Earthwise Herbal* (Berkeley: North Atlantic Books, 2008), 4.

10. Per Binde, *Bodies of Vital Matter* (Göteborg, Sweden: Acta Universitatis Gothoburgensis, 1999), 37.

11. Wikipedia, s.v. "thumos," accessed January 13, 2023.

12. Per Binde, *Bodies of Vital Matter* (Göteborg, Sweden: Acta Universitatis Gothoburgensis, 1999), 38.

13. Treccani, s.v. "sècco," accessed January 13, 2023.

14. Luisa Vertova, "La Morte Secca," *Mitteilungen des Kunsthistorischen Institutes in Florenz*, 36, no 1/2 (1992): 103–28.

15. Thomas Hauschild, *Power and Magic in Italy* (New York: Berghahn Books, 2011), 107.
16. Cassandra Leah Quave and Andrea Pieroni, "Ritual Healing in Arbëreshë Albanian and Italian Communities of Lucania, Southern Italy," *Journal of Folklore Research: An International Journal of Folklore and Ethnomusicology* (January 2005): 74.
17. Hauschild, "*Power and Magic in Italy*," 17.
18. Storl, *The Herbal Lore of Wise Women and Wortcunners*, 109.
19. Encyclopedia.com, s.v. "heliocentric theory," accessed January 13, 2023.
20. Dane Rudhyar, *The Astrologicial Houses* (New York: Doubleday, 1972), 5.
21. Graeme Tobyn, *Culpeper's Medicine* (Rockport, MA: Element Books Limited, 1997), 79.

7. Stregoneria and Benedicaria

1. M. Estellie Smith, "Folk Medicine among the Sicilian-Americans of Buffalo, New York," *Urban Anthropology* 1, no. 1 (Spring, 1972), 87–106.
2. Sabina Magliocco, "Spells, Saints, and Streghe," Rue's Kitchen (website), May 23, 2010.
3. Francesco Scaroina, "Tra terra e cielo: quando il popolo si faceva dottore," *Giornale Della Accademia di Medicina di Torino*, 2014, 101.
4. Scaroina, "Tra terra e cielo: quando il popolo si faceva dottore," 100.
5. Sabina Magliocco, "Spells, Saints, and Streghe: Witchcraft, Folk Magic, and Healing in Italy," Italiansrus (website), accessed February 28, 2023.
6. Cassandra Leah Quave and Andrea Pieroni, "Ritual Healing in Arbëreshë Albanian and Italian Communities of Lucania, Southern Italy," *Journal of Folklore Research: An International Journal of Folklore and Ethnomusicology* (January 2005): 57.
7. Quave and Pieroni, "*Ritual Healing in Arbëreshë Albanian and Italian Communities of Lucania, Southern Italy*," 57.
8. Quave and Pieroni, "Ritual Healing in Arbëreshë Albanian and Italian Communities of Lucania, Southern Italy," 59.
9. Sabina Magliocco, "Italian Cunning Craft: Some Preliminary Observations," *Journal for the Academic Study of Magic* 5, 103.
10. Wikipedia, s.v. *Aradia, or the Gospel of the Witches*, accessed February 28, 2023.
11. Francesca Gerardo, Marialaura Simeone, and Umberto Rinaldi, Leggenda sulle streghe di Benevento DOC—"A uno a uno le fil' cuntavano," YouTube video, Benevento, Italy, 2017.

12. Gerardo, Leggenda sulle streghe di Benevento DOC.

13. "The Witches of Benevento and the Magic Walnut Tree," Insolita Italia (website), accessed January 13, 2023.

14. Gerardo, Leggenda sulle streghe di Benevento DOC.

15. Marguerite Rigoglioso, "Stregoneria," Scribd, accessed January 13, 2023.

16. Angela Puca, "The Tradition of *Segnature*. Underground Indigenous Practices in Italy," *Journal of the Irish Society for the Academic Study of Religions*, 2019.

17. Fabrizio M. Ferrari, *Ernesto De Martino on Religion: The Crisis and the Presence* (London, Routledge, 2012), 78.

18. Scarlet Imprint, "Transgressing Angels, Entangled Bodies: Alkistis Dimech, Astro Magia 2021," YouTube video, December 3, 2021.

19. Jean de Blanchefort, *Riti e magie delle campagne*" (Cornaredo, Milan: Armenia, 2020), 23.

20. Frances M. Malpezzi and William M. Clements, *Italian-American Folklore* (Little Rock, AR: August House, 1992), 113.

21. Malpezzi and Clements, 114.

22. "Benedicaria: Una Tradizione stregonesca siculo-americana," Centro Studio Misteri Italiani (website), accessed January 13, 2023.

23. Agostino Taumaturgo, "The Things We Do: Ways of the Holy Benedetta" (self-published, CreateSpace, 2007), 12.

24. Taumaturgo, "The Things We Do," 128.

25. Taumaturgo, "The Things We Do," 129.

26. Paola Giovetti, *I guaritori di campagna* (Rome: Italy: Edizioni Mediterranee, 2016), 15.

27. Thomas Hauschild, *Power and Magic in Italy* (New York: Berghahn Books, 2011), 40.

28. Adalberto Pazzini, *La medicina popolare in Italia* (Stargatebook, 2019), 26.

29. Smith, "Folk Medicine among the Sicilian-Americans of Buffalo, New York," 87–106.

30. "Fascinazione: i riti, i simboli, le guaritrici, le affascinatrici, e le vittime," Fondazione Terra d'Otranto (website), accessed February 28, 2023.

31. Frederick Thomas Elworthy, *The Evil Eye* (Mineola, NY: Dover Publications, Inc., 2004), 8.

32. Leonard W. Moss and Stephen C. Cappannari, "Folklore and Medicine in an Italian Village," *The Journal of American Folklore* 73, no. 288 (April–June, 1960): 95–102.

33. Treccani, s.v. "sciogliere," accessed February 28, 2023.

34. Moss and Cappannari, "Folklore and Medicine in an Italian Village," 95–102.

35. James George Frazer, "The Golden Bough" (Oxford University Press, 1988), 26.

36. Elworthy, *The Evil Eye* (Mineola, NY: Dover Publications, Inc., 2004), 48.

37. Gabriel Peroni, Cleonice Bonalberti, and Adalbeto Peroni, *Le nostre nonne si curavano così* (Varese, Italy: Pietro Macchione Editore, 2008), 193.

38. Giovetti, *I guaritori di campagna*, 17.

39. Giovetti, *I guaritori di campagna*, 17.

40. Giovetti, *I guaritori di campagna*, 17.

8. Segnatura

1. Alice Imbalzano, "Segnare la malattia: Ricerca etnografica presso le guaritrici tradizionali nel parmense," (Thesis: Corso di Laurea Magistrale in Antropologia Culturale, Etnologia, Etnolinguistica, University of Venice, 2018), 5.

2. Imbalzano, "Segnare la malattia," 11.

3. "Occhio, malocchio, prezzemolo e finocchio . . . Chi sono i segnatori della Garfagnana?" Verde Azzurro Notizie (website), accessed January 15, 2023.

4. Andrea Romanazzi, *Stregoneria Popolare Italiana* (Sossano, Italy: Anguana Edizioni, 2022), 32–34.

5. Romanazzi, *Stregoneria Popolare Italiana*, 32.

6. "Perché la Segnatura è Magia Cristiana," YouTube video, accessed January 23, 2023.

7. Romanazzi, *Stregoneria Popolare Italiana*, 38.

8. Romanazzi, *Stregoneria Popolare Italiana*, 37.

9. Grazia and the Holy Wonderworkers

1. Frances M. Malpezzi and William M. Clements, *Italian American Folklore* (Little Rock: August House, Inc., 1992), 115.

2. Malpezzi and Clements, *Italian American Folklore*, 113

3. "Is It a Cult, or a New Religious Movement?" Penn Today (website), accessed January 25, 2023.

4. James T. Richardson, "Definitions of Cult: From Sociological-Technical to Popular-Negative," *Review of Religious Research* 34, no. 4 (June, 1993): 1.

5. Andrea Romanazzi, *Stregoneria Popolare Italiana* (Sossano, Italy: Anguana Edizioni, 2022), 37–38.

6. Romanazzi, *Stregoneria Popolare Italiana*, 37–38.

7. Per Binde, *Bodies of Vital Matter* (Göteborg, Sweden: Acta Universitatis Gothoburgensis, 1999), 115.

8. Binde, *Bodies of Vital Matter*, 150.

9. "Manna Falling from Heaven in Sicily," ABC News (website), accessed January 25, 2023.

10. Malpezzi and Clements, *Italian American Folklore*, 100.

11. Angela Puca, "The Tradition of *Segnature*. Underground Indigenous Practices in Italy," *Journal of the Irish Society for the Academic Study of Religions*, 2019.

12. Judika Illes, *Encyclopedia of Mystics, Saints, and Sages* (New York: HarperCollins, 2011), 95.

13. Illes, *Encyclopedia of Mystics, Saints, and Sages*, 442.

14. William Giovinazzo, "Our Lady of Mount Carmel," June 2020, La Gazzetta Italiana (website) , accessed January 25, 2023.

15. "Flower of Carmel—Flos Carmeli—You Are Our Mother," SpiritualDirection. com, July 16, 2015, accessed January 25, 2023.

16. Illes, *Encyclopedia of Mystics, Saints, and Sages*, 311.

17. "San Gennaro (Saint Januarius)," Italy Heritage (website), accessed January 25, 2023.

18. Andrea Mubi Brighenti and Mattias Kärrholm, "Domestic Territories and the Little Humans: Understanding the Animation of Domesticity," *Space and Culture*, October 2017.

19. Autori Vari, *Folklore: Antologia del fantastico sul folklore italiano*, ed. Alessandro Iascy and Alfonso Zarbo (Rome, Italy: Watson Edizioni, 2021).

20. Nelide Romeo, Olivier Gallo, and Giuseppe Tagarelli, "From Disease to Holiness: Religious-Based Health Remedies of Italian Folk Medicine (XIX-XX Century)," *Journal of Ethnobiology and Ethnomedicine*, 2015.

21. Romeo, Gallo, and Tagarelli, "From Disease to Holiness."

10. Preparations and Treatments

1. Paolo Luzzi, "The 'Garden of Simple' in Florence: Its Origin and Its Role in the Evolution of Modern Botany," (lecture, 11th Annual International Herb Symposium, 2013).

2. "Blog by Ambassador Mulhall on Black '47: Ireland's Great Famine and Its After-Effects," Embassy of Ireland, USA (website), December 3, 2018, accessed March 4, 2023.

3. James R. Ehleringer, John Casale, Donald A. Cooper, and Michael J. Lott,

"Sourcing Drugs with Stable Isotopes," Ehleringer Lab University of Utah (website), accessed March 4, 2023.

4. Sarah Everts, "Isotopes Mark the Spot," C&EN (website), accessed March 4, 2023.

5. Colleen Walsh, "What the Nose Knows," Harvard Gazette (website), February 27, 2020, accessed March 5, 2023.

6. Martha Henriques, "Can the Legacy of Trauma be Passed Down the Generations?" March 26, 2019, accessed March 5, 2023.

7. "Chrism Oil," Saints, Feast, Family (website), accessed January 30, 2023.

8. D. D. Emmons, "What Are the Three Holy Oils?" Simply Catholic (website), accessed January 30, 2023.

9. Daniele Piomelli and Antonino Pollio, "In upupa o strige: A Study in Renaissance Psychotropic Plant Ointments," *History and Philosophy of the Life Sciences*, 16 (1994): 241–73.

10. Edina Gradvohl, "Healing Kitchen," *Graeco-Latina, Brunnesia* 17 (2012): 1.

11. Kristina Killgrove "The Curious History of Easter Eggs from Birth to Burial," Forbes (website), March 26, 2016, accessed January 30, 2023.

12. Nelide Romeo, Olivier Gallo, and Giuseppe Tagarelli, "From Disease to Holiness: Religious-Based Health Remedies of Italian Folk Medicine (XIX–XX Century)," *Journal of Ethnobiology and Ethnomedicine*, 2015.

13. Vito Quattrocchi, Sicilian Benedicaria—Magical Catholicism (Lulu.com, 2006), 115.

14. Marion Woodman, *Leaving My Father's House* (Boston: Shambhala Publications, 1993), 25.

15. Luzzi, "The 'Garden of Simple' in Florence."

11. Protezione

1. Etymonline, s.v. "protection," accessed January 30, 2023.

2. Etymonline, s.v. "apotropaic," accessed January 30, 2023.

3. Ernesto De Martino, *Magic: A Theory from the South* (Chicago: Hau Books, 2001), 97.

4. Simonetta Falasca Zamponi, "Of Tears and Tarantulas: Folk Religiosity, de Martino's Ethnology, and the Italian South," *California Italian Studies* 5, no. 1 (2014).

5. Zamponi, "Of Tears and Tarantulas," 46–47.

6. "Are Corals Animals or Plants?" National Ocean Service (website), accessed February 1, 2023.

7. Sophie Chavarria, "Menstrual Blood: Uses, Values, and Controls in Ancient Rome," *Anthropologie et Histoire des Mondes Antiques*, 2022.

8. "How to Make a Roman Bulla," Torquay Museum (website), accessed February 1, 2023.

9. Micaela Balìce, "Brevi, devozionali e abitini: gli amuleti di Nostra Signora," Micaela Balice (website), accessed February 1, 2023.

10. Sabina Magliocco, "Italian Cunning Craft: Some Preliminary Observations," *Journal for the Academic Study of Magic* no. 5: 103.

11. Gabriel Peroni, Cleonice Bonalberti, and Adalbeto Peroni, *Le nostre nonne si curavano così* (Varese, Italy: Pietro Macchione Editore, 2008), 194.

12. Portafortuna

1. Etymonline, s.v. "divination," accessed February 1, 2023.

2. Liu Ming, "Cosmology and Introduction," lecture recorded April 24, 2011, Da Yuan Circle (website).

3. Wikipedia, s.v. "iatromantis," accessed February 1, 2023.

4. William Smith ed., "Sibyllini Libri," in *A Dictionary of Greek and Roman Antiquities* (London: John Murray, 1875), 1043–44.

5. Per Binde, *Bodies of Vital Matter* (Göteborg, Sweden, Acta Universitatis Gothoburgensis, 1999), 74.

6. "All about the Fava," Virtual Saint Joseph Altar (website), February 25, 2021, accessed February 1, 2023.

13. Dream Incubation

1. Gil H. Renberg, *Where Dreams May Come* (The Netherlands: Brill, 2017), 238.

2. Renberg, *Where Dreams May Come*, 259.

3. Renberg, *Where Dreams May Come*, 623.

4. Peter Thonemann, "An Ancient Dream Manual: Artemidorus," in *The Interpretation of Dreams* (Oxford: Oxford University Press, 2020), 41.

5. Edward Tick, *The Practice of Dream Healing* (Wheaton, IL: Quest Books, 2001), 17.

6. Wiktionary, s.v. "ἀσκέω," accessed March 2, 2023.

7. Tick, *The Practice of Dream Healing*," (Wheaton, IL: Quest Books, 2001), v.

8. Monika Błaśkiewicz, "Healing Dreams at Epidaurus: Analysis and Interpretation of the Epidaurian iamata," *Miscellanea Anthropologica et Sociologica* 15, no. 4 (2014): 54–69.

Basilico (Basil)

1. Mariangel Bisanti, *Le erbe dell nonne* (Rimini, Italy: Idealibri, 2010), 50.
2. "Consortium for the Protection of the PDO Genovese Basil," Genovesa Storico (website), accessed March 2, 2023.
3. Rosella Omicciolo Valentini, *Le erbe delle streghe nel medioevo* (Tuscania, Italy: Penne & Papiri, 2010), 69.

Alloro (Bay Laurel)

1. Gabriele Peroni and Mariangel Bisanti, *Le erbe dell nonne* (Rimini, Italy: Idealibri, 2010).
2. Wiktionary, s.v. "laurus," accessed February 13, 2023.
3. Wilhelmina Feemster Jashemski, *A Pompeian Herbal: Ancient and Modern Medicinal Plants* (Austin, TX: University of Texas Press, 1999), 62.
4. Nicholas Culpeper, *Complete Herbal and English Physician* (Glenwood, IL: Meyerbooks, 1990), 18.
5. Alam Khan, Goher Zaman, and Richard A. Anderson, "Bay Leaves Improve Glucose and Lipid Profile of People with Type 2 Diabetes," *Journal of Biochemistry and Nutrition* 44, no. 1 (January 2009): 52–56.
6. Gabriel Peroni, Cleonice Bonalberti, and Adalbeto Peroni, Le nostre nonne si curavano così (Varese, Italy: Pietro Macchione Editore, 2008), 114.
7. This is a traditional recipe given to me by oral transmission from Kara Wood.

Belladonna (Belladonna)

1. Rosella Omicciolo Valentini, *Le erbe delle streghe nel medioevo* (Tuscania, Italy: Penne & Papiri, 2010).
2. Hildegard von Bingen, *Physica* (Rochester, VT: Healing Arts Press, 1998), 32.
3. Wikipedia, s.v. Atropa belladonna, accessed February 21, 2023.
4. Rosella Omicciolo Valentini, *Le erbe delle streghe nel medioevo* (Tuscania: Penne & Papiri, 2010), 73.
5. "Belladonna Ointment: By Bane Folk," Ritual Craft (website), accessed February 21, 2023.

Canapa (Cannabis)

1. "Canapa in sud Italia: la storia dimenticata," Dolce Vita (website), accessed February 9, 2023.
2. Thomas Wrona, "Where the Word 'Cannabis' Comes From," The Cannigma (website), accessed February 9, 2023.

3. "Una storia "fatta" di canapa," Canapa Indutriale (website), accessed February 10, 2023.

4. "History of Cannabis," University of Sydney Lambert Initiative for Cannabinoid Therapeutics (website), accessed February 9, 2023.

5. "Oldest Evidence of Marijuana Use Discovered in 2500-Year-Old Cemetery in Peaks of Western China," Science (website), accessed February 9, 2023.

6. Anna Maria Mercuri, Carla Alberta Accorsi, and Marta Mazzanti, "The Long History of Cannabis and Its Cultivation by Romans in Central Italy (Pollen Records from Lago Albano and Lago di Nemi)," *Vegetation History and Archaeobotany* 11 (2002): 263–76.

7. The History of Herodotus, trans. George Rawlinson, book 4, The Internet Classics Archive (website), accessed February 2023.

8. Marguerite Rigoglioso, *The Cult of Divine Birth* (New York: Palgrave Macmillan, March 2011), 129.

9. William J. Broad, *The Oracle: Ancient Delphi and the Science Behind its Lost Secrets* (New York: Penguin Books, 2007), 101.

10. Christian Rätsch, *Marijuana Medicine: A World Tour of the Healing and Visionary Powers of Cannabis* (Rochester, VT: Healing Arts Press, 2001), 56.

11. Marc-Antoine Crocq, "History of Cannabis and the Endocannabinoid System," *Dialogues in Clinical Neuroscience* 22, no. 3 (September, 2020): 223–28.

12. Chris Bennett, "The Cannabis Infused Wine of Dionysus," *Cannabis Culture* (2020): 18.

13. Chris Bennett, "The Cannabis Infused Wine of Dionysus," *Cannabis Culture* (2020), 8.

14. Tammi Sweet, *The Wholistic Healing Guide to Cannabis: Understanding the Endocannabinoid System, Addressing Specific Ailments and Conditions, and Making Cannabis-Based Remedies*, (North Adams, MA: Storey Publishing, LLC, 2020), 65.

15. Gabriel Peroni, Cleonice Bonalberti, and Adalbeto Peroni, *Le nostre nonne si curavano così* (Varese, Italy: Pietro Macchione Editore, 2008), 189–90.

16. Rosella Omicciolo Valentini, *Le erbe delle streghe nel medioevo* (Tuscania: Penne & Papiri, 2010), 78–79.

Sambuco (Elder)

1. Gabriele Peroni, Cleonice Bonalberti, and Adalberto Peroni, *Le nostre nonne si curavano così* (Varese, Italy: Pietro Macchione Editore, 2008), 72;

Mariangel Bisanti, *Le erbe dell nonne* (Rimini, Italy: Idealibri, 2010), 302.

2. D. C. Watts, *Dictionary of Plant Lore* (Cambridge, MA: Academic Press, May 16, 2007).

3. Rosella Omicciolo Valentini, *Le erbe delle streghe nel medioevo* (Tuscania: Penne & Papiri, 2010), 159.

4. Anete Borodušķe et al., "Sambucus nigra L. Cell Cultures Produce Main Species-Specific Phytochemicals with Anti-Inflammatory Properties and in Vitro ACE2 Binding Inhibition to SARS-CoV2," *Industrial Crops and Products*, 186 (October 15, 2022).

5. Peroni, Bonalberti, and Peroni, *Le nostre nonne si curavano così*, 73.

6. Cassandra Leah Quave and Andrea Pieroni, "Ritual Healing in Arbëreshë Albanian and Italian Communities of Lucania, Southern Italy," *Journal of Folklore Research: An International Journal of Folklore and Ethnomusicology* (January 2005): 70.

Finocchio (Fennel)

1. "Fennel," University of Illinois Extension (website), accessed February 21, 2023.

2. "Giant Anise Fennel (*Ferula communis*)," Strictly Medicinal Seeds (website), accessed February 21, 2023.

3. "Fennel," Botanical.com, accessed February 21, 2023.

4. Wikipedia, s.v. "thyrsus," accessed February 21, 2023.

5. *Euripides, The Bacchae*, trans. William Arrowsmith (Yale University, 1967), 155.

6. Pliny the Elder, *The Natural History*, trans. John Bostock and H. T. Riley (London: Taylor and Francis, 1855), chapter 95, Perseus Digital Library (website), accessed February 20, 2023.

7. "Fennel," Botanical.com, accessed February 21, 2023.

8. Carlo Ginzburg, *The Night Battles: Witchcraft and Agrarian Cults in the Sixteenth and Seventeenth Centuries* (Baltimore: John Hopkins University Press, 1992), 22.

Aglio (Garlic)

1. Gabriele Peroni, Cleonice Bonalberti, and Adalberto Peroni, *Le nostre nonne si curavano così* (Varese, Italy: Pietro Macchione Editore, 2008), 173.

2. Biljana Bauer Petrovska and Svetlana Cekovska, "Extracts from the History and Medical Properties of Garlic," *Pharmacognosy Reviews* 4, no. 7 (January–June 2010): 106–10.

3. Petrovska and Cekovska, "Extracts from the History," 106–10.

4. Pliny the Elder, *The Natural History*, trans. John Bostock and H. T. Riley (London: Taylor and Francis, 1855), chapter 34, Perseus Digital Library (website), accessed February 20, 2023.

5. Homer, *Odyssey*, Perseus Digital Library (website), accessed February 20, 2023.

6. "Garlic," Ashkenazi Herbalism (website), accessed February 20, 2023.

7. "Garlic," Botanical.com, accessed February 20, 2023.

8. Peroni, Bonalberti, and Peroni, *Le nostre nonne si curavano così*, 194.

9. Peroni, Bonalberti, and Peroni, *Le nostre nonne si curavano così*, 194.

Altea or Malva (Mallow)

1. Gabriele Peroni, Cleonice Bonalberti, and Adalberto Peroni, *Le nostre nonne si curavano così* (Varese, Italy: Pietro Macchione Editore, 2008), 117; Mariangel Bisanti, *Le erbe dell nonne* (Rimini, Italy: Idealibri, 2010), 188.

2. Pliny the Elder, *The Natural History*, trans. John Bostock and H. T. Riley (London: Taylor and Francis, 1855), chapter 84, Perseus Digital Library (website), accessed February 20, 2023.

3. Graeme Tobyn, Alison Denham, and Margaret Whitelegg, *The Western Herbal Tradition: 2000 Years of Medicinal Plant Knowledge* (Amsterdam: Elsevier, 2011), 69.

4. Pliny the Elder, *The Natural History*, trans. John Bostock and H. T. Riley (London: Taylor and Francis, 1855), chapter 84, Perseus Digital Library (website), accessed February 20, 2023.

5. Edina Gradvohl, *"Healing Kitchen," Graeco-Latina, Brunnesia*: 17 (2012), 72.

6. Wilhelmina Feemster Jashemski, *A Pompeian Herbal: Ancient and Modern Medicinal Plants* (Austin, TX: University of Texas Press, 1999), 24.

7. Cassandra Leah Quave and Andrea Pieroni, "Ritual Healing in Arbëreshë Albanian and Italian Communities of Lucania, Southern Italy," *Journal of Folklore Research: An International Journal of Folklore and Ethnomusicology* (January 2005): 79.

8. Peroni, Bonalberti, Peroni, *Le nostre nonne si curavano così*, 117.

9. Pliny the Elder, *The Natural History*, trans. John Bostock and H. T. Riley (London: Taylor and Francis, 1855), chapter 84, Perseus Digital Library (website), accessed February 20, 2023.

Artemisia (Mugwort)

1. Gabriele Peroni, Cleonice Bonalberti, and Adalberto Peroni, *Le nostre nonne si curavano così* (Varese, Italy: Pietro Macchione Editore, 2008), 42.

2. Matthew Wood, *The Earthwise Herbal* (Berkeley: North Atlantic Books, 2008), 116.

3. The Free Dictionary, s.v. "mater," accessed February 20, 2023.

4. "Mugwort: John the Baptist's Girdle?," Sabbats and Sabbaths (website), accessed February 2023.

5. A. Pollio et al., "Continuity and Change in the Mediterranean Medical Tradition: Ruta spp. (rutaceae) in Hippocratic Medicine and Present Practices," *Journal of Ethnopharmacology,* 116 (2008): 469–82.

6. Rosella Omicciolo Valentini, *Le erbe delle streghe nel medioevo* (Tuscania: Penne & Papiri, 2010), 68.

7. Valentini, *Le erbe delle streghe nel medioevo,* 68.

8. Anne McIntyre, *Flower Power* (New York: Henry Holt and Company, 1996), 58.

9. John M. Riddle, *Goddesses, Elixirs, and Witches: Plants and Sexuality throughout Human History* (London: Palgrave Macmillan, 2010), 138.

Verbasco or Tasso Barbasso (Mullein)

1. Gabriele Peroni, Cleonice Bonalberti, and Adalberto Peroni, *Le nostre nonne si curavano così* (Varese, Italy: Pietro Macchione Editore, 2008), 157.

2. "Verbascum Thapsus: Verbasco—Tasso Barbasso—Barbasso," Summa Gallicana (website), accessed February 21, 2023.

3. Britta K. Ager, "Roman Agricultural Magic" (dissertation, University of Michigan, 2010).

4. M. Riaz, M. Zia-ul-Haq, and H. Jaafar, "Common Mullein, Pharmacological and Chemical Aspects," *The Brazilian Journal of Pharmacology* 23 (2013): 948–59.

5. Peroni, Bonalberti, and Peroni, *Le nostre nonne si curavano così,* 157.

Oliva (Olive)

1. Gabriele Peroni, Cleonice Bonalberti, and Adalberto Peroni, *Le nostre nonne si curavano così* (Varese, Italy: Pietro Macchione Editore, 2008), 123; Mariangel Bisanti, *Le erbe dell nonne* (Rimini, Italy: Idealibri, 2010), 218.

2. "Oliva," EtymoloGeek (website), accessed March 2, 2023.

3. Giovanna Parmigiani, "Ulìa," lecture at Ecological Spiritualities, Harvard Divinity School, April 27–30, 2022.

4. "The Origins of the Olive Tree Revealed," Scientific American (website), accessed March 2, 2023.

5. "The Olive Tree of the Acropolis," Atlas Obscura (website) accessed March 2, 2023.

6. Pliny the Elder, *The Natural History*, trans. John Bostock and H. T. Riley (London: Taylor and Francis, 1855), book 14, Perseus Digital Library (website), accessed February 20, 2023.

7. "The Olive Oil in the Hippocratic," Aenaon (website), June 16, 2014.

8. Howard E. LeWine, "Is Extra-Virgin Olive Oil Extra Healthy?" Harvard Health Publishing (website), November 1, 2021.

9. Victor R. Preedy and Ronald Ross Watson, eds., "The Mediterranean Diet," (Academic Press, 2020), 363–70.

10. Andrea Da Porto et al., "The Pivotal Role of Oleuropein in the Anti-Diabetic Action of the Mediterranean Diet: A Concise Review," *Pharaceutics*, 14, no. 1 (December 25, 2021): 40.

11. Peroni, Bonalberti, and Peroni, *Le nostre nonne si curavano così*, 200.

12. Peroni, Bonalberti, and Peroni, *Le nostre nonne si curavano così*, 200.

13. Hakim G. M. Chishti, *The Traditional Healer's Handbook* (Rochester, VT: Healing Arts Press, 1991), 353.

Prezzemolo (Parsley)

1. Mariangel Bisanti, *Le erbe delle nonne* (Rimini, Italy: Idealibri, 2010), 268.

2. "Parsley," Botanical.com, accessed February 21, 2023.

3. "Parsley—The Herb of Death," Nourishing Death (website), accessed February 21, 2023.

4. "Parsley," Legendary Dartmoor (website), accessed February 21, 2023.

5. "Parsley," Legendary Dartmoor (website), accessed February 21, 2023.

6. Wilhelmina Feemster Jashemski, *A Pompeian Herbal: Ancient and Modern Medicinal Plants* (Austin, TX: University of Texas Press, 1999), 76.

7. "Parsley: The Most Underrated Herb," Permies (website), accessed March 2, 2023.

8. Gabriele Peroni, Cleonice Bonalberti, and Adalberto Peroni, *Le nostre nonne si curavano così* (Varese, Italy: Pietro Macchione Editore, 2008), *34*.

Rosa (Rose)

1. Gabriele Peroni, Cleonice Bonalberti, and Adalberto Peroni, *Le nostre nonne si curavano così* (Varese, Italy: Pietro Macchione Editore, 2008), 146; Mariangel Bisanti, *Le erbe dell nonne* (Rimini, Italy: Idealibri, 2010), 290.

2. "Roses," Botanical.com, accessed March 2, 2023.

3. Claudia Müller-Ebling, Christian Rätsch, and Wolf-Dieter Storl, *Witchcraft Medicine*, (Rochester, VT: Inner Traditions, 1998), 149.

4. Monica H. Green, ed. and trans., *The Trotula: A Medieval Compendium of Women's Medicine*, (Philadelphia: University of Pennsylvania Press, 2001), 126.

5. Green, *The Trotula*, 129.

6. Wikipedia, s.v. "Rosa Mystica," accessed March 2, 2023.

7. Peroni, Bonalberti, and Peroni, *Le nostre nonne si curavano così*, 146.

Rosmarino (Rosemary)

1. Gabriele Peroni, Cleonice Bonalberti, and Adalberto Peroni, *Le nostre nonne si curavano così* (Varese, Italy: Pietro Macchione Editore, 2008), 108; Mariangel Bisanti, *Le erbe dell nonne* (Rimini, Italy: Idealibri, 2010), 292.

2. "Goddess of the Pillar: The Mythology of Upright Rosemary," Paghat (website), accessed March 2, 2023.

3. William Shakespeare, *Hamlet*, act 4, scene 5.

4. Nicholas Culpeper, *Complete Herbal and English Physician* (Glenwood, IL: Meyerbooks, 1990), 155.

5. "Rosemary," Methovalley Herbs (website), accessed March 2, 2023.

6. Matthew Wood, *The Earthwise Herbal* (Berkeley: North Atlantic Books, 2008), 428.

7. Mariangel Bisanti, *Le erbe dell nonne* (Rimini, Italy: Idealibri, 2010), 292.

8. Paolino Uccello, *Piante E Parole che Guariscono* (Canicattini Bagni, Sicily: Museo del Tessuto, dell'Emigrazione e della Medicina Popolare, 2012), 25.

9. Patricia Kaminski and Richard Katz, *Flower Essence Repertory* (Nevada City, CA: The Flower Essence Society, 1994 edition), 367.

10. Rosemary Gladstar, *Herbal Healing for Women* (New York: Simon & Schuster, 1993), 98–99.

Ruta (Rue)

1. Gabriele Peroni, Cleonice Bonalberti, and Adalberto Peroni, *Le nostre nonne si curavano così* (Varese, Italy: Pietro Macchione Editore, 2008), 153.

2. "Herb to Know: Common Rue," Mother Earth Living (website), accessed March 2, 2023.

3. Wilhelmina Feemster Jashemski, *A Pompeian Herbal: Ancient and Modern Medicinal Plants* (Austin, Texas: University of Texas Press, 1999), 33.

4. "Rue," Botanical.com, accessed March 2, 2023.

5. Rosella Omicciolo Valentini, *Le erbe delle streghe nel medioevo* (Tuscania: Penne & Papiri, 2010), 145.

6. Andrea Pieroni, Cassandra L. Quavec, and Rocco Franco Santorod, "Folk Pharmaceutical Knowledge in the Territory of the Dolomiti Lucane, Inland Southern Italy," *Journal of Ethnopharmacology* 95, nos. 2–3 (December 2004): 373–84.

7. Cassandra Leah Quave and Andrea Pieroni, "Ritual Healing in Arbëreshë Albanian and Italian Communities of Lucania, Southern Italy," *Journal of Folklore Research: An International Journal of Folklore and Ethnomusicology* (January 2005): 87.

Iperico (Saint John's Wort)

1. Gabriele Peroni, Cleonice Bonalberti, and Adalberto Peroni, *Le nostre nonne si curavano così* (Varese, Italy: Pietro Macchione Editore, 2008), 100; Mariangel Bisanti, *Le erbe dell nonne* (Rimini, Italy: Idealibri, 2010), 166.

2. Charles Killinger, *Culture and Customs of Italy* (Westport, CT: Greenwood Press, 2005), 118.

3. Carol Field, *Celebrating Italy* (New York: Harper Perennial, 2000), 92.

4. Geof Kron, "A Deposit of Carbonized Hay from Oplontis and Roman Fodder Quality," *Mouseion*, 3rd ser., 4 (2004): 275–331.

5. "Hypericum Perforatum: Saint John's Wort," Gaia Herbs (website), accessed February 20, 2023.

6. Rosella Omicciolo Valentini, *Le erbe delle streghe nel medioevo* (Tuscania: Penne & Papiri: 2010), 107–10.

Noce (Walnut)

1. Gabriele Peroni, Cleonice Bonalberti, and Adalberto Peroni, *Le nostre nonne si curavano così* (Varese, Italy: Pietro Macchione Editore, 2008), 101.

2. Etymonline, s.v. "walnut," accessed February 13, 2023.

3. Abha Chauhan and Ved Chauhan, "Beneficial Effects of Walnuts on Cognition and Brain Health," *Nutrients* 12, no. 2 (February 2020): 550.

4. Frederick G. Meyer, "Carbonized Food Plants of Pompeii, Herculaneum, and the Villa at Torre Annunziata," *Economic Botany* 34, no. 4 (Oct–Dec 1980): 401–37.

5. Pliny the Elder, *The Natural History*, trans. John Bostock and H. T. Riley (London: Taylor and Francis, 1855), book 23, chapter 77, Perseus Digital Library (website), accessed February 15, 2024.

6. "La legenda del Noce di Benevento ed altro . . . ," You Reporter (website), accessed February 13, 2023.

7. Peter Holmes, *The Energetics of Western Herbs* (Boulder: Snow Lotus Press, 2006), 714–17.

8. "Landscaping and Gardening around Walnuts and Other Juglone Producing Plants," PennState Extension (website), accessed February 15, 2023.

9. Cassandra Leah Quave and Andrea Pieroni, "Ritual Healing in Arbëreshë Albanian and Italian Communities of Lucania, Southern Italy," *Journal of Folklore Research: An International Journal of Folklore and Ethnomusicology* (January 2005).

10. Peroni, Bonalberti, and Peroni, *Le nostre nonne si curavano così*, 197.

11. Peroni, Bonalberti, and Peroni, *Le nostre nonne si curavano così*, 101.

12. "Il nocillo e la notte della 'Nzilla di Cerreto Sannita," Fremondoweb (website), accessed February 15, 2023.

13. Nicholas Culpeper, *Complete Herbal and English Physician* (Glenwood, IL: Meyerbooks, 1990), 190–91.

Index